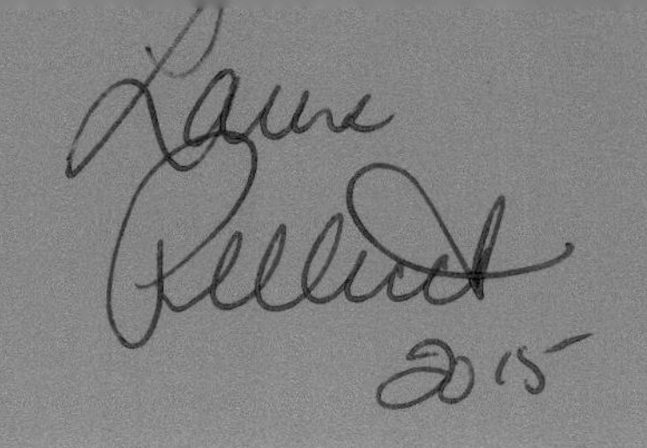

Interprofessional Health Care Practice

SUE COFFEY, RN, PHD, ASSOCIATE PROFESSOR

University of Ontario Institute of Technology

CHARLES ANYINAM, RN, MSC, PHD(c), PROFESSOR

Sally Horsfall Eaton School of Nursing, George Brown College

PEARSON

Toronto

To all of our loved ones,
here with us and beyond.

Managing Editor: Claudine O'Donnell
Senior Acquisitions Editor: Lisa Rahn
Marketing Manager: Michelle Bish
Program Manager: Darryl Kamo
Project Manager: Richard di Santo
Developmental Editor: Mary Wat
Production Services: Rashmi Tickyani, Aptara®, Inc.
Permissions Project Manager: Erica Mojzes
Text Permissions Research: Phyllis Padula, Aptara®, Inc.
Cover Designer: Alex Li
Cover Image: GettyImages (top-left, top-right, bottom-left);
Shutterstock (bottom-right)

Credits and acknowledgments for material borrowed from other sources and reproduced, with permission, in this textbook appear on the appropriate page within the text.

10 9 8 7 6 5 4 3 2 1 [WC]

Library and Archives Canada Cataloguing in Publication

Coffey, Sue, author
Interprofessional health care practice / Sue Coffey, RN, PhD, Associate Professor, University of Ontario Institute of Technology, Charles Anyinam, RN, MSc, PhD, Professor, Sally Horsfall Eaton School of Nursing, George Brown College.
Includes bibliographical references and index.
ISBN 978-0-13-209130-5 (pbk.)
1. Health care teams—Canada. 2. Interprofessional relations—Canada. 3. Medical care—Canada. I. Anyinam, Charles Andrews, author II. Title.
R729.5.H4C63 2014 C2014-904695-2
362.1068

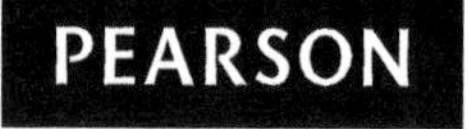

ISBN 978-0-13-209130-5

About the Authors

Dr. Sue Coffey is an award-winning nursing educator who has been practising nursing for 25 years, with a clinical focus in emergency nursing. Her research interests include access to higher education for non-traditional students, including internationally educated nurses and students in bridging programs, nurses' experiences in practice, and models of intra- and interprofessional practice. Dr. Coffey is the recipient of numerous awards and recognitions for excellence in nursing education, including the Leadership in Nursing Education (Academic) Award (Registered Nurses Association of Ontario, 2006); the Newcomer Champion Award (Ontario Ministry of Citizenship and Immigration, 2007); the Canadian Association of Schools of Nursing (CASN) Award for Excellence in Teaching (2008); and the Council of Ontario Programs in Nursing (COUPN) Award for Teaching Excellence (2009). She is currently the Director of the Nursing Program and an Associate Professor at the University of Ontario Institute of Technology.

Charles Anyinam is a PhD candidate in the critical disability studies program at York University. His dissertation work examines the workplace experiences of nurses with disabilities. His scholarly interests and research focus on diversity and disability within nursing and health care. He is an accomplished RN and educator with over a decade of teaching experience in nursing spanning across different models of undergraduate baccalaureate and post-registration nursing programs. Among many others, Charles has developed and taught courses focusing in the areas of transcultural nursing, nursing leadership and management, professional communication, and community nursing practice. He also has extensive experience as a leader within academic administration and faculty governance. Recognitions include the 2013 Registered Nurses Association of Ontario's (RNAO) Leadership Award in Nursing Education and the Dean's Teaching Award (Early Career), York University's Faculty of Health, 2009.

Brief Contents

Contents

Preface

Health care in Canada must transform quickly to address the increasingly complex and rapidly changing needs of a growing and diverse population of service users. At the same time, the system must manage health service expenditure and infrastructure issues while balancing these demands with those of non-health-related sectors. Over recent years, these challenges served as the catalyst for system-wide change.

As the 21st century began, the federal government provided funding to the provinces and territories for the development of broad programs of health care reform to deal with issues such as access to primary care and wait times. This major health care reform initiative demonstrated the need for health care professionals to work differently—to communicate, to consult, and to collaborate with each other. This book focuses on interprofessional practice (IPP), the health care practice approach that emerged from this realization.

IPP espouses the idea that in order to improve health care and efficiency in health service delivery, different professionals involved in providing care must work interdependently. Although the concept builds on decades of research and theories about the central role of teams and teamwork in health care delivery, IPP is novel and innovative. At no other point in the history of the Canadian health care system has an idea made such a significant impact in such a short period of time. There is already a sizable body of literature, including positive evaluative data related to various aspects of IPP. The term *IPP* (or its derivatives) has become commonplace, as has the implementation of IPP initiatives and IPP teams in health care settings. As the Canadian health care system continues to evolve, IPP will be central to the kinds of system-wide changes necessary to ensure effective and efficient health care for all Canadians.

While IPP offers much to patients, their support networks, professionals, organizations, and the system, there is no guide to IPP for learners and practitioners. Written for postsecondary students in health programs and for practitioners, this book provides an excellent start by equipping readers with the knowledge, understanding, resources, and tools to practise within an interprofessional context.

HIGHLIGHTS OF THIS BOOK

- *Opening Vignette:* Each chapter begins with a fictional vignette depicting a situation in a practice environment. Carrying the vignette through the chapter illustrates how concepts and ideas can be applied in practice.
- *Learning Outcomes:* Each chapter identifies learning outcomes, which provides a road map for reading as well as a basis for assessment.
- *Helpful Tools Boxes:* Providing practical advice, tips, or activities, this feature reinforces learning, or encourages the application of content to real-world or fictional situations.

- *Spotlight Boxes:* Showcasing real examples, this box demonstrates the application of a concept or idea in practice, most often in the Canadian context.
- *End-of-Chapter Summary:* To reinforce learning, a summary of key ideas and messages appears at the end of each chapter.
- *Review Questions and Application Exercises:* At the end of each chapter, readers find review questions for study and discussion purposes, and application exercises that require thinking critically about the topics included in the chapter.
- *Key Terms and Glossary:* Key terms introduced for the first time in the textbook are highlighted in bold and defined. A list of new key terms also appears at the end of each chapter, and definitions can be located in the glossary at the end of the book.

Four parts organize the textbook's 11 chapters, with each part focusing on a specific topic area related to IPP. Each chapter within a part explores a different aspect of the topic.

- Part I of the textbook introduces the reader to the background of the movement toward IPP. Chapter 1 introduces the reader to the context for IPP and presents an overview of the approach. Chapter 2 provides a general framework intended to help readers to organize and understand IPP.
- Chapters 4 to 7 make up Part II, and emphasize the major concepts central to IPP and where to start in applying these concepts to practice situations. The chapters in this section explore specific aspects of the organizing framework introduced in Chapter 2. Chapter 3 focuses on teams, team processes, and teamwork as the context within which IPP occurs. In Chapter 4, the relationship dimension of the framework is examined, focusing particularly on the roles and relationships of health care professionals in IPP and interprofessional communication. Chapter 5 focuses on collaboration, a central concept in IPP and a core element found within the process dimension of the organizing framework. Chapter 6 addresses problem solving and its relationship to conflict and negotiation. Finally, Chapter 7 discusses leadership within the context of IPP.
- Part III concentrates on the contexts within which IPP is taught, practised, and evaluated, and tackles key issues and complexities of IPP. Chapter 8 examines interprofessional education (IPE), an important area of development in the collaborative practice movement. Chapter 9 brings clarity to policy and regulation questions and issues related to IPP. Chapter 10 provides an overview of the ways in which evaluation of IPP has been approached and the emerging outcomes of IPP initiatives.
- Part IV contains the final chapter of the text, Chapter 11, which explores future directions related to IPP, with particular attention to intersectoral collaboration, a concept that expands on IPP.

As a final note, as you read though the book, you will notice that some ideas, concepts, and material are discussed in more than one chapter. This occurs for two reasons.

First, the material is foundational to many concepts and ideas. In each instance, that concept or idea is viewed from a different perspective. For example, several chapters refer to key policy documents released between 2002 and 2005 (e.g., First Ministers Accords, the Romanow Report, and the Health Council of Canada inaugural report). These documents outline the health reform agenda between the federal government of Canada and the provinces and territories and set the stage for the context within which the IPP movement flourished. However, each chapter focuses on these materials from a different viewpoint.

Second, some ideas and concepts are applied often in IPP. As a result, they are discussed several times in different contexts and using different examples, so that the reader may develop a good understanding of these foundational concepts and readily apply them.

It is our hope that this book offers readers the opportunity to learn about past and present situations in the Canadian health care system and elsewhere in the world that led to the promotion of IPP. The book explores both the robustness of health care services and delivery in Canada and the challenges we face in continuing to provide health care to an aging and increasingly complex population. IPP is at the centre of dealing with such challenges, with a view of collaboration that moves from the individual or team level to that of collaboration across sectors. Interprofessional practice is the key—an innovative approach to health care reform and renewal at all levels.

CONTENT OPTIONS

CourseSmart

CourseSmart goes beyond traditional expectations—providing instant, online access to the textbooks and course materials. Save time with a digital eTextbook that provides the ability to search for the most relevant content at the very moment needed. CourseSmart can make life a little easier. Visit **www.coursesmart.com**.

Pearson Custom Library

For enrollments of at least 25 students, you can create your own version of this textbook by choosing the chapters that best suit your own course needs. To begin building your custom text, visit **www.pearsoncustomlibrary.com**. You may also include your own original content, or mix and match Pearson content. Contact your local Pearson representative to get started.

ACKNOWLEDGMENTS

This text would not have been possible had it not been for the support, encouragement, and love of our family and friends.

We wish to acknowledge the superb contributions of the contributors, acknowledged experts in the themes of their chapters. Additionally, we extend our sincere gratitude to all of our colleagues who provided support and acted as sounding boards for our ideas.

Special appreciation is expressed to Michelle Sartor, now Executive Director, Strategic Partnerships at Pearson North America, for initiating the writing of the text, believing strongly in our vision, and providing ongoing support and encouragement. We wish to also acknowledge the excellent team at Pearson Canada, including Senior Acquisitions Editor Lisa Rahn and Developmental Editor Mary Wat for their tremendous encouragement and hard work behind the scenes to produce this text.

Finally, the authors and Pearson Canada would like to thank the many professors who provided feedback on the manuscript at various stages, including both the following and others who chose to remain anonymous:

Brad Armstrong, ACP, York Region Advanced Care Paramedic
Instructor, Continuing Education, Georgian College

Susan Brajtman, RN, PhD
Associate Professor, School of Nursing, University of Ottawa

Andrea Brandt, RN, BScN, MN
School of Health and Wellness, Georgian College

Pat Chornaby, RN, BHScN
Practical Nursing, Conestoga College

Vernon Curran
Faculty of Medicine, Memorial University

Sherry Espin
Daphne Cockwell School of Nursing, Ryerson University

Dr. Carole Ewashen
University of Calgary

Ruby Grymonpre, PharmD, FCSHP
Professor, Faculty of Pharmacy, IPE Coordinator, University of Manitoba

Corinne Hart, RN, PhD
Associate Professor, Daphne Cockwell School of Nursing, Ryerson University

Michelle Hughes, RN, BScN, MEd
Professor, Daphne Cockwell School of Nursing, Ryerson University; Collaborative Nursing Degree Program, George Brown College; School of Community & Health Studies, Centennial College

Gary Kapelus, DSP, MBA
Professor and Coordinator, Interprofessional Health Studies, George Brown College

Marian Luctkar-Flude, RN, MScN
School of Nursing, Queen's University

Ivy Oandasan
Family and Community Medicine, University of Toronto

Sharon Paton
Daphne Cockwell School of Nursing, Ryerson University

Linda J. Patrick, RN, PhD
Associate Professor, Faculty of Nursing, University of Windsor

Dr. Pammla Petrucka
College of Nursing, University of Saskatchewan

Katherine Poser, RN, BScN, MNEd
School of Health Sciences, BScN Program, St. Lawrence College (Kingston Campus)

Sharon Ronaldson
Langara College

Kathy L. Rush, PhD, RN
University of British Columbia Okanagan

Part I
Introduction to Interprofessional Practice

In recent years, a common goal has emerged at local, provincial, national, and international levels. There is consensus that the Canadian health care system must undergo change based on more effective and efficient ways to deliver care. Escalating costs over the past two decades, combined with decreasing available resources to provide health care, means that in Canada we are spending more on health care than we can afford. Additionally, the health care experience for many Canadians is not what it should be, with calls from both patients and health care providers for more seamless systems of care and mechanisms for providers to work together in more positive ways. As a result, a new health care delivery model is being proposed, based on the concept that highly integrated care provided by various professionals working to their full scope of practice leads to optimal (a) health care experiences for patients and their families, (b) practice experiences for health professionals, (c) health care outcomes, and (d) use of health care resources. The pressure of current system challenges, including high delivery costs, limited budgets, and shortages of health care workers, brings us to a time of opportunity. We find ourselves in a position where we are able to create a new vision of practice that places the patient, family, or community at the centre of care and is based on a fully participatory, team-oriented approach.

Part I of this book introduces the reader to the context for the current movement toward the collaborative care approach, commonly referred to as interprofessional practice (IPP). In Chapter 1, we define IPP, discuss its foundational concepts, and outline key factors driving us toward this approach. Chapter 2 presents a general framework for organizing and understanding IPP. Recognizing that there are a number of different ways to explore IPP, the framework is intended as a tool for readers to examine basic concepts inherent to IPP, to consider their IPP experiences, and to deconstruct factors in situations where IPP is involved.

Chapter 1

Introduction to Interprofessional Practice

It's just after 2 a.m. on a busy night shift in the emergency department of a midsized urban teaching hospital. Jennie, the charge nurse for the overnight shift, begins making her way around the various treatment areas.

She enters the Resuscitation Room (RR) and sees Chen, a respiratory therapist, and Nuzhat, a registered nurse who's working as the float nurse, intently attending to their patient.

Jennie: Do you have a moment to update me?

Nuzhat: Yes, things are settling down here. I came in to help because the two RR nurses are swamped. Mr. Papas suffered a myocardial infarct tonight. His wife called 911 and while the paramedics were treating him, he began experiencing acute respiratory distress and required intubation. The paramedics did a great job of stabilizing him, but I've had my hands full in here trying to get his thrombolytics and other drips started. Chen has come down to help set up the ventilator and adjust the settings.

Jennie: Thanks, Chen, we can use all the help we can get.

Chen: I know they had an empty bed up in the Cardiac Care Unit. I'll see if I can speed things up to transfer Mr. Papas up there.

Jennie: We'll be ready to go as soon as we have a green light from them. Anything you need from me, Nuzhat?

Nuzhat: Yes—can you find his wife in the waiting room?

Jennie: Will do. I'm heading out to triage and the waiting room as soon as I check with the other staff in here.

As Jennie heads to the triage desk, she notes the waiting room is almost full. Salvatore, the triage nurse, is interviewing a mom with a crying toddler on her lap. She watches as he gives the little girl stickers and gently places a sling on her left arm before turning to Jennie.

Jennie: What's up?

Salvatore: With the little one? I'm pretty sure it's a fracture. The wait to go back to the ambulatory area is over two hours. It's so frustrating to send her to the waiting room knowing that what she needs right now is an x-ray and something for pain. I've explained to her mother that we will try to have her daughter assessed as quickly as possible by a physician and that I anticipate she will require x-rays. I've also asked the mom to let me know if there are any changes and I'll keep checking in on them.

Jennie: You're right. We've had standing orders in place in the ER for years, but we need to expand what we're able to do. The hospital's Interprofessional Practice Committee has been looking into the risks and benefits of expanding our range of standing orders. Why don't you join the committee?

Salvatore: Me? I don't have time for that and I don't have any confidence that real change will happen.

Jennie: Change definitely won't happen without expert input, and you have a lot to offer. Think about it, Sal. In the meantime, I'll find one of the residents to assess that toddler. What else do I need to know about the patients waiting out here?

After listening to a quick overview of the patients, Jennie is about to head off when Salvatore calls after her.

Salvatore: And where the heck is the float nurse? I haven't seen her for an hour and it's *busy* out here. She better not be off in the break room ...

Jennie: She's busy in the RR. As soon as she transfers her patient to CCU, I'll ask her to come out to help you.

As she turns to leave, Jennie hears Salvatore mumble something under his breath about his colleague. With so much going on, she decides to ignore the comment for now, promising herself to return to this conversation in a quieter moment.

Entering the Ambulatory Treatment Area, Jennie heads over to the Reception Desk. Amina, the unit clerk, is simultaneously entering orders and answering the phone. A quick look around reveals a small waiting room full of patients and all of the available cubicles occupied. Jennie can hear a somewhat boisterous patient, sounding intoxicated, protesting that he doesn't require any treatment and insisting that he's ready to leave.

As Jennie readies to follow the trail of voices, she hears a familiar voice. It's Heather, the X-Ray Department porter. Within a few short moments, Heather is able to change the tone of the exchange from one of conflict to one of jovial banter. Jennie breathes a small sigh of relief and mentally notes how often Heather is effective in these types of situations.

Just as Jennie is wondering where everyone is, Iyabo, a second-year medical resident, emerges from a treatment room.

Jennie: Hi, Iyabo, how's the night going back here?

Iyabo: Is it always like this on the night shift? We haven't stopped and everyone's in a bad mood. Can you talk to your nurses about making sure patients who need to be assessed on stretchers are changed into gowns? I don't have time to be doing my work and everyone else's work too and I'm getting fed up!

Jennie: It's a tough night for everyone and we're all struggling to keep up. You're right that patients who need to be assessed without their clothes on should be changed into gowns as soon as we find a stretcher for them. But that's not just to get them ready for you. Is this an issue you've experienced before tonight?

Iyabo: I'm really noticing it tonight ... I guess I haven't worked enough shifts to say for sure. But we worked differently on my last rotation on the surgical unit.

Jennie: The ER is different from a surgical unit. I think we'll make more progress seeing how the team in this area can pull together than we would by blaming each other. There's no question you need some more help. I think Jim, the unit aid, can help to get patients ready and provide some assistance to both you and the nurses. I'll find him and ask him to come to this area as soon as he's free.

Iyabo: Any help is worth a shot.

Jennie: Speaking of help, while we're waiting for Jim, can I get your help in seeing a toddler in the waiting room so we can get her to X-Ray and give her something for pain? The x-ray technologist who's working tonight is fantastic with kids. If you can see her and write some orders, we'll get her over there for some films pronto.

Iyabo: As soon as I wrap up with this charting, I'll go find Salvatore.

Jennie thanks the medical resident and heads off to complete her rounds and locate Jim. As she passes the ER physician for the night shift, she stops to connect.

Jennie: How are you doing, Dan?

Dan: I've had better shifts, but I've also had worse. How's the department?

Jennie: We're strained, but coping. We're pulling together and that's making all the difference. But it's not always easy, and when the dust settles we need to look at strategies for improving patient flow and enabling everyone to work to their full scope of practice. We always say this in moments of crisis, but then fail to follow through. This time, we need to ensure that we follow up.

Dan: I'm with you. Maybe we can push to make this a priority for the Interprofessional Practice Committee. But first, let's get through this night!

Learning Outcomes

AFTER STUDYING THIS CHAPTER, YOU SHOULD BE ABLE TO:

1. **Define interprofessional practice.**
2. **Describe the core concepts inherent in interprofessional practice approaches.**
3. **Explain how health care team approaches form the foundation for the current interprofessional practice movement.**
4. **Describe trends and events in health care policy and practice over the past decade that have led to the promotion of interprofessional practice as a Canadian health care renewal strategy.**
5. **Discuss the relationship between interprofessional education and interprofessional practice.**

INTRODUCTION

THE OPENING VIGNETTE CALLS OUR ATTENTION TO THE NEED FOR ALL OF THE MEMBERS OF the health care team to work together and communicate effectively in order to provide the highest quality, client-centred care. As each of the members of the health care team in the opening vignette works to provide the best possible care to his or her patients, the need to collaborate with each other and negotiate about shared priorities is critical. Health care environments are busier than ever, with more complex patient issues. There are also a multitude of organizational and systemic issues at play, including a shortage of educated health care professionals and the broader economic dilemma of ever-increasing health care costs at the same time that provincial and federal budgets for health care are decreasing. Understandably, this context may leave health professionals feeling frustrated and unsatisfied with their work. One need look no further than print media, newscasts, or fictionalized television shows for common portrayals of burnout and frustration among health care professionals. Many health care professionals and researchers are recommending restructuring the way we provide health care, and specifically how the various health care professions work together. For example, in the opening vignette, there are several instances where the various health care professionals, such as the nurse and the respiratory therapist, work as a team to provide collaborative, client-centred care. Patient satisfaction and positive health outcomes are enhanced through a concerted and coordinated effort by all members of the team working to their full scope of practice. This type of practice is called **interprofessional practice (IPP)**. Interprofessional practice is an approach to practice "designed to promote the active participation of each discipline in patient care. It enhances patient and family-centred goals and values, provides mechanisms for continuous communication among caregivers, optimizes staff participation in clinical decision-making within and across disciplines and fosters respect for disciplinary contributions of all professionals" (Health Canada, 2003).

This chapter focuses on introducing the reader to this emerging approach. We will define IPP and related concepts and examine the context within which IPP has emerged in Canada and internationally. We will also discuss the current status of efforts to develop and integrate IPP within the Canadian health care system. Finally, we will review what is currently known about the benefits and challenges of this approach to health care delivery.

DEFINING INTERPROFESSIONAL PRACTICE

In virtually all health care sectors across the nation, there is widespread consensus that the future of Canadian health care design and delivery must be built upon team-oriented, IPP approaches. The concept of IPP is seen as an integral component of efforts to establish, maintain, and improve the health of Canadians and provide quality patient-centred care (Braithwaite & Travaglia, 2005a, 2005b). In the past, health care professionals were often educated, and subsequently practised, within a profession-specific model (i.e., physicians learned almost exclusively in classrooms with other physicians and then collaborated most effectively in their practice with other physicians; pharmacists learned with other pharmacists and then collaborated most effectively with other pharmacists; etc.) In this model, often referred to as *silos of knowledge*, health care professionals were seen as possessing a wealth of knowledge related to their own field of practice, but not as effective in sharing that knowledge and collaborating across professional perspectives.

While Greenfield, Nugus, Travaglia, and Braithwaite (2010) point out the challenges in transitioning to interprofessional learning and IPP, the benefits are indisputable. Enhanced teamwork through IPP practice has been shown to benefit virtually all stakeholder groups. Chapter 10 will provide an overview of research findings related to implementation of IPP. However, in summary, emerging evidence points to shorter wait times for care, increased satisfaction with the health care provided, greater access to a broader range of services, and better health outcomes for patients. Health care providers report increased job satisfaction, decreased stress and burnout, improved working environments, and the opportunity to work within their full scope of practice. Health care organizations describe increased efficiency and greater capacity to provide quality care for more patients, improved staff recruitment and retention with decreased turnover, and better patient safety. Within the health care system as a whole, evidence reveals overall increased access to the system, better ability to develop quality improvement and accountability measures, and increased potential to coordinate all aspects of health care. If we consider the opening vignette, we see a consistent focus on trying to ensure that health care providers work in collaboration and are able to practise to their full scope, while patients receive the best possible health care.

Although there is little doubt that IPP is hugely beneficial, it also has many complexities (D'Amour, Ferrada-Videla, San Martin Rodriguez, & Beaulieu, 2005; Greenfield et al., 2010). Therefore, it is important that IPP be both well defined and clearly understood. A number of definitions in use today attempt to explain the idea of IPP.

Table 1.1 Common Terms and Definitions for Interprofessional Practice in Health Care

Term Used	Definition	Author
Interprofessional collaborative patient-centred practice	"A practice orientation designed to promote the active participation of each discipline in patient care. It involves the continuous interaction of two or more professions or disciplines, organized into a common effort, to solve or explore common issues with the best possible participation of the patient."	Curran, 2007
	"... is designed to promote the active participation of each discipline in patient care. It enhances patient and family-centred goals and values, provides mechanisms for continuous communication among caregivers, optimizes staff participation in clinical decision-making within and across disciplines and fosters respect for disciplinary contributions of all professionals."	Health Canada, 2003
Interprofessional collaborative practice	"... is guided by shared values, a common purpose or care outcome, mutual respect, and effective communications [and] optimizes participation in clinical decision-making within and across professions. It evolves over time, requiring the flexibility to add or subtract health team members based on the needs of the individual clients. It must be supported through policy, protocols, and procedures at all levels of decision-making, including government, professional associations, regulatory bodies and health care organizations."	Health Professions Regulatory Network, 2008

Table 1.1 provides an overview of the definitions currently found within the literature. You'll notice that while there are variations in the terms used, the key elements are the same. There is widespread agreement on the core concepts of collaboration, teamwork, decision making, and communication, with a focus on improved patient quality of care as the desired outcome.

Core Concepts of Interprofessional Practice

Core concepts encapsulated by IPP include collaboration, teamwork, communication, decision making, and person-centred care. In this section, we provide a brief introduction to these concepts and discuss their relationship to IPP. Subsequent chapters of this text will explore these concepts in greater detail.

Collaboration D'Amour and colleagues (2005) assert that the concept of collaboration is an important element of IPP that must be well understood if IPP activities and initiatives are to meet targeted outcomes, such as improved patient care. At a basic level, collaboration involves two or more persons coming together around a common goal. Within the literature related to IPP, the concept of collaboration is described in more complex ways. Oandasan and colleagues (2006) define **collaboration** as "a process that requires relationships and interactions between health professionals regardless if they perceive themselves as part of a team" (p. 4). Their review of the literature highlights the relationship between collaboration and teamwork and identifies five underlying concepts of collaboration: sharing, partnership, power, interdependency, and process. In the opening vignette, we see a simple example of collaboration between Jennie, the ER nurse in charge, and Iyabo, the ER resident. Iyabo's request to ensure that nurses assist in having patients ready to be assessed when she goes in to see them, and Jennie's request to have a toddler in the waiting room evaluated for a possible fracture, are both important. By working together to solve the individual and systemic challenges to providing timely and appropriate health care, health professionals are able to accomplish more, and patients experience better care.

Teamwork When we see health professionals working interdependently to provide care for clients, we are witnessing teamwork. **Teamwork** is a goal-oriented and relationally based process that relies heavily on cooperation and collaboration in pursuit of a common goal to ensure success. In the chapter vignette, we saw Nuzhat and Chen working together to provide care for Mr. Papas. While Nuzhat focused on starting important medications to treat Mr. Papas' myocardial infarct, Chen set up the ventilator and adjusted the settings. By cooperating and collaborating together as a team, the nurse and respiratory therapist were able to accomplish the required tasks critical to Mr. Papas' care in a timely fashion. Oandasan and colleagues (2006) identify teamwork as important to the integration of IPP into health care delivery in Canada. In the context of IPP, teamwork requires that health care professionals share information, possess an understanding of team functioning, and apply these ideas to enhance patient-centred care. In Chapter 3 we focus on teams and teamwork.

Communication When we refer to **communication**, our focus is on the transmission of and response to information. Effective communication is essential to the success of IPP. Health care professionals must develop communication skills that transmit concise, timely, and important information about patients and issues related to decision making, while also promoting relationships among themselves. In the vignette, we see a focus on communication both among health professionals and between health care providers and the patient. For example, the triage nurse Salvatore shares with the Charge Nurse Jennie his assessment of a pediatric patient in the waiting room. He also shares what he has communicated to the toddler's mother. A key factor related to effective communication in IPP involves the notion of communication styles. **Communication styles** refer to how individuals use both verbal and nonverbal communication to signal to others how they should interpret messages. The communication styles of health care professionals are often honed through professionalization processes, leading to diverse and sometimes opposing approaches to communication that may become a barrier to collaboration.

Decision Making When we select an alternative from an existing set of options, we are engaging in **decision making** (Myers & Anderson, 2008). We can think of decision making as the mechanism that individuals and teams use to make choices. In IPP, decision making occurs at both the individual and the collective level. The role of the patient is an important aspect of the discussion about decision making in the IPP context. Patient involvement in decision making has been dubbed *shared decision making* and has been linked with quality of health care. Decision making is further explored in Chapter 6.

Person-Centred Care A cornerstone of IPP is the idea that the person or patient is at the centre of care. Person-centred care is an approach to health care practice that diverges from the traditional paternalistic model in which patients are seen as passive recipients of health care that is solely determined by the practitioner. In **person-centred care** (or *patient-centred care*), patients are not acted upon, but rather supported to be fully involved in their own care to the extent that they choose (Canadian Interprofessional Health Collaborative [CIHC], 2009). Key features of person-centred care include listening to the needs of clients/patients and their families and engaging with clients/patients and families as members of the health care team (CIHC, 2009; Registered Nurses' Association of Ontario [RNAO], 2009). The movement to person-centred care is part of a global trend toward humanizing health care, recognizing the importance of placing the patient/family at the centre of care and ensuring that their voice is heard.

BACKGROUND: THE EMERGENCE OF INTERPROFESSIONAL PRACTICE

Why is there such growing momentum toward IPP? One need look no further than a local newscast to hear stories of escalating health care costs and widening gaps between available resources and increasing needs. In the federal election of 2011, health care was cited as the single most important issue for the majority of Canadians surveyed. In these times of economic challenge, it is more essential than ever to consider how we deliver health care services and if there are ways to maximize our resources. At the same time, there is an equal focus on the need to continue to improve the quality and efficacy of the care we provide while supporting the ongoing development of a health care system at both the national and provincial levels. So where do we turn in our search for effective innovation? A review of health care delivery models and trends reveals an extensive focus on the integration of a collaborative, team-based approach to providing health services as a means to (a) ensure information is shared effectively among all relevant health care providers in any given situation, (b) reduce replication of service through improved communication, and (c) ensure resources are utilized most appropriately. As discussed previously in this chapter, providing care through an IPP model has been shown to improve the patient experience, lead to better patient outcomes, and support more positive work experiences for providers. Understanding the evolution of IPP is important as we continue to refine this approach.

Health Care Team Approaches as the Precursor to Interprofessional Practice

Teams play an important role in today's health care system, but the focus on how individual providers can work together effectively to provide comprehensive care is not new. Baldwin (2007) and Schmitt (1994) trace the development of interdisciplinary health care teams internationally from the turn of the century. Examples include (a) those achieved through multidisciplinary medical teams in World War II, (b) United States President Johnson's conception of The Great Society in the 1960s that included community health centres designed to meet the needs of the poor and underserved, and (c) the notable advances made in the United Kingdom in areas such as interprofessional geriatric units. In 1972, the Institute of Medicine in the United States held a conference titled Education for the Health Team. As a result of the enthusiasm generated from this gathering, a decade of funding for early projects aimed at interprofessional educational experiences followed. While much of this funding had ceased by the early 1980s, the stage had been set for the next wave in health care reform in North America and beyond.

The move to a focus on the interactions and relationships of health professionals has increased as our health care system has evolved through the 20th century. The creation of a national system of health care in Canada (medicare) and a number of changes that occurred in the health care system in the United States in the 1980s have often been called the "health care revolution." This revolution shined the spotlight on how health care professionals can best provide care that is comprehensive, seamless, and most efficacious. Current issues including the aging of the North American population, and new perspectives on the influence of social-psychological aspects of health care have resulted in a growing sensitivity to the complex nature of health. These issues have also resulted in an emphasis on the need for health care professionals to work effectively and collaboratively both with other health care providers and with patients to improve health outcomes.

The Canadian Perspective on Interprofessional Practice

In order to understand how the movement toward IPP fits within the context of health care delivery in Canada, it is important to understand the basic structure of the Canadian health care system. Fundamentally, our system was designed to ensure that all Canadians have equal access to health services. To this end, the Canadian system, known as "medicare," is reflective of the culture of our nation. It is a national system of health care insurance that is publicly funded through both federal and provincial/territorial contributions, and provides access to universal, comprehensive coverage for medically necessary hospital and physician services. The five core principles of the *Canada Health Act* are (Health Canada, 2010):

- public administration (i.e., administered on a nonprofit basis),
- comprehensiveness (i.e., all medically necessary services are insured),

- universality (i.e., uniform service coverage for all),
- accessibility (i.e., reasonable access to medically necessary hospital and physician services without financial or other barriers for all insured individuals), and
- portability (i.e., coverage for all insured persons when they move to another province or territory within Canada and when they travel abroad).

There is widespread consensus that the future of health care in Canada must continue to reflect our values as a nation as embedded in these five principles. However, the current context of health care delivery and the factors driving us toward change must be acknowledged.

A fundamental shift in the Canadian health care delivery status quo occurred in 2002 when Commissioner Roy Romanow, Q.C., released a report on the status and future direction of health care in Canada. The report, *Building on Values: The Future of Health Care in Canada*, included recommendations around the need for a comprehensive strategy focusing on the development and evaluation of plans for the health care workforce in Canada (referred to as a *health human resources strategy*). Notable among its recommendations was the need to prepare health care professionals to work together more effectively, beginning with the adoption of interprofessional education.

As we review below the critical events over the last decade promoting IPP, it is important to note that we expect this type of innovation to continue. Consequently, it is anticipated that policy and practice documents will continue to evolve to reflect this dynamic, growing field.

Health Care Policy Repeated calls for a move to IPP have been driven by national and provincial/territorial policy initiatives. In the past decade, two major federal government reports have clearly identified the need to create enhanced teamwork in health care delivery. These reports have set the stage for the movement toward IPP as a national priority. In the Health Council of Canada's (HCC) inaugural report, *Health Care Renewal in Canada: Accelerating Change* (2005a), three relevant recommendations speak directly to the need for collaboration and the removal of barriers to effective IPP. Specifically, the report calls for:

- accelerating the movement to new delivery models that have proven successful,
- removing the regulatory barriers between the various health professions to address the division of labour among them, and
- changing education and training models to reflect the vision of multidisciplinary teams (HCC, 2005a).

A national policy summit was held in 2005 as well. The HCC brought together over 120 key stakeholders to tackle the issue of health human resources. In the final report, *Modernizing the Management of Health Human Resources in Canada: Identifying Areas for Accelerated Change* (2005b), two policy recommendations addressed the need to move toward IPP approaches as a priority. The need to expand opportunities for interprofessional education was identified, along with recommendations for university health sciences programs to become involved and the development of funding for various learning and practice opportunities. Additionally, the issue of liability as it relates to health care professionals who are working collaboratively was identified as a priority area of focus (see Chapter 9 for more discussion of this issue). Both of these major policy directions were the result of foundational work in the preceding years. As a result, the provinces and territories followed with significant policy initiatives focusing on regional issues. Consistent across these initiatives is a clear message that the stability of the Canadian health care system is dependent upon our willingness to embrace both systemic and provider innovations based on an IPP approach.

Emerging Best Practices in Interprofessional Practice Internationally, advances in the adoption of IPP hold important clues to the directions we might take here in Canada. In the United States, the use of interprofessional teams to improve the delivery of care for persons suffering with chronic diseases by applying clinical guidelines is considered a best practice. In the United Kingdom, the National Health Service undertook widespread system reforms that resulted in most primary care groups adopting interprofessional team practice. Based on the success of this transition, the Primary Health Care Strategy was created in New Zealand, which focuses on providing universal access to primary health care services using an IPP approach. Finally, in Australia, interprofessional teams were established to respond to specific patient populations, including those in rural and remote regions. All of these examples support the transition to IPP as a means to ensure improved patient outcomes, enhanced health human resources utilization, and increased satisfaction with the health care system.

In Canada, innovations are under way that show the hallmarks of emerging best practices here as well. For example, in British Columbia, the College of Health Disciplines at the University of British Columbia (UBC) compared and contrasted 15 existing competency frameworks to look for consistencies and inconsistencies, overlap, and discrepancies. This resulted in the creation of the Competency Framework for Interprofessional Collaboration (2008), the intent of which is to support learning for health and human services professionals through the identification of three areas of competency: (a) interpersonal and communication skills, (b) patient-centred and family-focused care, and (c) collaborative practice (including decision making, roles, team functioning, and quality improvement).

In addition to the emerging focus on competencies, there are projects that focus on the development of guidelines, collaborations, and practice innovations. Spotlight 1.1 summarizes some examples that are representative of the significant advances being made in the development and identification of best practices in IPP over the last decade.

Despite the progress we have made to date, a readymade road map to IPP does not exist. However, after many decades of speculation, there is now a clearly emerging international consensus around the necessary elements required to promote IPP. Two key messages from the World Health Organization's (WHO) *Framework for Action on Interprofessional Education and Collaborative Practice* (2010) focus specifically on the role that interprofessional education plays in laying the foundation for successful IPP. **Interprofessional education (IPE)** "occurs when two or more professions learn with, from and about each other to improve collaboration and the quality of care" (Centre for the Advancement of

Helpful Tools 1.1

Best Practice Guidelines for IPP

Toolkits and guidelines are emerging as a means to support the development of competencies related to IPP. These resources also help to ensure that health care providers from all disciplines are engaged in evidence-informed practice related to IPP. Below are a few examples of available materials for specific health disciplines.

- **Medical laboratory technologists.** The College of Medical Laboratory Technologists of Ontario (CMLTO) has developed a document titled *Collaboration Practice Guidelines and Guidebook*. This resource is intended to assist medical laboratory technologists to collaborate with other health care professionals to support optimal patient outcomes. The guidelines can be accessed as a PDF file from the CMLTO's website by searching on "guidelines" (www.cmlto.com).
- **Practitioners working in primary health care.** The Enhancing Interdisciplinary Collaboration in Primary Health Care (EICP) Initiative has developed a collaboration toolkit whose aim is to provide practical tools, advice, and examples to organizations involved in primary care in order to build or sustain interdisciplinary primary health care teams. The toolkit can be accessed on the EICP Initiative website (www.eicp.ca/en).
- **Health professionals.** The Registered Nurses' Association of Ontario has developed a set of practice guidelines titled *Developing and Sustaining Interprofessional Health Care: Optimizing Patient Organizational and System Outcomes.* They focus on supporting health professionals to develop excellence in key areas salient to IPP, so that they are able to contribute to better patient care and healthy workplace environments. The guidelines provide health professionals (and administrators and educators) with the best available evidence about IPP. The RNAO's BPG on collaboration may be accessed as a PDF file from their website (www.rnao.org).

Interprofessional Education [CAIPE], 2002). As we move forward into a future where health care design and delivery must be collaborative, it is increasingly apparent that (a) interprofessional education is a prerequisite to preparing health care workers who are collaborative-practice-ready (WHO, 2010) and (b) "interprofessional education enables effective collaborative practice which in turn optimizes health-services, strengthens health systems and improves health outcomes" (WHO, 2010, p. 18).

The Interprofessional Education Movement

Chapter 8 of this text will explore in detail what we have learned about interprofessional education (IPE) to date and discuss possible future directions. However, a very brief summary of national and international trends and recommendations in IPE will be presented in order to set the stage for greater understanding of the current status of IPP. This will also help reinforce why learning about IPP and participating in IPE are important.

Spotlight 1.1

Examples of Interprofessional Practice Projects

- The development of the Canadian Interprofessional Health Collaborative (CIHC), funded by Health Canada until 2012 when it became an incorporated, not-for-profit organization, has made a significant contribution to policy development. The CIHC works with health policymakers and educational institutions to support patient-centred, collaborative care provided by various health professionals working in teams. The CIHC (2010) also works to identify and profile best practices in research, interprofessional education, and collaborative practice.
- The Health Professions Regulatory Network in Nova Scotia was formed to create a forum for the regulatory bodies of all health professions in that province to address regulatory issues. In 2008, the Network published a policy statement on interprofessional collaborative practice, identifying principles of interprofessional collaborative practice and associated outcomes (Health Professions Regulatory Network, 2008).
- Bringing together 10 national health care associations, a health care coalition, health professionals, and key stakeholders in Canada's primary health care system, the Enhancing Interdisciplinary Collaboration in Primary Health Care (EICP) Initiative focuses on creating conditions for health professionals to work together to produce the best health outcomes for individuals and families. The resulting *Framework for Interdisciplinary Collaboration in Primary Health Care* focuses on creating the practice context in which interprofessional practice may be implemented within primary health care settings.
- The Calgary Health Region, in partnership with the University of Alberta, University of Calgary, Capital Health, Southern Alberta Institute of Technology (SAIT), Bow Valley College, and Mount Royal College, undertook a project entitled Creating an Interprofessional Learning Environment Through Communities of Practice: An Alternative to Traditional Preceptorship. The focus of this three-year project is to implement a lateral mentoring framework that deemphasizes hierarchies and creates communities of practice, bringing together members of multiple professional groups in teaching and learning roles. Expected results from this project include the sharing of best approaches to interprofessional education and practice, increased numbers of health care practitioners trained to provide patient-centred collaborative care, and increased numbers of educators able to teach and mentor clinically within an interprofessional perspective.
- The University of New Brunswick, in partnership with the Dalhousie University Faculty of Medicine, New Brunswick Community College, and Atlantic Health Sciences Corporation including the St. Joseph's Community Health Centre, undertook a program entitled Interprofessional Education Using Simulations of Patient Centred Chronic Disease. The objectives of the project were to employ simulated care experiences created around chronic disease scenarios to develop a model of health care education geared to supporting students to practice in collaborative, patent-centred environments. Anticipated outcomes for this project include the production of an increased numbers of professionals trained in collaborative patient-centred practice focusing specifically on working with patients experiencing chronic diseases.

Recognizing that changes to the way we educate health care providers are key to making more systemic changes, the WHO conducted an international survey of interprofessional education practices in 2008. Close to 400 respondents from 42 countries, representing fields of health care practice, education, research, and administration, provided information about the status of interprofessional education in their respective jurisdictions. Interprofessional education was reported to take place as part of basic educational programs most often among nurses and midwives, with 16% of learners participating in some form of interprofessional education. Next most likely to take part in interprofessional education as part of their curriculum were physicians (10.2%) and physiotherapists (10.1%), followed close behind by social workers (9.3%), occupational therapists (8.9%), and pharmacists (7.7%) (WHO, 2010). As we face a global shortage of health care workers estimated at 4.3 million professionals, innovative strategies to mitigate the crisis are essential. Interprofessional collaborative practice has been identified as a singularly important strategy that has applicability across jurisdictions, with great potential for creative, context-driven utilization. At the same time, research and policy analysis dating back to the mid-1960s has identified a clear link between effective IPE and effective IPP (WHO, 2010).

Consistent with the WHO focus, one important component of Canada's national strategy to address health human resources issues is the Interprofessional Education for Collaborative Patient-Centred Practice (IECPCP) Strategy (Health Canada, n.d.). This is a pan-Canadian health human resources strategy designed to facilitate health care system change. The goal is to ensure that providers are able to work effectively within the team structure of the evolving health care system. Specific objectives of the IECPCP initiative include:

- promoting and demonstrating the benefits of interprofessional education for collaborative patient-centred practice,
- increasing the number of educators prepared to teach from an interprofessional collaborative patient-centred perspective,
- increasing the number of health professionals trained for collaborative patient-centred practice before and after entry-to-practice,
- stimulating networking and sharing of best educational approaches for collaborative patient-centred practice, and
- facilitating interprofessional collaborative care in both education and practice settings (Curran, 2007).

At this point, it is important to note that much progress has been made in the emerging field of IPP, with more under way. The growing health human resources crisis and the need to strengthen health care systems and promote improved patient outcomes supports adoption of IPP as a cornerstone of health care. To that end, this book aims to add a user-friendly resource to this exciting movement toward innovation. It should not be considered a step-by-step "how to" guide for IPP. The enactment of IPP is far too complex for such a simplistic approach. Instead, it will present, explore, and examine key aspects of IPP. Throughout, our goal is to provide a means for the reader to understand and develop an approach to practice that it is consistent with the definition and outcome measures of IPP.

CONCLUSION

This chapter provides an overview of IPP as an emerging approach to health care in Canada. IPP builds on earlier international development of team-based approaches to health care throughout the 20th century and includes key concepts such as teamwork, communication, decision making, and person-centred care. Within an IPP approach, the patient is placed at the centre of care and seen as a member of the health care team, while a more seamless, comprehensive, and efficacious system of care is promoted. Citing positive outcomes for both the recipients of health care and providers, IPP has the potential to improve both the health and the health care experience of Canadians. It also has the potential to improve the efficiency of the Canadian system, making more effective use of providers by reducing redundancy and supporting full scope of practice. Creating mechanisms by which providers are both educated together and subsequently work together effectively is an important component of the IPP movement in Canada.

SUMMARY

- Health care environments are moving toward IPP. Interprofessional practice is an orientation to health care delivery designed to promote the active participation of each discipline and the patient in health care.
- IPP is founded on principles of patient- and family-centred practice. Concepts such as collaboration, teamwork, communication, and decision making are essential to IPP.
- The stage has been set in Canada for IPP as a result of a number of key policy developments. Over the past decade, government recommendations at the provincial and federal level have called for a movement toward a more fully integrated, IPP approach to the delivery of health care.
- Although the IPP approach is considered relatively new, its roots can be traced back to practice innovations in World War II and through the health care revolution of the 1960s, 1970s, and 1980s in the United States and Canada.
- There is consistent evidence to suggest that IPP leads to improved patient outcomes, including improved patient satisfaction with health care received.
- Emerging data consistently point to interprofessional education approaches as an effective precursor to IPP. The movement toward interprofessional education is growing, with evidence pointing to the advantages of health care workers who are collaborative-practice-ready (WHO, 2010).
- Nationally, the pan-Canadian IECPCP strategy is designed to facilitate health care system change to **ensure** that health care providers are able to work together optimally.

Key Terms

collaboration
communication
communication styles
decision making
interprofessional education
interprofessional practice
person-centred care
teamwork

Review Questions

1. Identify and define the core concepts of IPP.
2. Identify and describe important contextual factors that have led to the current call for a movement toward IPP as a necessary health care innovation.
3. Summarize the emergence of the current IPP movement.
4. Describe the relationship between interprofessional education and interprofessional practice.

Application Exercises

1. *Interprofessional Practice*
   This exercise is intended to help you to become familiar with the concept of IPP. Reflect on a health care environment in which you are currently either practising or completing a practicum experience and consider the following questions. If you are currently not practising or not in a placement, consider a previous practice environment or placement that you experienced.
   a. What types of regulated and unregulated health care professionals can you identify in your practice environment?
   b. Consider the definition of IPP and the characteristics of the team-based practice approach that it requires. These characteristics include a focus on collaboration, teamwork, communication, decision making, and person-centred care. How does the clinical practice approach in your health care environment demonstrate or not demonstrate these characteristics? Would you describe the care provided as interprofessional practice? Why or why not?
2. *Interprofessional Education Opportunities*
   In this chapter, you read about interprofessional education as an important element of developing interprofessional practice skills. What examples of formal interprofessional education initiatives are in place at your educational institution or the health care setting in which you work? What examples of informal interprofessional education opportunities can you identify?

Additional Resources

Electronic Documents

Building on Values: The Future of Health Care in Canada (Romanow Report)
http://dsp-psd.pwgsc.gc.ca/Collection/CP32-85-2002E.pdf
Shared Scope of Practice Model Working Paper for British Columbia
www.health.gov.bc.ca/leg/hpc/review/shascope.html

Websites

Provincial or Territorial Healthcare Legislation/Professional Regulatory Bodies

Alberta

www.health.alberta.ca/professionals/regulatory-colleges.html

British Columbia

www.health.gov.bc.ca/professional-regulation

Manitoba

http://web2.gov.mb.ca/laws/statutes/1998/c03298e.php

New Brunswick

www.welcomenb.ca/content/wel-bien/en/immigrating_and_settling/working/foreign_qualification_recognition/health-related_regulatedoccupations.html

Newfoundland

www.gov.nf.ca/publicat/gsl/occreg.htm#C

Northwest Territories

www.hss.gov.nt.ca/professional-licensing

Nova Scotia

http://novascotia.ca/dhw/professionals.asp

Nunavut

www.gov.nu.ca/health

Ontario

www.regulatedhealthprofessions.on.ca/WHOWEARE/default.asp

Prince Edward Island

http://96.30.40.192/~peihsc/wp-content/uploads/2010/12/health_careers_on_pei_sm.pdf

Quebec

www.professions-quebec.org/index.php/en/element/visualiser/id/11

Saskatchewan

www.health.gov.sk.ca/professional-associations

Yukon

www.hss.gov.yk.ca/health_professionals.php

Additional Readings

Barrett, J. (2007). *Analysis and synthesis report PHC: Interprofessional collaboration, chronic disease management, and health promotion and disease prevention, activities, processes and tools*. Toronto, ON: Ontario Ministry of Health and Long-Term Care.

Barrett, J., Curran, V., Glynn, L., & Godwin, M. (2007). *CHSRF synthesis: Interprofessional collaboration and quality primary healthcare*. Ottawa, ON: Canadian Health Services Research Foundation.

References

Baldwin, D. C. (2007). Some historical notes on interdisciplinary and interprofessional education and practice in health care in the USA. *Journal of Interprofessional Care, 21*(S1), 23–37.

Barr, H., Freeth, D., Hammick, M., Koppel, I., & Reeves, S. (2000). *Evaluation of interprofessional education: A UK review of health and social care*. Centre for the Advancement of Interprofessional Education (CAIPE)/The British Educational Research Association (BERA). Retrieved from http://www.caipe.org.uk

Braithwaite, J., & Travaglia, J. (2005a). *The ACT health interprofessional learning and clinical education project: Background discussion paper #2. Interprofessional practice*. Canberra, AU: Braithwaite and Associates and ACT Health Department.

Braithwaite, J., & Travaglia, J. (2005b). *Inter-professional learning and clinical education: An overview of the literature*. Canberra, AU: Braithwaite and Associates and ACT Health Department.

Canadian Interprofessional Health Collaborative (CIHC). (2009). *What is patient-centred care?* Retrieved from http://www.cihc.ca/files/CIHC_Factsheets_PCC_Feb09.pdf

Canadian Interprofessional Health Collaborative (CIHC). (2010). *A national interprofessional competency framework* [PDF document]. Retrieved from http://www.cihc.ca/files/CIHC_IPCompetencies_Feb1210.pdf

Centre for the Advancement of Interprofessional Education (CAIPE). (2002). *Defining IPE*. Retrieved from http://www.caipe.org.uk/about-us/defining-ipe

College of Health Disciplines & Interprofessional Network of BC. (2008). *The British Columbia competency framework for interprofessional collaboration.* Vancouver, BC: Authors.

Curran, V. R. (2007). *Collaborative care*. Ottawa: Health Canada.

D'Amour, D., Ferrada-Videla, M., San Martin Rodríguez, L., & Beaulieu, M. D. (2005). The conceptual basis for interprofessional collaboration: Core concepts and theoretical frameworks. *Journal of Interprofessional Care, 19*(S1), 116–131.

D'Amour, D., & Oandasan, I. (2005). Interprofessionality as the field of interprofessional practice and interprofessional education: An emerging concept. *Journal of Interprofessional Care, 19*(S1), 8–10.

Greenfield, D., Nugus, P., Travaglia, J., & Braithwaite, J. (2010). Auditing an organization's interprofessional learning and interprofessional practice: The interprofessional praxis audit framework (IPAF). *Journal of Interprofessional Care, 24*(4), 436–449.

Health Canada. (n.d.). *Health care system: Interprofessional education for collaborative patient-centred practice.* Retrieved from http://www.hc-sc.gc.ca/hcs-sss/pubs/hhrhs/2006-iecps-fipccp-workatel/index-eng.php

Health Canada. (2010). *Canada's health care system (Medicare).* Retrieved from http://www.hc-sc.gc.ca/hcs-sss/medi-assur/index-eng.php

Health Canada. (2003). *First Ministers' accord on health care renewal*. Ottawa: Author.

Health Council of Canada (HCC). (2005a). *Health care renewal in Canada: Accelerating change*. Toronto, ON: Author.

Health Council of Canada (HCC). (2005b). *Modernizing the management of health human resources in Canada: Identifying areas for accelerated change. Report from a national summit*. Toronto, ON: Author.

Health Professions Regulatory Network (2008). *Position statement on interprofessional collaborative practice*. Nova Scotia: Author.

Myers, S. A., & Anderson, C. M. (2008). *The fundamentals of small group communication*. Thousand Oaks, CA: Sage Publications.

Oandasan, I., Ross Baker, G., Barker, K., Bosco, C., D'Amour, D., Jones, L., ... Way, D. (2006). *Teamwork in healthcare: Promoting effective teamwork in healthcare in Canada: Policy synthesis and recommendations*. Ottawa, ON: Canadian Health Services Research Foundation.

Registered Nurses' Association of Ontario (RNAO). (2009). *Nursing best practice guidelines: Client centred care supplement*. Toronto: Author.

Romanow, R. (2002). *Building on values: The future of health care in Canada*. Ottawa: Government of Canada Publications.

Schmitt, M. (1994). USA: Focus on interprofessional education, practice, and research. *Journal of Interprofessional Care, 8*(1), 9–18.

World Health Organization (WHO). (2010). *Framework for action on interprofessional education and collaborative practice*. Geneva: Author.

Chapter 2

Dimensions of Interprofessional Practice

Andrew Lang is a 43-year-old man, diagnosed with human immunodeficiency virus (HIV) when he was in his early twenties and currently living with acquired immune deficiency syndrome (AIDS). He describes the last two decades of his life as a "roller coaster of hope and disappointment." Andrew lives at home with his long-time partner Tam, who remains HIV-negative. He is no longer able to work, has difficulty mobilizing at times, and has been hospitalized three times during the last four months for serious AIDS-related complications. In the last week, he has experienced two falls while at home alone.

Today, Andrew and Tam have a meeting at Oakridge House, a specialty community-based hospital that focuses on compassionate HIV/AIDS care. Oakridge House provides comprehensive, coordinated services to clients in their 15-bed residential unit. A wide variety of outpatient services are also provided, including a home hospice program and many community-based support and treatment options. In the past, both Andrew and Tam have accessed services provided by Oakridge House. Andrew has participated in HIV/AIDS support groups on and off for more than 10 years. He has also taken part in nutrition counselling and holistic therapy information and educational sessions. Tam has participated in support groups for caregivers of persons with AIDS. Both Andrew and Tam describe feeling understood and cared for by the team at Oakridge House.

Andrew and Tam begin their appointment with Claire, a social worker. After his last admission to hospital six weeks ago, Andrew decided that he would no longer seek treatment that would prolong his life. He describes to Claire that he feels at peace with his choice, but he worries about the responsibility for his care that Tam has had to shoulder. Andrew shares that they are seeking to access whatever support is available to them and asks Claire for a summary of the services that Oakridge House offers.

Claire explains how health care is structured at Oakridge House. She tells them that care is provided through a team made up of various health care professionals who work together. Claire informs Andrew and Tam that she and the other team members will share information and create opportunities for consultation and dialogue, to ensure that all available options and services are considered. She explains that Andrew and his support network are considered members of the team as well, and that all decisions about what kind of care is required, who provides it, and where it happens are made collaboratively. Andrew asks who on the team makes the final decision when there is a disagreement about the best option and notes that having a say in his care is really important to him. Claire explains that, like other groups of people with different opinions, the team doesn't always agree on everything. However, team members work to understand each other's perspectives, respect each other's specialized knowledge and skill, and build consensus.

Claire says she would like to review with Andrew and Tam the information they have already provided to Oakridge House in preparation for this meeting. This includes Andrew's medical details and a summary of what their hopes are in terms of the care and services they will be able to access. But before proceeding, she notes that Andrew has a black eye and a very large bruise on the right side of his face and asks what happened. Tam informs her that he had arrived home from work two days ago to find Andrew on the floor, having fallen earlier that afternoon and unable to get himself up. He had encouraged Andrew to seek medical treatment to make sure he was all right, but had respected Andrew's adamant refusal to go back to the hospital. Claire takes the time to clarify Andrew's perspective. Together, they determine that while he is willing to be assessed by a health care professional, his fear that seeking treatment would lead to an admission against his wishes has been uppermost in his mind. Claire explains that seeking treatment from any of the team members at Oakridge House, including physicians, nurses, physiotherapists, counsellors, dieticians, and holistic care practitioners, does not mean Andrew will lose the ability to direct the decision making about his care.

Learning Outcomes

AFTER STUDYING THIS CHAPTER, YOU SHOULD BE ABLE TO:

1. **Explain the importance of an organizing framework to interprofessional practice.**
2. **Discuss the three dimensions that are central to most interprofessional practice situations.**
3. **Describe what contextual factors are and how they impact interprofessional practice.**
4. **Analyze an interprofessional practice situation using the problem identification and resolution process.**

INTRODUCTION

IN CHAPTER 1, WE MADE THE CASE THAT THE MOVEMENT TO INTERPROFESSIONAL PRACTICE (IPP) is the single most important health care change on the horizon. The above vignette provides us with an opportunity to begin to see the various aspects of IPP. The situation also invites us to consider how we might organize information in a meaningful and useful way.

In this chapter, we introduce an organizing framework intended to help health professionals understand the dimensions of IPP and approach their practice in a way that results in the desired outcomes of IPP. This framework is just one of a multitude of ways to consider the dimensions of IPP. Our intent in describing it is to provide a structure that can be used by both novice and experienced health care professionals in examining the various elements involved in practice situations. Identifying and exploring the factors involved in any situation enables us to engage more effectively as health professionals within the context in which we find ourselves. The framework may be thought of as a helpful first step in making sense of all the information to be considered in any given situation.

AN ORGANIZING FRAMEWORK FOR INTERPROFESSIONAL PRACTICE

IPP can be conceptualized as having many dimensions. It involves the coming together of health care providers, each possessing specialized knowledge and life and practice experiences. At the same time, these professionals must navigate their way through the complex contextual factors in any given practice situation. Such factors are often experienced differently depending upon one's personal and/or professional experience and perspective. Despite these differences, what is commonly shared among health care professionals is a desire to provide the best possible care to their patients/clients, be they individuals, families, groups, or communities. When we examine the many aspects of IPP, the contexts within which it occurs, and the individuals involved (e.g., patients and their support networks, as well as the health care providers representing many professions), four key observations emerge.

Observation 1: IPP involves a number of complex and interrelated processes. Many key concepts related to IPP, such as collaboration, teamwork, and communication, are processes. **Processes**, as summarized by Ellis and Fisher's (1994) classic definition, involve actions that occur in the progression toward some goal and within a given period of time. For example, teamwork in health care requires the coordination of actions within the period of time when care is planned, provided, and evaluated. IPP involves complex interactions of multiple processes occurring simultaneously.

There is growing consensus around the process-orientation of IPP (e.g., Clements, Dault, & Priest, 2007; Oandasan et al., 2006; Weaver, 2008; Xyrichis & Lowton, 2008). In a groundbreaking systematic review of collaborative practices in health care, San Martin Rodríguez, Beaulieu, D'Amour, and Ferrada-Videla (2005) identify that interprofessional collaboration in health care practice is almost always conceptualized as a process, often leading to the development of frameworks for interaction. These authors note that "the success of initiatives to develop and consolidate collaborative practices in healthcare teams ... depends on factors that are based in interpersonal factors (interactional determinants), [and] in processes inside the organization (the organizational determinants)" (p. 144).

Observation 2: IPP is relationship-driven and depends on the collaboration of the people involved in any health-related situation, including patients. Relationships are a central theme of IPP. Certainly the provision of comprehensive patient-centred care is process-driven and relies on task completion to meet desired outcomes. However, it is the relationships between patients (and their support networks) and the professionals involved in providing care that constitute the glue holding everything together. Relationships maintain team function and cohesion. They also form the foundation upon which process-driven tasks are accomplished. Smith, Stone, and Bull (2008) note that the relationships involved in IPP are complex and the focus shifts as the needs of patients and their families emerge and change. In turn, this changing priority of needs determines the composition of the members of the team involved in providing the required care.

Across the professional literature, the development of healthy professional relationships is seen as fundamental to practice. Positive relationships between care providers and patients (including their support networks) are seen as fundamental to achieving desired outcomes. Equally important are the relationships among the various health professionals involved (Mahmood-Yousuf, Munday, King, & Dale, 2008; Stenner & Courtenay, 2008). Keyton's (1999) overview of the central role of relationships in achieving desired goals of team practice continues to be widely cited in the literature. Keyton identifies three main reasons why relational factors are critical:

- Relational issues are inextricably interwoven with team tasks and processes. Tasks, for example, cannot be accomplished without the development of some form of connection between members.
- There is an expressive and emotive quality in all teams. Team and group membership help meet interpersonal needs. Being a member of a team makes us feel needed and important.
- The members of teams are interdependent. As a result, the relationship between any two individuals affects all team members.

Additionally, there is a growing body of literature citing the centrality of relationships to effective IPP. Emerging areas of focus include (a) the nature and importance of the relationships involved in IPP (e.g., Stenner & Courtenay, 2008), (b) the specific relational aspects identified as important to IPP (e.g., D'Amour, Ferrada-Videla, San Martin Rodríguez, & Beaulieu, 2005; McCallin & Bamford, 2007), and (c) the evaluation of tools to facilitate the relational components of IPP (e.g., Mahmood-Yousuf et al., 2008).

Observation 3: The practice of IPP is task-oriented, with a multitude of task-related components contributing to the provision of comprehensive health services. Health care service delivery is task-driven (Soubhi, 2010). Tasks are an important component of the work of health care professionals. The task aspects of IPP often focus on elements such as (a) role clarification and assignment of responsibility, (b) the division of labour, (c) coordination among members of the IPP team, and (d) other factors contributing to effective completion of the defined objective.

In IPP, the team of professionals who are collaborating provides a set of services, requiring different and specialized tasks to be completed. Often, only professionals who have received educational preparation in order to be able to safely and competently undertake these activities perform these tasks. Sometimes the task to be completed is psychomotor in nature, such as assisting a patient who has mobility limitations to transfer from lying in bed to sitting in a chair. In other situations, the task involves development and planning, such as assessing a patient for mobility needs and then determining a plan for teaching the patient and his or her support network how to safely move from a bed to a chair. Regardless of the exact nature of a task, there is often more than one team member who possesses the knowledge, skill, and judgment required. Thus, it is essential to be aware of the overlapping competencies that the professionals possess when considering the task component of IPP. In many situations, we need to determine which member of the team should take the lead. For example, an occupational therapist, a personal support worker, a registered nurse, a registered practical nurse, a physiotherapist, or many other professionals on the team could easily take the lead in assisting a patient to transfer, depending on the exact nature of the situation. As Soubhi (2010) points out, when considering the focus of any task-oriented situation, health care professionals must determine what actually needs to be done (e.g., help the patient to transfer). They must then organize the interdependent elements of the task (i.e., assign the right person to assist with the transfer at the right time, using the right assistive devices with the appropriate knowledge, skill, and judgment).

Further, the nature of the tasks required to provide comprehensive and concerted care to patients is emergent. It often only becomes known as the needs and issues of the patient, as well as the processes involved in caring for him or her, unfold. In IPP, as the composition of the team changes in response to patient preferences, health needs, and external constraints, tasks may vary to include those that fall outside the normal routines of team members (Smith et al., 2008). This shifting of responsibilities is an example of the flexibility inherent in health care service delivery and should be considered one of the strengths of IPP.

Observation 4: There are many contextual factors that may be unique to a practice situation or environment. Within any given practice situation, there are unique factors related to the patient, the health professional(s), the practice environment, and even the health care system. Some of these contextual factors may be known at the outset (e.g., we may be aware that an elderly patient lives alone and will require discharge planning that takes this fact into account). Other contextual factors may emerge as we provide health care services. For example, we may discover that this elderly patient has two children who are pushing for very different discharge scenarios: one advocating a long-term-care facility and one desiring to see his parent return home with supports. Another common area in which we may see contextual factors impinging on health care delivery relates to the diminishing availability of resources, from equipment to health professionals; this is becoming a more and more significant concern in health care.

Bringing Everything Together

On the basis of the observations described above, we have broadly categorized the various components of IPP into three interrelated dimensions: (a) process dimension, (b) relationship dimension, and (c) task dimension. All of these are situated within a backdrop of complex and constantly evolving contextual factors. Considered together, these dimensions and coexisting contextual factors represent a framework that can be used by health care practitioners to analyze IPP situations through an organized and fluid process. This process of uncovering key elements occurring in any given situation is essential to bringing clarity to practice. It also helps to illuminate individual and team issues that are present or likely to emerge. By examining the process dimension, the relationship dimension, the task dimension, and contextual factors in any given situation, we are able to identify individual and group perspectives that will support the provision of the best possible health care.

The ultimate goal of the organizing framework is to create an approach by which health care providers are able to engage in IPP. This happens in the moment and at the point of service, as well as during long-term health care planning activities. The organizing framework integrates perspectives, traditionally considered oppositional, that focus on the outcome of health care and on the processes involved in providing it. In so doing, it enables us to create a holistic view in which the most relevant elements present within a given situation are examined (see Figure 2.1).

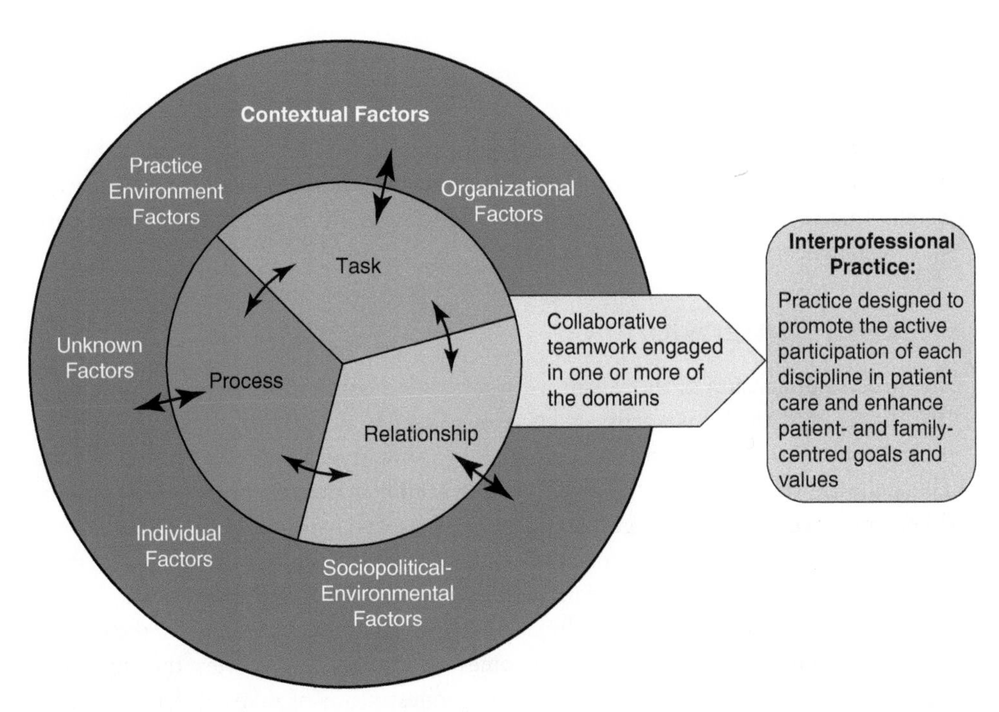

Figure 2.1 Organizing Framework for IPP

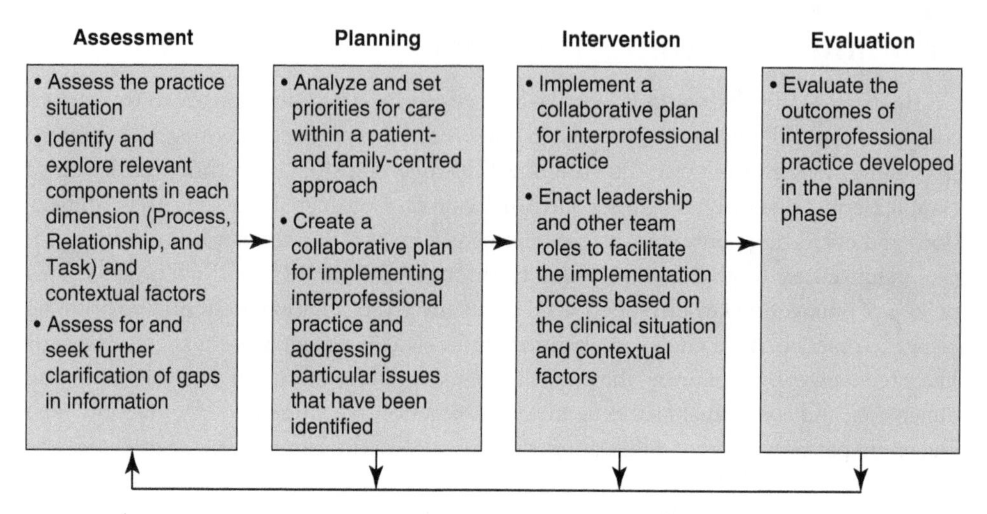

Figure 2.2 Problem Identification and Resolution Process

We have also provided a problem identification and resolution process consistent with other basic problem-solving approaches (see Figure 2.2). The intent of this process is to further assist the reader to appreciate how this framework might be applied in health care practice situations.

DIMENSIONS OF IPP

In this section, we turn our attention to the dimensions of IPP that are organized by the framework. To demonstrate how the framework may be used within a practice situation, we will first review each of the dimensions and then return to the opening vignette to illustrate application of these ideas.

Process Dimension

The **process dimension** of the organizing framework describes the "how" of engaging in IPP. Recall that earlier we defined the term *process* as actions that take place in the progression toward the completion of a goal or task within a particular period of time. This definition suggests that there are four essential elements in a process: (a) actions, (b) progression of time, (c) change that occurs over time, and (d) outcomes or results. A process is not a fixed sequence of events; rather, it is dynamic, frequently consisting of many elements that interact, change, and influence each other (Ellis & Fisher, 1994).

Our growth and development as human beings is an excellent example of the interaction of many processes to produce the outcomes we observe. We can view the physiological functioning of our bodies as a complex orchestration of many different cellular processes, leading to larger body system processes, and affecting overall developmental processes. To illustrate this point, consider Jamie, an 18-month-old toddler who is eating a snack. As Jamie eats his cheese and crackers, multiple interrelated processes are set into motion. At the body-system level, processes for breaking down the food into digestible components begin through chewing in the mouth and mechanical grinding and release of digestive enzymes in the stomach. One outcome of this complex process of digestion is the absorption of nutrients that are the basic building blocks for cellular growth and differentiation. This is yet another biological process, which occurs at a more micro level. At the same time, psychological and cognitive processes are also under way. Jamie is learning to feed himself and to begin to have an impact on his environment. As he plays with his food, sometimes dropping it on the floor for the family dog to eat, cognitive processes around learning are initiated.

Within any given situation, countless overlapping processes may be identified and explored. Often the challenge is to determine which are most relevant to the desired outcome. Consider Jamie again for a moment. His mother is concerned that his weight is low for his age and height. She wonders if it is more important to provide him with food that is more easily digested (i.e., supporting the digestive process) or to decrease his level of distraction and help him to focus on putting food in his mouth rather than on the floor (i.e., supporting the cognitive/psychological process). Both digestion and cognition are likely highly relevant to this situation. As is typically the case in health care settings as well, the answer is often a combination of strategies that simultaneously have an effect on multiple processes.

In a similar way, there are a multitude of processes at play within a health care organizational system and among the collaborative actions of health care professionals working toward achieving IPP. As with our growth and development, individual professionals engaged in IPP are sometimes not aware of all the processes under way that result in the outcomes they observe and achieve. For example, some of the processes that occur within an IPP team, such as how members interpret the information and messages they receive, operate automatically. Understanding how to utilize processes in such a way that they help us to attain the optimal results seems obvious. However, it is not always as apparent as we may assume. If not well thought out, a team's choices regarding the processes they are utilizing within a given situation may lead to poor team performance, low productivity, and even errors that affect the well-being of patients. IPP efforts involving teams and teamwork require an understanding of how to appropriately engage in the multitude of processes required to attain desired outcomes. Table 2.1 provides a description of four basic categories of processes commonly seen in IPP.

The opening vignette of this chapter demonstrates two examples of processes common in IPP:

- *Problem-solving* is illustrated when Claire engages with Andrew and Tam to determine the underlying reason for Andrew's resistance to seeking medical treatment for the injuries he sustained from his recent falls. Her ability to help Andrew to identify and verbalize the source of his resistance is the first step in successful resolution of this issue. Secondly, Claire's openness to Andrew's perspective about

Table 2.1 Process Dimension Categories

Process Category	Description
Personal or person-to-person processes	■ Reflect an individual's preferred information processing style. ■ Individuals typically favour some approach to interacting with and responding to events and information to which they are exposed. ■ For example, one broad categorization of individual information processing preferences describes whether a person is most comfortable with verbal information (auditory processing), written information (visual processing), or tactile information (kinesthetic processing).
Team processes	■ Describe the mechanisms by which teams function and are organized in order to ensure that work is accomplished. ■ Team processes are most effective when they take into account both personal processes of members and higher level profession-specific and organizational processes. ■ For example, within some teams, decision making occurs through a hierarchical, top-down approach, while in other teams input from all team members is considered.
Profession-specific processes	■ Describe processes that are specific to each regulated health care profession. These processes are commonly associated with a particular profession through legislation or specialized education. ■ Also includes processes that may be common across a range of professions, but are tailored by each profession on the basis of scope of practice, professional standards, and codes of practice (e.g., physical assessment). ■ For example, health legislation may indicate what types of activities may be delegated from one health professional to another and the process for this delegation of responsibility.
Organizational or health care system-specific processes	■ Refer to processes that are unique to an organization or to the health care sector, as compared to other organizations or sectors. ■ For example, the process for formal consultation of additional types of health care providers, such as certain types of medical specialists in a given clinical situation, may occur along implicit organizational processes or explicit health care system processes. Health care system processes also include accreditation and government reporting requirements. Internal organizational processes include specific policies in place within a given health care setting.

decision making related to his care options allows her to work collaboratively with him to find an acceptable alternative solution to avoiding health care. In this way, Claire and Andrew collaborate around problem solving, each bringing important information and perspectives.

- *Conflict resolution* is described as Claire shares with Andrew and Tam the Oakridge House IPP team's approach to differing perspectives. Instead of expecting all team members to agree, the IPP team members focus on trying to understand each other's viewpoints and appreciating the specialized knowledge and skill of all of the other team members. This is a somewhat idealized portrayal, but it is important in its focus on a foundation of respect.

Relationship Dimension

The **relationship dimension** of the organizing framework encompasses variables related to the interpersonal realm of health care practice; the "who" of IPP. When we consider the relationship dimension, we are concerned with the people involved in the situation at hand. This dimension consists of elements such as people, roles, perceptions, emotions, values and beliefs, communication styles, leadership and membership approaches, group dynamics, and group climate.

Within the relationship dimension, it is not only professional roles (e.g., an addiction counsellor, a paramedic, a nurse, a physician, a social worker) that are relevant. It also matters who people are as persons and professionals, their self-concept, and their identity within the context of a team. Health care professionals participating in IPP bring with them multiple characteristics and perspectives, including personal elements such as perceptions, emotions, and values and beliefs. Additionally, because the patient and their support network are a part of the team, the relationships between them and the health care professionals providing care are equally significant.

Within this dimension, we also consider elements associated with the relationships involved in IPP. This includes variables such as communication styles, methods, and approaches; leadership and membership styles; and relational dynamics and conflict. Given these multiple factors, it is not a surprise that the relationship dimension often poses the greatest challenge for professionals engaging in IPP.

Returning to the opening vignette, many of the elements of the relationship dimension can be identified, including the following:

- *People and roles* involved in the situation include the patient (Andrew), his partner (Tam), and a health professional (Claire, a social worker). In the vignette Clair also discusses the various professional team members who will be involved in the care provided to Andrew and his support network. Each of these people brings a unique perspective and life and professional experiences. When enacting a professional role, each of the team members also brings common role-defined characteristics, such as empathy, patience, and integrity.
- *Values and beliefs* are depicted from a personal and professional perspective in the vignette. Andrew shares that being involved in decisions about his own care is most important to him. Claire also demonstrates professional values and beliefs related to patient-centred care when she collaborates with Andrew and Tam, seeking solutions to the situation at hand that meet everyone's desires.

- *Leadership and membership styles* emerge as Claire, Andrew, and Tam begin to form a care team. In the exchange described in the vignette, we see a somewhat formal type of leadership role being enacted by Claire as the professional assigned to begin the collaborative partnering process with Andrew and Tam. However, in IPP, health professionals and patients commonly engage in leadership and membership role enactment that is more fluid and informal. This is evident in the vignette as Claire works collaboratively with Andrew and Tam, exploring with them their past experiences and their hopes for the care that Oakridge House is able to provide. Claire also provides options for next steps, permitting Andrew and Tam to make decisions that best meet their needs.

Task Dimension

The **task dimension** consists of variables representing the work that needs to be undertaken in order to provide patient care. The task dimension is the "what" of IPP. Variables found within this dimension include actions, behaviours, and desired outcomes. It is often within this dimension that the goals for patient care are illuminated.

One of the most important elements to consider along the task dimension is temporality, or the time frame for achieving the desired outcome. Short-range, midrange, and long-range goals may be identified within given health care situations. Understanding how these goals fit together in creating a comprehensive, interprofessional plan of care for each client is essential. In traditional hospital-based acute care, short-range goals often take highest priority, as the focus is on helping patients get to the point of either discharge home or transfer to a long-term-care or rehabilitation setting for further recovery. As we consider the broader concept of health, we need to focus not only on recovery from the acute phase of an illness or injury but also on the care patients access within the community setting. Care in the community is often associated with mid-term and long-range goals related to persistent or chronic health concerns. For example, in the opening vignette, Andrew and Tam accessed support group and counselling services through Oakridge House to meet mental health related mid-term goals such as improved coping and stress reduction. Moving forward from this point in the vignette, it would be important to explore the types of services available to Andrew in relation to rehabilitation and potentially palliation to meet his long-range goals.

A full list of all possible task dimension elements might extend almost endlessly and would certainly be tedious to compile, even when we consider only the tasks that one type of health professional on a team might perform in a specific context (e.g., all the tasks an activation coordinator might perform in working with residents in a long-term-care facility). It is, however, worth noting a few important elements in order to appreciate the focus of this dimension within the larger picture of the organizing framework. The task dimension includes activities and behaviours that we perceive to be part of our professional roles. The types of elements found within this dimension include temporality, skilled care, skilled assessments, knowledge application including patient teaching, and patient advocacy.

Once again, the opening vignette is a helpful tool in exploring this dimension. Many task dimension elements are identifiable in the scenario. A few are described below:

- *Temporality* (or time frame) becomes more apparent as the situation involving Andrew and his partner, Tam, unfolds. Initially, one might assume that Claire, Andrew, and Tam are meeting to create a plan for Andrew's immediate care given his recent experience with multiple falls. However, as Andrew shares with Claire his concerns about maintaining control over decisions about his ongoing care, it is apparent that a long-term vision of what priorities will underpin his care choices and the approach the team takes will be essential.
- *Provision of skilled care and performance of skilled assessments* were demonstrated throughout the scenario. Throughout the interview, Claire's expert performance of skilled social-work care in her partnering with Andrew and Tam is very apparent. She is also in a position to make arrangements, should Andrew agree, for another type of health care provider to undertake a focused health assessment in relation to his recent falls.
- *Patient advocacy* is one of the cornerstones of professional health care practice, and it is reflected in the mission of Oakridge House, the approach taken by Claire, and the support provided by Andrew's partner, Tam.

Contextual Factors

The three core dimensions of the organizing framework for IPP (process, relationship, and task) share a reciprocal relationship with a number of **contextual factors**. These include factors specific to the practice environment, to the individual (both the patient and the professional), and to the organization. Additionally, the inclusion of unknown factors is intended to capture those factors within the environment or the situation that are not tangible or were not identifiable at the outset. Contextual factors may be categorized as practice environment factors, organizational factors, individual factors, sociopolitical factors, and unknown factors. Some examples of contextual factors in the opening vignette that may shape IPP and ultimately the care Andrew will receive are identified as follows:

- *Practice environment factors* in this situation include the availability of specific interprofessional team resources (e.g., a well-developed interprofessional team with established team functioning norms).
- *Organizational factors* include issues of funding for the organization, organizational structure, and lines of communication. Understanding how decision making takes place outside of a single interprofessional team and within the broader organization may be important.
- *Individual factors* may include the other spheres of Andrew and Tam's lives, as well as those of the professionals who are collaborating with them.

Applying the Organizing Framework

The organizing framework we have presented may serve a number of useful purposes for health professionals working toward IPP. First, it provides a means to support individuals or teams of health professionals to engage in IPP by enabling them to organize and analyze the many aspects of a given health care situation. In those health care environments where more formal IPP teams exist, the organizing framework also presents a perspective for viewing teams and teamwork. From a developmental perspective, for example, the framework may be used to guide and support team development. As the interprofessional team develops, the interactions between specific elements of the three dimensions may be emphasized, highlighting areas in which team members may focus their attention. For example, as the team that will collaborate with Andrew and Tam forms, elements of the relationship dimension intersecting with the processes involved in Andrew's care may come into focus.

It is important to remember that while we have focused on each of the dimensions of the framework one at a time through the use of this chapter's vignette, in the real world of health care practice there is overlap and fluidity among the dimensions of IPP. Elements from each dimension may be relevant to any given situation, and the intersection of multiple factors is often the hallmark of the complex health care situations that we experience on a daily basis.

CONCLUSION

This chapter provides an organizing framework for IPP. This framework includes the process dimension, the task dimension, and relationship dimension. Each of these dimensions is typically represented in IPP situations, while their relative significance in any given situation varies. These three dimensions are viewed from within a backdrop of complex contextual factors, which are unique to the situation. The organizing framework is intended to create an approach that will support health care providers in IPP situations to provide care in the moment and at the point of care. It is also useful in promoting reflective approaches necessary to enhance longer term health care planning purposes.

SUMMARY

- IPP involves dynamic and intersecting processes and is both complex and contextually based. As a result, it is unlikely that a how-to user manual can be developed to instruct health professionals in implementing and practising IPP. However, there is a growing body of knowledge from which to develop approaches to successfully practise interprofessionally.
- The organizing framework presented in this chapter is one tool that may help to bridge the gap between conceptualizing and practising IPP.

- The organizing framework emerges from key observations in the literature that hold that IPP is task-oriented, process- and relationally driven, and influenced and modified by many contextual factors.
- The framework consists of three dimensions (process–relationship–task), each with specific elements. The organizing framework also takes into account the influence of a number of contextual factors that include individual, sociopolitical, and environmental factors.

Key Terms

contextual factors
processes
process dimension
relationship dimension
task dimension

Review Questions

1. Identify the three dimensions that are included in the organizing framework described in this chapter, and describe why an approach such as this might be beneficial in health care practice.
2. Describe two elements that would be found in each of the process, relationship, and task dimensions.
3. Discuss what contextual factors are and how they may influence IPP.
4. Describe how examination of the process, relationship, and task dimensions of the opening vignette enables you to uncover more information than would be the case if you just read the scenario alone.

Application Exercises

1. Imagine in the opening vignette that Andrew further shares with Claire and other members of the IPP team that his greatest concern is loss of control over what will happen to him if he seeks medical treatment for events such as his recent falls. Apply the problem identification and resolution process to consider how to address his concern.
2. Identify a practice situation that you have experienced involving various members of the health care team as you respond to the following questions.
   a. Applying the organizing framework for IPP, identify as many process-, relationship-, and task-dimension elements as you can.
   b. Identify which are the most relevant elements in each of the dimensions.
   c. Describe which dimension was most central in the situation and why.
   d. Identify the contextual factors in this situation, and consider how they might have influenced what was happening.
   e. Describe what insights may be gained by analyzing this event.

Additional Resources

Websites/Organizations

Journal of Interprofessional Care (may be accessed through institutional library online resources)
http://informahealthcare.com/loi/jic

Journal of Research in Interprofessional Practice and Education (may be accessed through institutional library online resources)
www.jripe.org/index.php/journal

Additional Readings

Meads, G., Ashcroft, J., Barr, H., Scott, R., & Wild, A. (2005). *The case for interprofessional collaboration: In health and social care*. Oxford, UK: Wiley-Blackwell.

References

Clements, D., Dault, M., & Priest, A. (2007). Effective teamwork in healthcare: Research and reality. *Healthcare Papers 7*(Spec. Issue), 26–34.

D'Amour, D., Ferrada-Videla, M., San Martin Rodríguez, L., & Beaulieu, M. D. (2005). The conceptual basis for interprofessional collaboration: Core concepts and theoretical frameworks. *Journal of Interprofessional Care, 19*(S1), 116–131.

Ellis, D. G., & Fisher, B. A. (1994). *Small group decision making: Communication and the group process* (4th ed.). New York: McGraw-Hill.

Keyton, J. (1999). Relational communication in groups. In L. R. Frey (Ed.), *The handbook of group communication theory & research* (pp. 192–222). Thousand Oaks, CA: Sage.

Mahmood-Yousuf, K., Munday, D., King, N., & Dale, J. (2008). Interprofessional relationships and communication in primary palliative care: Impact of the Gold Standards Framework. *British Journal of General Practice, 58*, 256–263.

McCallin, A., & Bamford, A. (2007). Interdisciplinary teamwork: Is the influence of emotional intelligence fully appreciated? *Journal of Nursing Management, 15*(4), 386–391.

Oandasan, I., Ross Baker, G., Barker, K., Bosco, C., D'Amour, D., Jones, L., ... Way, D. (2006). *Teamwork in healthcare: Promoting effective teamwork in healthcare in Canada. Policy synthesis and recommendations*. Ottawa: Canadian Health Services Research Foundation.

San Martin Rodríguez, L., Beaulieu, M. D., D'Amour, D., & Ferrada-Videla, M. (2005). The determinants of successful collaboration: A review of the theoretical and empirical studies. *Journal of Interprofessional Care, 19*(S1), 132–14.

Stenner, K., & Courtenay, M. (2008). The role of inter-professional relationships and support for nurse prescribing in acute and chronic pain. *Journal of Advanced Nursing, 63*(3), 276–283.

Smith, T., Stone N., & Bull, R. (2008). Chapter 12: Strengthening interprofessional practice. In S. Liaw & S. Kilpatrick (Eds.), *A textbook of Australian rural health* (pp. 165–176). Canberra: Australian Rural Health Education Network.

Soubhi, H. (2010). *Problem solving: What is the residue?* Retrieved from http://jripe.wordpress.com

Weaver, E. T. (2008). Enhancing multiple disciplinary teams. *Nursing Outlook, 56*(3), 108–113.

Xyrichis, A., & Lowton, K. (2008). What fosters or prevents interprofessional teamworking in primary and community care? A literature review. *International Journal of Nursing Studies, 45*(1), 140–153.

Part II
Foundations of Interprofessional Practice

Part II of this book is designed to help the reader develop greater understanding of the concepts central to interprofessional practice (IPP) and begin to apply these ideas to practice situations. The knowledge base pertaining to IPP is immense and continues to grow. However, we believe the topics in Part II provide the necessary foundation on which both new and experienced health professionals can begin to work interprofessionally.

To this end, Chapter 3 focuses on teams, team processes, and teamwork as the context within which most aspects of IPP occur. Chapter 4 examines the elements that make up the relationship dimension of the IPP organizing framework. In particular, it explores the roles and relationships of health care professionals in IPP and focuses specifically on interprofessional communication. The core concept of collaboration, an element found within the process dimension, is the focus of Chapter 5. In Chapter 6 we turn our attention to problem solving and its relationship to conflict and negotiation. Finally, in Chapter 7, we discuss leadership within the context of IPP. It is important to note that although the task dimension and contextual factors of the organizing framework are not the focus of any specific chapter of Part II, these elements and their relationship to the other dimensions are interwoven throughout the chapters.

Chapter 3
Teams and Teamwork

A team comprising various health care professionals who work in a complex continuing care and rehabilitation centre is meeting for the first time. The team has been brought together to revitalize the centre's Employee Orientation Program after consistent feedback indicating that newly hired staff felt it failed to meet their needs. Apart from a few details that were provided when they were approached to volunteer, the members of the team know little about the project when they first meet.

The team consists of Julie, a physiotherapist, Yuhong, a registered practical nurse, Kelly, a registered nurse, David, a respiratory therapist, Helen, a physician, Phil, a rehabilitation therapist, and Sally, the director of education for the hospital. As might be expected of a team meeting for the first time—with the exception of David and Sally, the members have never worked together in any capacity—they are both excited and nervous. However, most of them have been part of similar teams, with varying degrees of success. Yuhong and Julie have worked in unproductive teams with poor interpersonal dynamics.

Sally is chairing this first meeting. As an administrator with knowledge and expertise in the area of education, she sees her role as that of team leader/facilitator. She has prepared a presentation that describes the Employee Orientation Program and the issues that have been identified with it. As a means of generating new ideas to improve the program, Sally's plan is to engage the team in a brainstorming activity. However, as the meeting gets under way, it quickly derails from her agenda.

Sally: Thanks, everyone, for your brief introductions. Now that we all know who's who, let's get started. I've prepared a slideshow outlining the current orientation program and the feedback we have received to date.

David: Sally, thanks for putting this together, but I was thinking maybe we should spend a little more time getting to know each other before we jump into the meat of the project. What do you think?

Sally: Well ... OK. What does the rest of the team think?

Yuhong: I don't think we really need to do that. We're all pretty busy and this is a time-limited project, so we need to use our time wisely. Let's save the chit-chat for coffee breaks and get on with the work. I think we should let Sally finish telling us about the project, then plan what we are going to do and who is doing what.

Julie: I agree with Yuhong. We need very clear roles. The last time I was part of a team project, it dragged on for ages because there was lack of clarity in tasks and roles and only a few people did the work. We would get side-tracked by social conversation and others would goof around.

Phil: I hear what you're saying, Julie, but I think it's important to get to know each other if we're going to work together as a team for the next several weeks. I think we can spare a few minutes to get acquainted!

Yuhong: What does it matter who we are? I don't see how that contributes to what we have been asked to do.

Sally: OK, I think there are some really valid points here on both sides, and it's clear that we're all passionate about doing a good job and meeting our goal. How about we start by going around the table and each person can briefly offer his or her perceptions and experiences of orientation, both in general and here? We can learn a bit about each other and begin to tackle the issues related to the orientation program at the same time.

Learning Outcomes

AFTER STUDYING THIS CHAPTER YOU SHOULD BE ABLE TO:

1. **Define a health care team and teamwork.**
2. **Identify and describe key concepts related to teams and teamwork.**
3. **Explain how interprofessional teams differ from other types of health care teams.**
4. **Describe how teams and teamwork influence IPP and health care outcomes.**
5. **Recognize facilitators and barriers to team effectiveness within a team-based situation or activity.**

INTRODUCTION

TEAMS, TEAMWORK, AND THE PROCESSES INVOLVED IN THIS TYPE OF INTERACTION ARE important core concepts in interprofessional practice (IPP). Within the literature, teamwork is identified as the main context within which IPP occurs (D'Amour, Ferrada-Videla, San Martin-Rodriguez, & Beaulieu, 2005). In IPP, varying degrees of teamwork take place. These distinctions are reflected in the different types of teams that can be identified within today's health care settings. They range from very informal ones that are nonspecific in function to formal ones with clearly defined functions such as the project team in the opening vignette.

Every one of us has likely been in a situation similar to the one in the vignette, in which we saw members of a team meeting for the first time to work on a problem. In these team-related situations, the problems to be solved and the interactions and processes between the members of the team may be equally complex. In the vignette, this complexity is revealed in the different perspectives that members share about how to establish the team and begin their work. Team members are able to acknowledge the importance of working together to renew the centre's program. However, they lack clarity about how to proceed and engage with each other. The vignette also touches on the kinds of or lack of processes that can occur within a team. Team processes and structures are fundamental to team function and effectiveness (Drinka & Clark, 2000). They have both direct and indirect effects on the ability to meet a team's objectives. If a team in health care, or any other area, is to function effectively, it must actively focus on developing and establishing processes and structures, rather than leaving these to chance.

This chapter aims to help the reader develop knowledge and understanding of the key concepts and processes related to teams and teamwork, promoting participation as a member of IPP team. We begin with a review of key concepts such as team development and norms. We then examine teams and teamwork as the context for IPP. Finally, we identify and discuss attributes and issues that influence the effectiveness of teams, and ultimately the outcomes of IPP.

DEFINING A HEALTH CARE TEAM AND TEAMWORK

Teams play an important role in today's health care system. The shift in focus toward team-based practice has increased as our health care system has evolved over the past several decades. As was noted in Chapter 1, both historical factors, such as the creation of medicare in Canada, and present-day factors (e.g., current population health issues and the global shortages of health professionals) have been the driving forces behind this trend. Although creating consensus around the definitions of teamwork-related ideas has been challenging (Drinka & Clark, 2000), it is possible to synthesize them using common features of the various conceptualizations within the literature.

In this text we define a **health care team** as an organized system consisting of interdependent health care professionals who provide care. This happens as they engage in processes and develop structures to guide actions and encourage collaborative problem solving and decision making. A health care team takes into consideration the expectations of both the patient(s) being cared for and the organization or system in which care is provided. As defined in Chapter 1, teamwork is a goal-oriented and relationally based process. In the context of IPP, it constitutes the interactions and relationships between health professionals who work together to address the patient's care needs (Oandasan et al., 2006). Mickan and Rodger (2005) identify the key components of teamwork as (a) agreed-upon objectives, (b) shared and agreed-upon responsibilities, (c) clearly defined boundaries and roles, and (d) sharing of information, learning opportunities, and resources. Teamwork involves coordination, cohesion, and leadership. Consequently a number of conditions, behaviours, and attitudes can be expected when engaging in it (Poulton, 2003):

- Team members are mutually dependent upon each other.
- Team members gain from working together to achieve patient-centred care.
- Team members have an awareness of when it is best to engage in teamwork.
- Team members perceive themselves as working together to achieve patient-centred care.
- Team members foster the likelihood of shared decision making through the open sharing of information.

Types of Health Care Teams

It is important to consider the research that has explored the types of teams found in health care environments and the characteristics and outcomes of effective teamwork in those environments (e.g., D'Amour et al., 2005; Oandasan et al., 2006). Additionally, there has been considerable attention paid to the type of team-based practice needed to achieve the goals of improving patient outcomes, maintaining the principles of medicare, and managing the fiscal and other realities of our health care system (e.g., Hayward, Forbes, Lau, & Wilson, 2000). Similar driving forces underscore efforts related to the development of team-based approaches within health care systems outside of Canada (Sampson & Marthas, 1990).

Numerous terms are used to differentiate the types of teams and the level of engagement and interaction that occurs within them in health care environments. In many instances, these terms are not clearly defined and are used interchangeably (D'Amour et al., 2005). Table 3.1 provides a summary of the most frequent types of health care teams described in the literature.

Consider for a moment the team in the opening vignette. Which type of team listed in Table 3.1 do you think it most closely resembles? On the basis of the characteristics of the team and their stated goals, we would conclude that it is a project team. The members have been brought together to achieve the specific goals of evaluating and redeveloping the hospital orientation program. Therefore, the life of the team is short-term, with an expectation that it will disband once those goals are achieved.

Response to Team-Based Approaches

Historically, the response from health care professionals to team-based approaches has been mixed, including confusion, the emergence of hidden agendas, and even outright resistance and rejection. Often these responses stem from concerns that they will have to relinquish their professional autonomy (Drinka & Clark, 2000). A common concern among nurses, for example, is that team-based approaches may represent hierarchically structured processes that leave them little decision-making authority. On the other hand, professionals who have traditionally held greater decision-making authority and

Table 3.1 Commonly Described Types of Health Care Teams

Type of Team	Description
Project team/ working group	Short-term; membership consists of one or many professions/ disciplines/departments that come together to solve a problem or meet objective(s) and then disbands; team often elects a formal leader.
Multidisciplinary team	Involves situations in which different types of professionals interact on a limited basis and may not engage with each other; professionals work and make decisions independently but in parallel to provide care for patients or to complete a project; team utilizes structures that facilitate coordination of their work.
Interdisciplinary/ interprofessional team	Members of this type of team are from more than one profession/ discipline; the team works interdependently with a stronger emphasis on team dynamics, shared ownership, common goals, and common decision-making processes; members open up professional boundaries in order to effectively share responsibilities, collaborate, and engage in integrated activities to address problems and provide care; leadership is appropriate to issues and/or expertise required. There is debate over which term, *interdisciplinary* or *interprofessional*, should be used to describe this type of team. This debate centres on which disciplines should be considered professionals.
Transdisciplinary team	Type of practice characterized by an evolved level of interdependency and trust among members; professional boundaries and territories are opened, roles and skills are transferrable across disciplines; members of the team share information, knowledge, skills, and responsibilities across disciplinary boundaries to meet shared and agreed-upon goals and objectives.

responsibility, such as physicians, may view team approaches as a threat to their status and position. Both of these perspectives reflect deeper, historically rooted, and generally unhealthy professional territorial issues. It is essential to uncover and resolve these issues and biases in order to work collaboratively.

Team-based approaches neither disenfranchise health care professionals nor require that they give up autonomous practice. While the majority of clinical situations require health care providers to interact with each other, thus engaging in a team-based approach, there will be times when they need to act and make decisions autonomously. Autonomous practice and IPP are but two of a number of different methods of practice. In any given workday, practitioners are often engaging in a range of independent and interdependent health care activities. D'Amour and colleagues (2005) emphasize that team-based approaches fall within a broader continuum of professional autonomy that is capped on one end by health care professionals practising independently yet parallel to each other and on the other by highly autonomous teams. Determining in which circumstances one should utilize a certain method of practice requires that the health care professionals involved have an understanding of the various available methods.

KEY CONCEPTS RELATED TO TEAMS

Current conceptualizations of health care teams and the various ways that professionals often work together in health care environments have their roots in the fields of organizational studies and sociology. This literature reveals many conceptions of why people form teams, how teams develop and work effectively, and the nature of the systems within which they operate. Key concepts necessary for an understanding of teams in IPP include team development, communication, norms, and normative pressure. These concepts are broadly categorized as team processes.

Team Processes

Team processes might be thought of as the "how" of IPP—the sets of steps or actions enacted by health care professionals, working in teams and engaged in teamwork, that result in the outcomes of IPP. Unlike individual processes, which often take place in the background and are not detectable (e.g., thinking), team processes are the largely visible and tangible behaviours team members engage in as they enact IPP. Within the process dimension of the organizing framework for IPP described in Chapter 2, team processes are prominent elements.

Descriptions of the following three key team processes are presented: (a) team development, (b) communication (which will be further discussed in Chapter 4), and (c) the development of team norms and normative pressures. As you read about these processes and additional ones that will be introduced later in this text, it is important to keep in mind that they are not mutually exclusive. Rather, they impact health care situations and team interactions to varying degrees in all kinds of contexts. Further, the individual processes of each team member also influence these team processes. For example, in the opening vignette the thought processes and personal communication style of each team member may influence the communication structure of the team in a positive or negative direction.

Helpful Tools 3.1 presents an exercise involving the problem identification and resolution process introduced in Chapter 2. The exercise is intended to help you apply what you learn about team processes.

Team Development The development of a team is a fundamental process that often structures, organizes, and influences other processes involved in IPP, including communication and decision making. A team's development may be conceptualized in much the same manner as our individual development as human beings. Like individuals, teams progress through their own developmental stages and reach milestones. Analogously to theories of human development, several theoretical approaches to understanding how teams function and develop over time have been proposed. Although these theories are not perfectly applicable and should be considered more as exemplars or ideal

Helpful Tools 3.1

Applying the Problem Identification and Resolution Process

In this activity, you will apply your knowledge of team processes to the opening vignette of this chapter. You will use the problem identification and resolution process tool introduced in Chapter 2, which is designed to enable you to analyze a situation by focusing on the process–relationship–task organizing framework for IPP. The tool includes four phases by which to consider a practice situation: assessment, planning, intervention, and evaluation.

In this activity we focus on the assessment phase. Recall that this phase involves:

- collecting data
- identifying and exploring relevant components/issues within each dimension (process, relationship, and task) and contextual factors
- assessing for and seeking further clarification of gaps in information

Activity Steps

Review the opening vignette again and consider, if you were a member of the project team, how you would assess the situation. Answer the following questions:

1. What information (data) is available and what is unknown?
2. What are the issues in the vignette? Thinking about the processes described in this chapter and Chapter 2, which are relevant?
3. What is the problem in the situation? Provide a succinct statement of the problem.

representations, they still provide us with a way to describe and analyze the stages through which health care teams might progress. They can also provide insight into how individual members engage within the team context, and how teams interact within the health care system and with each other.

There are a multitude of relevant theories that describe how teams develop and change, but most include consideration of:

- the critical issues teams experience
- the work or task of teams, and the relationships and interactions between the members
- the order or manner in which the team's critical issues are thought to occur
- consideration of issues related to authority as the first priority, along with leadership and member-to-member relationships

Among the theories related to team development, the most commonly used describe a linear, sequential progression through stages or phases, from initiation or beginning to termination or closure. Bruce Tuckman's (1965) Stages of Group Development is the best-known and perhaps most influential of these models. Reference to Tuckman's model is commonplace today in environments where teams and teamwork are a focus. Tuckman arrived at it in 1965 through a synthesis of the literature on group development. He initially described

Table 3.2 Tuckman's Stages of Group Development

Stage/Component	Description
Forming	In this initial stage, group members learn about each other and the tasks to be completed.
Storming	This stage notes that group members will engage each other in arguments and vie for status and authority in the group as they become more comfortable with each other. This is notably a period of tension and conflict within the group.
Norming	In this stage, group members establish norms—the implicit or explicit rules about how they will behave and achieve their goal. They identify forms of communication that will or will not help with the task at hand.
Performing	In this stage, the group is ready to work together toward meeting their goal and completing tasks. It looks for effective and efficient ways to get things accomplished. The members focus on ways in which to build functional relationships among each other.
Adjourning	In this stage, the group prepares to dissolve as it completes its tasks and projects end.

Source: Tuckman, B. W. (1965). Developmental sequence in small groups. *Psychological Bulletin, 63*(6), 384–399; Sampson, E. E., & Marthas, M. (1990). *Group process for the health professions* (3rd ed.). Albany, NY: Delmar Thompson Learning.

four group developmental process stages (*forming*, *storming*, *norming*, and *performing*). Each of these stages included two main types of developmental issues a group must address: (a) task issues and (b) interpersonal issues. A fifth stage, *adjourning*, referring to group termination after the desired goals are met, was added in a subsequent revision to the model.

Tuckman's stages are described in Table 3.2.

Critique of Linear Models of Team Development Linear, sequential models of team development, such as Tuckman's Stages of Group Development, Fisher's (1970) Model of Decision Emergence in Groups, and Tubbs' (1995) System Model have met with some criticism. Sampson and Marthas (1990) suggest that so-called linear theories should be thought of more as developmental spirals. That is to say, teams don't just move in one direction, meeting objectives and then moving forward. Rather, they progress and grow through multiple cycles, interacting in complex situations, often revisiting similar issues and yet addressing them differently on the basis of new learning.

Team Development and IPP Teams Many considerations of the process of team development are pertinent to the operation of IPP teams, such as:

- Health care team development is a dynamic and iterative process.
- Health care teams move through phases that are partially time-ordered and interconnected. However, these phases do not necessarily occur in lockstep.

- Health care teams form as a result of people (including patients and their support networks), resources, and plans or intentions coming together as an interconnected and interrelated system.
- The main focus of a health care team's existence is the progressive pursuit of goals and identified needs that centre on persons, groups, and/or communities.
- Health care teams may exist indefinitely (i.e., as long as there is a need for care) or they may exist only for a finite period of time, after which they terminate.
- The development of a health care team is influenced by a number of internal and external factors.

Developmental Analysis of Teams A general understanding of how a team develops is invaluable to achieving the goals set by a health care team. A developmental understanding provides information with which to assess behaviours observed in a team. It also enables members to guide and evaluate the outcomes of processes, including aspects of the team's performance.

The opening vignette of this chapter describes a number of observable behaviours that are open to various interpretations. For example, during the discussion about how the meeting should proceed, team members express divergent views, and the dialogue suggests that some members, such as Yuhong, are frustrated. On the surface, it may seem logical to conclude that the team is not functioning well and that poor team member relations are developing. We might also attribute characteristics to individual members, for example deciding quickly that Sally is an ineffective leader. However, analysis from a team development perspective provides an alternative explanation that might transform the team and its processes. This approach suggests that the team in the vignette is in the forming stage. The majority of team development theories note that this stage is characterized by an orientation in which the team deals with issues of coming together and trying to get to know each other. A team in this stage is also mainly concerned with the defining its purpose. In this light, the behaviours described in the vignette may be interpreted differently, and seen to be quite typical of a team that is just forming. This viewpoint might provide information that helps the team get past this stage and address their main goal: revising the Employee Orientation Program.

Communication Communication is said to be a predictive feature of the potential success of a team. Effective communication is essential in IPP for many reasons, not the least of which is that it facilitates achievement of patient-centred goals. In Chapter 1, we introduced the concept of communication, making the case that it is integral to IPP. In this chapter we explore the aspects of communication salient to teams and teamwork.

In all teams, there is a structure related to how members communicate. The **communication structure** of a team refers to the pattern of communication that exists such as who talks to whom (Keyton, 2002). Communication within a team is dependent on factors such as the type of team that exists and what objectives or tasks are to be accomplished. For example, a formal team with specifically defined objectives and tasks is more likely to have a predictable and rigid communication structure. This structure may also change as a team moves through developmental stages before stabilizing.

Centrality (whether a central position exists) and efficiency (how well the structure facilitates transmission of information) are important features of communication structures (Sampson & Marthas, 1990). In general, teams with open and free communication between all members, or an "all channels" pattern, lack a central position. This pattern tends to lengthen other team processes (e.g., decision making), may lead to communication that is complex, and may result in information overload and confusion (Borkowski, 2005; Keyton, 2002). However, teams with an "all channels" structure are more likely to make accurate and sound judgments and have team members who are satisfied because they experience a higher level of participation (Beebe & Masterson, 2009).

Researchers Bavelas (1948, 1950) and Leavitt (1951) first described four basic communication structures that exist in teams, later expanded upon by additional authors (e.g., Longest, Rackich, & Darr, 2000). These structures are: line, Y, circle, and star (see Figure 3.1). It is important to note that rarely in a real world situation do teams adhere to these rigid structures. However, understanding the structures helps us conceptualize the general communication patterns within teams to which we belong. For example, a study conducted by Bokhour (2006) focusing on the communication practices of two health care teams in a long-term-care facility revealed that they used various communication structures depending on their goals and objectives. The study also found that a structure similar to the "all channels" pattern was most effective for accomplishing goals such as coordination and joint decision making about patient care.

It is important for health care professionals engaging in IPP to have an understanding of communication and how it is structured within a team. Information about patterns of communication can assist team members to effectively and efficiently communicate with each other. An awareness of communication patterns may also help a team to navigate through the stages in their development, prevent unnecessary conflict, and appropriately problem-solve. Consider the communication processes evident in the opening vignette. A team member with an understanding of communication would likely observe that the communication structure of the team is complex. The communication pattern changes during a single meeting, highlighting the concepts of centrality and efficiency. The communication structure toggles between having a central position (Sally, the team leader) and open and freely directed communication between members. At the start of the meeting, the communication structure resembles the "star" pattern, with Sally at the centre (see Figure 3.1). However, as the team struggles to identify the tasks of the meeting, the communication structure begins to resemble the "all channels" variety. It shifts back to the "star" pattern when Sally suggests a solution to the conflict. If we were to observe the team over a longer period, we would likely note overall changes from meeting to meeting. This understanding of the team's communication structure can be shared among the team members in order to provide insight and assist them in stabilizing the team and focusing on their goals.

Norms and Normative Pressure **Norms**—standards or expectations of appropriate behaviour, attitudes, and even perceptions—are present in all teams (Sampson & Marthas, 1990). Norms will vary widely in extensity (the degree to which they extend) and explicitness depending on the purpose and structure of a team (Forsyth, 2006).

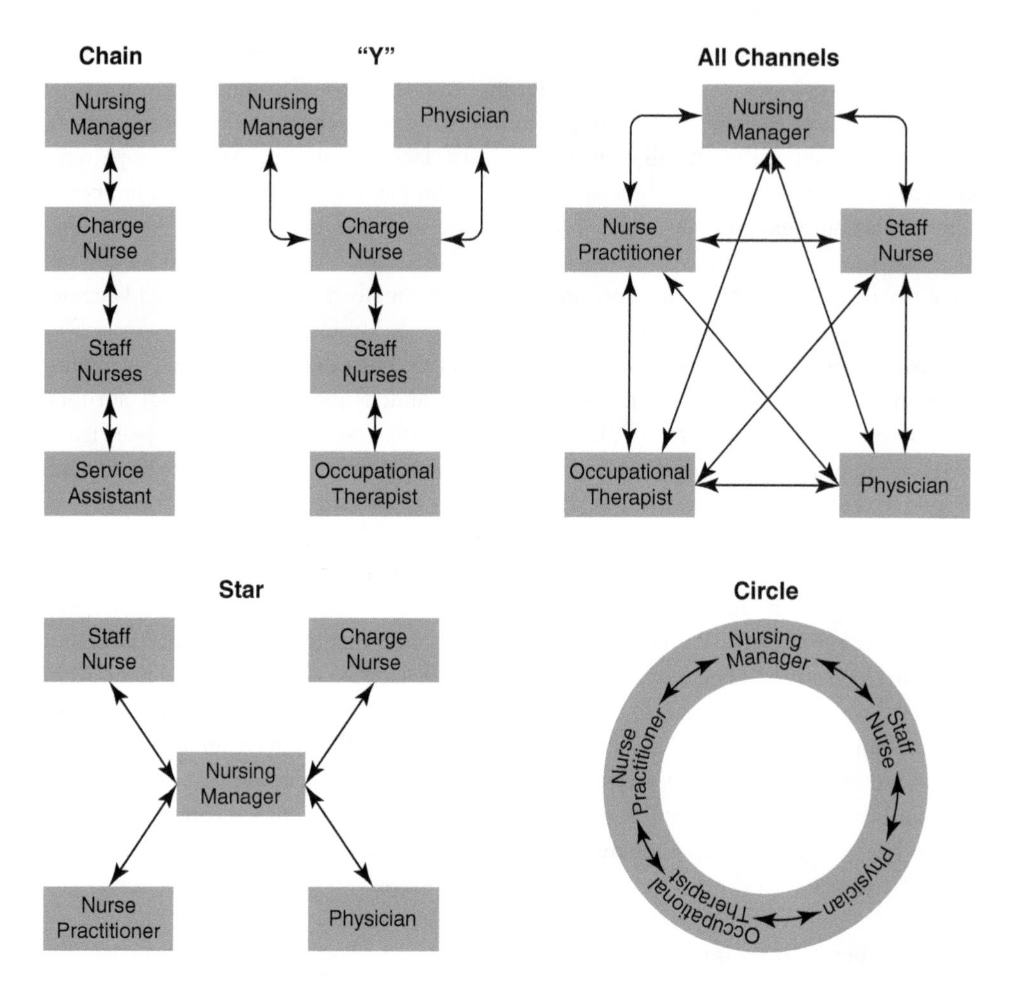

Figure 3.1 Examples of Basic Communication Structures

Within IPP teams, the content of norms largely focuses on role-related activities and issues and less on the personal and private lives of team members. They may concern how members interact with each other and their patients, the formality of relationships among/between members and patients, and the tasks in which members engage. The individual professions to which health care team members belong also have their own sets of norms. One common explicit component of profession-specific norms is a set of practice standards. Another is a code of ethics articulated for each regulated health profession.

Regardless of how explicit norms may be, they would be ineffective without mechanisms to ensure conformity. The term **normative pressure** refers to how a team enforces the norms it has established. Normative pressures encourage compliance and discourage deviation. All teams exert some degree of normative pressure. Within formal teams, such as IPP health care teams, norms are usually enforced through mechanisms clearly articulated and communicated through documentation and instruction. For example, hospitals and other health care organizations commonly describe expected conduct and practice in written policies and procedures. The norms are both documented and communicated through educational programs and formal orientations. Additionally, the regulatory bodies of professions such as medicine, pharmacy, and occupational therapy enforce standards of practice through complaint and disciplinary regulations and procedures supported by government legislation.

Norms and normative pressures are important because they reduce uncertainty within teams, supporting team cohesiveness and functioning. They are a determinant of the effectiveness of a team and can strongly influence its identity and the processes, such as communication, that take place within it (Myers & Anderson, 2008). More specifically, norms and normative pressures serve essential functions for IPP teams (Myers & Anderson, 2008; Sampson & Marthas, 1990), including:

- *Task functions*. Norms and normative pressures allow teams to organize and coordinate their activities so that they meet their goals.
- *Maintenance functions*. Norms and normative pressures related to maintenance issues and team processes such as attendance and decision making serve to keep teams intact and progressing toward goals.
- *Social reality functions*. Norms and normative pressures provide social definitions and interpretations of reality that are shared within a team or group.

This chapter began with a vignette in which team members are working to develop norms about how they will relate to each other (social reality functions) and what the goals of the team and roles of each member will be (task and maintenance functions). This effort, although initially challenging for the team, will serve to reduce the anxiety members might feel about working together and to provide clearer direction toward meeting their overall goal of revising the orientation program.

In conclusion, it should be noted that when norms are highly hierarchical, extensive, rigid, and tied to factors such as power and status, they can be harmful to health care teams, giving rise to tension and conflict. Undetected and unresolved issues can lead to further problems.

Observing and Analyzing Teams

If health care professionals are to be effective in the teams in which they work, they must be able to assess and evaluate key characteristics and processes that are important to team practice. There are many ways to observe and analyze team processes. To help you get started, we have provided some basic approaches in Helpful Tools 3.2.

Having reviewed the definitions and basic elements of teams and teamwork within the context of health care, in the next section we move to a focus on IPP teams and effective teamwork in health care environments. We explore the extent to which IPP teams

Helpful Tools 3.2

Observing and Analyzing Teams

A comprehensive approach to observing and analyzing team processes may involve:

- initial assessment of the structures, norms, and roles of the team
- focus on your own individual contributions and reflection upon how you relate to yourself and others in the group
- journalling consistently about the team's progress in meetings, identifying the goals set, issues that arise, and developmental milestones
- utilizing a theoretical perspective as a guiding framework
- documenting critical incidents

When observing and analyzing a team, try to follow these simple rules:

- Be systematic.
- Separate observation and interpretation.
- Support interpretations (with body of observed evidence or theoretical perspectives).
- Remember interpretations are hypotheses and theories, not fact.
- Consider carefully how you use what you have observed or interpreted.
- Start with yourself!

and teamwork have been integrated into health care settings in Canada and internationally. We also examine the determinants of an effective team and successful teamwork. Finally, we review briefly the literature identifying barriers to teamwork and suggested interventions to overcome these obstacles.

IPP TEAMS AND TEAMWORK IN HEALTH CARE ENVIRONMENTS

Integration of IPP Teams and Teamwork in Health Care Environments

If we are to practise interprofessionally and meet desired health care outcomes, working successfully within teams is a necessary component. There is a growing body of literature identifying the essential role of teams and teamwork in health care, with calls from government agencies and health care professions for continued work to advance the role of teams. Some highlights are:

- In Canada, several key government documents/reports call for improved teamwork in health care (e.g., Commission on the Future of Healthcare in Canada, 2002; Health Council of Canada, 2005; Commission on Medicare, 2001; Herbert, 2005; Oandasan et al., 2006).
- In the United States, agencies such as the Joint Commission on Accreditation of Healthcare Organizations (JCAHO) have espoused the benefits of teamwork and

integrated standards that promote effective teamwork. The agency more recently underscored the importance of teams and teamwork, reporting that 70% of patient adverse events in the United States are related to ineffective teamwork and communication among health practitioners (Lujan, 2010).

- Across the United Kingdom, public forums such as the Bristol Inquiry (Department of Health, 2002) and government polices/documents have put emphasis on interprofessional working and the need to move toward teamwork (Larkin & Callaghan, 2005).
- In Australia and New Zealand and in member states across the European Union, there is growing consensus supporting interprofessional teams and teamwork. Government policy promoting interprofessional team practice among health care professionals is emerging (Oandasan et al., 2006; Tope & Thomas, 2007).
- Finally, in Canada and internationally, researchers have explored the literature on the effectiveness of teams and teamwork (e.g., Lemieux-Charles & McGuire, 2006), examining various aspects of teamwork that contribute to effective IPP and attaining desired outcomes (e.g., Fay, Borrill, Amir, Haward, & West, 2006; Larkin & Callaghan, 2005; Mickan & Rodger, 2005; Simpson, 2007; Undre, Sevdalia, Healey, Darzi, & Vincent, 2006).

Unfortunately, despite the evidence supporting the need for teams in health care, the integration of effective teams and teamwork within health care environments requires more than just assembling the different professionals. To this end, more recently, there has been a significant drive toward strengthening Canadian health care delivery through initiatives that foster IPP teams and teamwork. Much of the investment in these initiatives has occurred on a large scale and at the systems level. However, it is important to remember that the current focus on IPP teams and teamwork has been an ongoing phenomenon, building in waves for the past century in Canada and elsewhere (Day, 2013; Drinka & Clark, 2000; Ryan, 1996, 2008). Additionally, it should be noted that collaborative engagement has been occurring on a smaller scale in individual health care units and organizations for some time.

IPP Team-Based Initiatives in Canada and Internationally Numerous activities focused on developing and implementing teams and facilitating teamwork in health care settings point to their potential impact. On the basis of their synthesis of projects related to primary health care delivery in Canada, Oandasan and colleagues (2006) identified several best practices that facilitate teamwork. These include clarifying the role of all members of the team and improving communication and partnerships among its members. Spotlight 3.1 highlights the GF Strong ALS Team as an example of exemplary teamwork that results. Oandasan and colleagues also reported that teamwork is most often implemented in five key areas:

- Aboriginal communities
- care of disease- or diagnosis-based groups (e.g., mental health services, diabetic care)
- demonstration projects exploring new primary health care practice models

Spotlight 3.1

Exemplary Teamwork: The GF Strong ALS Team

The Amyotrophic Lateral Sclerosis (ALS) Centre Team of the GF Strong Rehabilitation Centre of British Columbia is an example of a highly engaged team of health care professionals committed to IPP outcomes such as improved patient care. GF Strong is a transdisciplinary outreach resource team made up of professionals from the disciplines of social work, nursing, occupational therapy, speech-language pathology, dietetics, and physiotherapy. It provides province-wide comprehensive consultative services to people with ALS and works in consultation with specialists in physical medicine, rehabilitation, and neurology. Additionally, it partners with several organizations, including the ALS Society of British Columbia, the Provincial Respiratory Outreach Program, and Technology for Independent Living. In 2003, the team was the recipient of the ALS Society of Canada's Exceptional Support Service Award.

- remote primary care centres that provide services for specialized populations
- academic institutions and teaching hospitals engaged at the practice and organizational levels

Below are descriptions of a number of the efforts focused on developing, implementing, and supporting teams and teamwork. This listing, while not exhaustive, does give a sense of the progress that has been made to improve teamwork for IPP.

- Health Canada's *Interprofessional Education for Collaborative Patient-Centred Practice (IECPCP) Strategy* has funded educational initiatives across Canada aimed at developing IPE curriculum and improving care delivery/health outcomes. A number of these projects supported IPP team skills development among health care professional students and post-licensure professionals (e.g., *Creating Interprofessional Collaborative Teams for Comprehensive Mental Health Services*, University of Western Ontario; *Cultivating Communities of Practice for Collaborative Care*, Cancer Care Nova Scotia; *Creating an Interprofessional Learning Environment Through Communities of Practice: An Alternative to Traditional Preceptorship*, Calgary Health Region, Research Initiatives in Nursing & Health) (Health Canada, 2008).
- Province-wide initiatives include Saskatchewan's use of facilitator training to help build IPP team approaches (Med-Emerg International Inc. & Centre for Strategic Management, 2004). In the province of Ontario, HealthForceOntario's Interprofessional Care/Education Fund (ICEF) provides funding for programming that supports innovation in health education or health care projects that promote and build interprofessional teams (HealthForceOntario, 2013).
- Illustrating the application of their approach to achieving a high-performing health system in Canada, the Health Council of Canada (HCC) (2013) calls for improving the effectiveness and functioning of IPP teams. Central to this call was

a focus on capacity building as a means of accelerating Canada's primary health care commitments initiated through the 2003 and 2004 health accords.

- International examples include reforms in the National Health Service (NHS) in the United Kingdom that have resulted in the vast majority of primary care groups adopting interprofessional team-based practice and teamwork approaches (Tope & Thomas, 2007).

Team Effectiveness

Understanding what makes a team effective and acquiring the tools and strategies that will assist teams to engage in successful collaboration are essential as we strive to continually improve the quality of care in our health care system.

There is a significant body of literature in the field of organizational studies about team effectiveness that can be applied, albeit cautiously, to the teams in which we are interested. There is also a growing body of health care–specific literature to inform us about effective teams. Taken as a whole, this literature reveals that what determines team effectiveness and what indicators we use to measure it often depend on the types of teams we are concerned with (Cohen & Bailey, 1997; Mathieu, Maynard, Rapp, & Gilson, 2008). It also suggests that many factors influence effectiveness, including the structural aspects of the team, the context within which the team completes its objectives, and the interactional processes that occur among the team members (Mathieu et al., 2008; Oandasan et al., 2006). Lastly, the literature suggests several approaches to assessing and enhancing team effectiveness. These are outlined in this section.

To define **team effectiveness**, we might take the approach of identifying the outcome(s) or product(s) expected and using them as indicators of a team's success, which provides us with a guide for enhancing the effectiveness of our own teams. Another way to define team effectiveness is to identify the components, attributes, and processes we would expect to observe in an effective team. With these criteria, we could analyze our team and determine if we exhibit these attributes and what factors may be influencing the team's ability to be effective. Several models of team effectiveness (both specific to and outside of health care) that focus on outcome measures have been proposed, including Hackman's Model of Team Effectiveness, the Integrated (Healthcare) Team Effectiveness Model, and Heinemann and Zeiss' Model of Team Performance (see Spotlight 3.2).

A widely accepted approach to determining the effectiveness of health care teams includes the use of subjective and objective outcome measures. Objective outcome measures include those related to clinical data (e.g., patient satisfaction with the care provided), organizational data (e.g., indicators of efficiency such as length of patient stay), and patient behaviours (e.g., maintenance of treatment regimens following discharge). Subjective measures consist of the attitudes and beliefs of team members and may include assessments of team functioning and efficiency from the perspective of team members (Oandasan et al., 2006).

Heinemann and Gardner (as cited in Heinemann & Zeiss, 2002) have identified components or processes of effective teams, including: (a) collaboration, (b) communication,

Spotlight 3.2

Team Effectiveness Models

A number of team effectiveness models have been proposed. Below we describe three, each of which presents a different perspective on how to structure and evaluate team effectiveness.

- Hackman's (1990) Model of Team Effectiveness identifies three relevant dimensions: (a) the generation of a high-quality outcome or product, (b) the workability or viability of the members of the team into the future, and (c) the team's contribution to the well-being and professional growth of its members. Hackman's model also identifies a number of influential factors, including the configuration and composition of the team (e.g., size, skill sets of individuals), team norms, and how the work of the team is designed (e.g., decision-making capacity, level of interdependence).
- Lemieux-Charles and McGuire's (2006) Integrated (Healthcare) Team Effectiveness Model (ITEM) is rooted in organizational studies. The model is tailored specifically to health care and articulates the relationship between task design, team processes, team psychosocial traits, and outcomes. In the model, the objective and subjective measures of team effectiveness are identified through reflection and response to several questions relating to the components of the model. The responses a team provides to these questions are used to help them improve their teamwork effectiveness.
- Heinemann and Zeiss' (2002) Model of Team Performance articulates the concept of best team practice, which centres on health care team effectiveness. It proposes that team effectiveness is defined within four domains: (a) structure (membership and hierarchal organization of the member), (b) context (relationship of the team to the larger organization), (c) process (how the team progresses, functions, and is shaped by factors such as communication patterns and power structures), and (d) productivity (the impact of teams and what outcomes they produce). This model is helpful in organizing outcome measures and promoting and enhancing team effectiveness.

(c) cooperation, (d) maintaining cohesiveness, (e) being committed to the team, (f) coordinating efforts, (g) having a common plan, (h) consensus decision making, (i) the sense that a contribution is being made, (j) caring for each other, (k) confronting problems directly, and (l) engaging in conflict management. These occur in the context of maintaining consistency with one another and the environment surrounding the team. A team might apply these components or processes in their assessment of their own effectiveness. In the project team of the opening vignette, some of these components and processes are identifiable. Based on the actions of the team members, we might conclude that the project team is struggling to establish effective communication and that members are currently experiencing low levels of cooperation and coordination of efforts. Referring back to the previous discussion regarding effectiveness, the dissatisfaction expressed by some team members may be interpreted as subjective evidence of the team's lack of effectiveness at this point in their development.

As a final note, in assessing the effectiveness of a team it is important to take into consideration factors internal (e.g., stage of team development) and external (e.g., environment of the organization) to the team (Lemieux-Charles & McGuire, 2006). In the opening vignette, an internal factor that might impact effectiveness is the team's early stage of development. An external factor might be the workloads of some of its members.

Barriers to and Facilitators of Team Effectiveness

Research focused on the characteristics of team effectiveness, barriers to effective teamwork, and initiatives to facilitate teamwork provide direction to improve team effectiveness. Team members who have an understanding of the barriers to and facilitators of team effectiveness are able to better position themselves as effective members and contribute more to meeting the objectives of IPP.

Barriers to Team Effectiveness Challenges to developing and optimizing effective teams and teamwork for IPP include:

- *Professional identity*. Silos of practice that have developed through professional identity formation may result in professionals guarding boundaries of practice. This sometimes also takes the form of protecting authority and status within the health care environment. The result may be a reluctance to participate in teams and engage in collaborative interactions (Fay et al., 2006; Hall, 2005; Mickan & Rodger, 2005; Wagner, 2004).
- *Differences in attitude*. Conflicts may arise due to differing and even negative attitudes toward teams and teamwork (Robinson & Cottrell, 2005; Tunstall-Pedoe, Rink, & Hilton, 2003). In a phenomenon called *in-grouping*, professionals might also harbour negative attitudes about other professional groups (Sampson & Marthas, 1990) fostered by professional identity socialization (Hall, 2005; Robinson & Cottrell, 2005). These attitudes may contribute to a poor climate in and poor functioning of the team.
- *Blurring of roles*. A lack of clarity on one another's roles within the team may act as a barrier to teamwork by fostering confusion, tension, and rivalry (Hall, 2005; Larkin & Callaghan, 2005). Role ambiguity may also lead to unclear lines of accountability and responsibility (Norman & Peck, 1999). Knowledge of each member's professional roles and responsibilities, behaving in accordance with these roles, and open negotiation of roles are necessary for team building. They also encourage greater team productivity and effective teamwork.
- *Preconceptions and assumptions*. Teams in health care environments often exist under the assumption that members have the capacity to engage in team-based practice. There is also the expectation that members will be able to transition from their silo-oriented thinking and adjust their practice accordingly, such that they effectively collaborate with other professionals to bring about particular patient outcomes (Barrie, 2004). However, health care professionals often lack the skills to effectively engage in teamwork (Hall, 2005).
- *Lack of clarity of goals, policies, and outcomes*. These can lead to confusion among professionals who may interpret ambiguous policies differently and act in a manner counterproductive to the intended outcomes. A lack of clear patient and team goals

may lead to ineffective care, lack of efficiency, and member dissatisfaction (Øvretveit, Mathias, & Thompson, 1997; Villeneau, Hill, Hancock, & Wolf, 2001).

- *Differing approaches and procedures*. In teams where professionals are not working from the same base in terms of their approaches and care priorities, there is a greater likelihood of poor collaboration (Thomassy & McShea, 2001).
- *Systems barriers*. These include regulatory and legislative frameworks that contribute to silos of practice, as well as inconsistent governmental policies and funding that discourage collaboration (Oandasan et al., 2006).

Facilitators of Team Effectiveness Within the literature, many facilitators to effective teams and teamwork have been articulated. The following list is just a sampling of some of the many facilitators that have been identified at the practice, organization, and health care system levels:

Practice Level

- High levels of contact and interaction among team members (e.g., frequent team meetings, common documentation system, regular patterns of communication) (Fay et al., 2006; Mickan & Rodger, 2005; Molyneux, 2001; Villeneau et al., 2001)
- Common values and purpose, and clearly articulated norms and tasks (Oandasan et al., 2006; Mickan & Rodger, 2005; San Martin-Rodriguez, Beauliey, D'Amour, & Ferrada-Videla, 2005; Thylefors, Persson, & Hellstrom, 2005)
- Supportive structures and encouraging and positive atmospheres and climates (Thylefors et al., 2005)
- Effective interpersonal and group process/dynamic skills (e.g., respect for other professionals, role clarity, effective conflict resolution, shared accountability and responsibility, good communication patterns, high levels of collaboration and coordination, awareness of group process) (San Martin-Rodriguez et al., 2005; Poultin & West, 1999; Sampson & Marthas, 1990; Vinokur-Kaplan, 1995)
- Team leadership (Mickan & Rodger, 2005)

Organizational Level

- Culture of commitment to IPP teams and teamwork (Oandasan et al., 2006; Robinson & Cottrell, 2005)
- Adoption of policies that promote and support IPP and integration of core competencies for IPP
- Providing structures and resources that support teamwork (e.g., management structures, leadership training) (Oandasan et al., 2006; San Martin-Rodriguez et al., 2005)

Systems Level

- Legislative and regulatory reform responsive to trends in the practice environment, which fosters organizational autonomy to address barriers in the approaches taken by the professionals engaging in IPP

- Addressing key liability issues related to roles and responsibility in performing shared tasks
- Changes to education and accreditation processes (e.g., interprofessional education; accreditation standards for IPP) (Oandasan et al., 2006)

CONCLUSION

We are all fortunate to be engaging in health care practice during a time of such positive change. As we move more fully into integrating IPP, it is important to appreciate the many deep roots from which this new approach to health care delivery grew. Extensive research focusing on teams and teamwork highlights that working collaboratively within an interprofessional team is the most effective and most satisfying approach for both patient and practitioner. In this chapter we reviewed in detail what we know about teams and teamwork. This information sets the stage and provides a strong foundation as we progress to the exploration of specific topics related to IPP.

SUMMARY

- It is widely accepted that teams and teamwork are essential to the care of patients. Recent efforts to renew and improve our health care system in Canada have focused attention on IPP. Teams and how they work effectively are a key component of IPP.
- Various types of teams exist in health care environments. The type of team and its membership within a given environment is contingent on a number of factors such as the purpose and function of the team and the setting. Teams involving health care professionals working together to provide patient care are described along a continuum of collaboration.
- The most common types of health care teams are project team/working group, multidisciplinary, interprofessional, and transdisciplinary.
- To effectively work in teams, health care professionals must have an understanding of the basic characteristics and concepts related to a team.
- Team processes are enacted by members in order to obtain the desired outcomes. Team processes include team development, communication, norms, and normative pressure.
- Across Canada and internationally there is growing support for the integration of IPP teams into the health care system at all levels. In Canada, funding from federal and provincial agencies has been provided for a number of innovative projects and initiatives in this respect.
- Although considerable emphasis has been put on IPP teams/teamwork, and action has been taken to make effective teams a mainstay in our health care system,

barriers exists that must be systematically addressed. These barriers exist at the levels of the individual professional, the organization, and the broader health care system and context in which IPP is situated.

- Working to uncover and understand these barriers and setting directions for improving teamwork will contribute to the IPP agenda.

Key Terms

communication structure
health care team
normative pressure
norms
team effectiveness
team processes

Review Questions

1. Why are teams and teamwork important to IPP?
2. Describe the common types of teams that are found in health care environments.
3. Identify and define the stages of Tuckman's Stages of Group Development theory.
4. What is the relationship between norms and normative pressure?
5. How can we assess the effectiveness of teams in health care environments?
6. Identify three barriers and three facilitators to IPP teams and teamwork.

Application Exercises: Communication Interaction Diagrams

How communication is structured within an interprofessional team can provide clues about how other processes are structured and about the overall climate within a team. An interaction diagram using data collected over a period of time is a helpful tool for discovering the patterns or networks present. It provides information about who is communicating with whom, and the frequency and direction of communication.

This exercise walks you through the steps of creating an interaction diagram and provides questions to help you analyze it. Try to create one the next time you are in a group or team setting. After completing your diagram, review and respond to the analysis questions provided below.

1. Draw a chart showing where every member of your team is sitting using a circle or square to represent each person. Make sure your arrangement on paper resembles the actual position of every member of the team/group. Label each circle or box with the person's name, and on the side write any other important information such as his/her role.
2. Whenever a member addresses another specifically, use an arrow to indicate that communication. The arrow should start from the speaker and point to the receiver. If the receiver or another member responds, draw an arrow in the opposite direction.
3. Keep a tally of the number of interactions that occur between different members.
4. Also keep a tally off to the side of the number of times team members openly address the entire team.

Analysis Questions

1. Describe the communication structure of your team on the basis of your diagram(s). Consider your diagram and the various types of communication structures discussed in this chapter.
   a. Does the communication pattern you have drawn indicate a central position (i.e., is one member or a sub-team of members receiving and sending most of the communications)?
   b. Which of the basic structures of communication (line, Y, circle, and star) does your diagram resemble most?
   c. Who is speaking to whom most often? Are there members who did not openly communicate with others?
   d. Were there any instances of one-way communication? Were there many instances in which members addressed the entire team?
2. What hypotheses about your team are you able to make on the basis of your analysis of your communication diagram?
3. Does the communication structure provide clues about other processes under way in your team (e.g., team development)?
4. What does this activity add to your general understanding of your team?

Additional Resources

Websites

Canadian Interprofessional Health Collaborative
www.cihc.ca

HealthForceOntario
www.healthforceontario.ca

Additional Readings

Hedley, G. D., & Kass, R. (2007). *How to observe your group* (4th ed.). North York, ON: Captus Press.

Sampson, E. E., & Marthas, M. (1990). *Group process for the health professions* (3rd. ed.). Albany, NY: Delmar Thompson learning.

References

Barrie, S. (2004). A research based approach to generic graduate attributes policy. *Higher Education Research and Development, 23*(3), 261–75.

Bavelas, A. (1948). A mathematical model for group structures. *Applied Anthropology, 7*, 16–30.

Bavelas, A. (1950). Communication patterns in task-oriented groups. *Journal of Acoustical Sociology of America, 22*, 725–730.

Beebe, S. A., & Masterson, J. T. (2009). *Communication in small groups: Principles and practice* (9th ed.). New York, NY: Allyn & Bacon.

Bokhour, B. G. I. (2006). Communication in interdisciplinary team meetings: What are we talking about? *Journal of Interprofessional Care, 20*(4), 349–363.

Borkowski, N. (2005). *Organizational behaviour in healthcare*. Sudbury, MA: Jones and Bartlett Publishers, Inc.

Cohen, S. G., & Bailey, D. R. (1997). What makes teams work: Group effectiveness research from the shop floor to the executive suite. *Journal of Management, 23*(4), 238–290.

Commission on Medicare. (2001). *Caring for medicare: Sustaining a quality system*. Regina, SK: Author.

Commission on the Future of Healthcare in Canada. (2002, November). *Building on values: The future of healthcare in Canada: Final report*. Saskatoon, SK: Author.

D'Amour, D., Ferrada-Videla, M., San Martin-Rodriguez, L., & Beaulieu, M. D. (2005). The conceptual basis for interprofessional collaboration: Core concepts and theoretical frameworks. *Journal of Interprofessional Care, 19*(S1), 116–131.

Day, J. (2013). *Interprofessional working: An essential guide for health and social professionals* (2nd ed.), pp. 14–210. Andover, UK: Cengage Learning EMEA.

Department of Health. (2002). *Learning from Bristol: The Department of Health's response to the report of the public inquiry into children's heart surgery at the Bristol Royal Infirmary 1984–1995*. Retrieved from https://www.gov.uk/government/uploads/system/uploads/attachment_data/file/273320/5363.pdf

Drinka, J. K., & Clark, P. G. (2000). *Healthcare teamwork: Interdisciplinary practice and teaching*. Westport, CT: Auburn House.

Fay, D., Borrill, C., Amir, Z., Haward, R., & West, M. A. (2006). Getting the most out of multidisciplinary teams: A multi-sample study of team innovation in health care. *Journal of Occupational and Organizational Psychology, 79*, 553–567.

Fisher, B. A. (1970). Decision emergence: Phases in group decision making. *Speech Monographs, 37*(1), 53–66.

Forsyth, D. R. (2006). *Group dynamics* (4th ed.). Belmont, CA: Thomson/Wadsworth.

Hackman, J. R. (1990). *Groups that work (and those that don't): Creating conditions for effective teamwork*. San Francisco, CA: Jossey-Bass.

Hall, P. (2005). Interprofessional teamwork: Professional cultures as barriers. *Journal of Interprofessional Care*, *19*(S1), 188–196.

Hayward, R., Forbes, D., Lau, F., & Wilson, D. (2000). *Strengthening multidisciplinary healthcare teams: Final evaluation report*. Edmonton, AB: Alberta Health and Wellness.

Health Canada. (2008). *Pan-Canadian health human resource strategy: 2007–2008 annual report*. Ottawa, ON: Author.

Health Council of Canada (HCC). (2005). *Healthcare renewal in Canada: Accelerating change*. Toronto, ON: Author.

Health Council of Canada (HCC). (2013). *Better health, better care, better value for all: Refocusing health care reform in Canada*. Retrieved from http://www.healthcouncilcanada.ca

HealthForceOntario. (2013). *Interprofessional care/education funding programs and projects*. Retrieved from http://www.healthforceontario.ca/UserFiles/file/PolicymakersResearchers/ICEF-2008-2009-feb-2011-en.pdf

Heinemann, G. D., & Zeiss, A. M. (2002). *Team performance in healthcare: Assessment and development*. New York, NY: Klewer Academic Publishers.

Herbert, C. P. (2005). Editorial. Changing the culture: Interprofessional education for collaborative patient-centred practice in Canada. *Journal of Interprofessional Care, 19*(S1), 1–4.

Keyton, J. (2002). *Communicating in groups: Building relationships for effective decision making* (2nd ed.). Boston, MA: McGraw-Hill.

Larkin, C., & Callaghan, P. (2005). Professionals' perceptions of interprofessional working in community mental health teams. *Journal of Interprofessional Care, 19*(4), 338–346.

Leavitt, H. J. (1951). Some effects of certain communications patterns on group performance. *Journal of Abnormal and Social Psychology, 46*, 38–50.

Lemieux-Charles, L., & McGuire, W. L. (2006). What do we know about healthcare team effectiveness? A review of the literature. *Medical Care Research and Review, 63*(3), 263–300.

Longest, B. B., Rackich, J. S., & Darr, K. (2000). *Managing health services organizations* (4th ed.). Baltimore, MD: Health Professionals Press, Inc.

Lujan, J. (2010). Promoting an interprofessional teamwork culture. *The Internet Journal of Allied Health Sciences and Practice, 8*(3).

Mathieu, J., Maynard, M. T., Rapp, T., & Gilson, L. (2008). Team effectiveness 1997–2007: A review of recent advancements and a glimpse into the future. *Journal of Management, 34*(3), 410–476.

Med-Emerg International Inc. & Centre for Strategic Management (2004). *Team development and implementation in Saskatchewan's primary healthcare sector.* Regina, SK: Saskatchewan Health.

Mickan, S. M., & Rodger, S. A. (2005). Effective healthcare teams: A model of six characteristics developed from shared perceptions. *Journal of Interprofessional Care, 19*(4), 358–370.

Molyneux, J. (2001). Interprofessional teamworking: What makes a team work well? *Journal of Interprofessional Care, 15*(1), 29–35.

Myers, S. A., & Anderson, C. M. (2008). *The fundamentals of small group communication*. Thousand Oaks, CA: Sage Publications.

Norman, I. J., & Peck, E. (1999). Working together in adult community mental health services: An interprofessional dialogue. *Journal of Mental Health, 8*(3), 217–314.

Oandasan, I., Ross Baker, G., Barker, K., Bosco, C., D'Amour, D., Jones, L., ... Way, D. (2006). *Teamwork in healthcare: Promoting effective teamwork in healthcare in Canada. Policy synthesis and recommendations*. Ottawa: Canadian Health Services Research Foundation.

Øvretveit, J., Mathias, P., & Thompson, T. (1997). *Interprofessional working for health and social care*. London, UK: Macmillan Press Ltd.

Poulton, B. (2003). Teamwork and team development in healthcare social care. In D. Watkins, J. Edwards, & P. Gastrell (Eds.), *Community Health Nursing: Frameworks for Practice* (2nd ed.). Edinburgh: Bailliere Tindall.

Poulton, B. C., & West, M. A. (1999). The determinants of effectiveness in primary healthcare teams. *Journal of Interprofessional Care, 13*(1), 7–18.

Robinson, M., & Cottrell, D. (2005). Health professionals in multi-disciplinary and multi-agency teams: Changing professional practice. *Journal of Interprofessional Care, 19*(6), 547–560.

Ryan, D. P. (1996). A history of teamwork in mental health and its implications for teamwork training and education in gerontology. *Educational Gerontology: An International Quarterly*, *22*(5), 411–431.

Ryan, D. P. (2008). Inter-professional practice in health care [PowerPoint slides]. Retrieved from http://giic.rgps.on.ca/inter-professional-practice

Sampson, E. E., & Marthas, M. (1990). *Group process for the health professions.* (3rd ed.). Albany, NY: Delmar Thompson learning.

San Martin-Rodriguez, I., Beaulieu, M., D'Amour, D., & Ferrada-Videla, M. (2005). The determinants of successful collaboration: A review of theoretical and empirical studies. *Journal of Interprofessional Care, 19*(S1), 132–147.

Simpson, A. (2007). The impact of team processes on psychiatric case management. *Journal of Advanced Nursing, 60*(4), 409–418.

Thomassy, C. S., & McShea, C. S. (2001). Shifting gears: Jump-start interdisciplinary patient care. *Nursing Management, 32*(5), 40.

Thylefors, L., Persson, O., & Hellstrom, D. (2005). Teams types, perceived efficiency and team climate in Swedish cross-professional teamwork. *Journal of Interprofessional Care, 19*(2), 102–114.

Tope, E., & Thomas, E. (2007, February). *Health and social care policy and the interprofessional agenda. The first supplement to creating an interprofessional workforce: An education and training framework for health and social care in England* London, UK: Department of Health.

Tubbs, S. (1995). *A systems approach to small group interaction.* New York, NY: McGraw-Hill.

Tuckman, B. W. (1965). Developmental sequence in small groups. *Psychological Bulletin, 63*(6), 384–399.

Tunstall-Pedoe, S., Rink, E., & Hilton, S. (2003). Student attitudes to undergraduate interprofessional education. *Journal of Interprofessional Care, 17*(2), 161–172.

Undre, S., Sevdalia, N., Healey, A. N., Darzi, A., & Vincent, C. A. (2006). Teamwork in the operating theatre: Cohesion or confusion? *Journal of Evaluation in Clinical Practice, 12*(2), 182–189.

Villeneau, L., Hill, R. J., Hancock, M., & Wolf, J. (2001). Establishing process indicators for joint working in mental health: Rationale and results from a national survey. *Journal of Interprofessional Care, 15*(4), 229–340.

Vinokur-Kaplan, D. (1995). Treatment teams that work (and those that don't): An application of Hackman's group effectiveness model to interdisciplinary teams in psychiatric hospitals. *Journal of Applied Behavioural Sciences, 31*(3), 303–327.

Wagner, E. (2004). Effective teamwork and quality of care. *Medical Care, 42*(11), 1037–1039.

Chapter 4
Professional Roles and Relationships

Golnaz Nahmet and her husband Farzan have recently immigrated to Canada from Iran, setting up home in British Columbia. After an uncomplicated pregnancy, Golnaz gave birth to their first child Parishad, born eight days ago. Following an overnight stay in hospital, Golnaz and Parishad were discharged and the family has been settling in. For the last day or so, Golnaz has noticed increased fussiness and the baby seems not to be nursing very well. Parishad seemed on two occasions to be gasping for air, which had Golnaz and Farzan worried, but uncertain about whether they were just inexperienced in knowing how babies behave.

To be on the safe side, the new parents decide to take Golnaz back to see her pediatrician, even though she had been for a well-baby check the day after discharge from hospital. After listening to their concerns and examining the baby, the pediatrician shares with Golnaz and Farzan that she believes she may have heard a heart murmur. While Parishad looks well, the pediatrician would like the baby to be examined by a pediatric cardiologist at the local children's hospital. The pediatrician assures the worried parents that she will call the hospital to let the staff know that the baby will be arriving shortly with her parents.

The family spends the next several hours moving through the emergency department and the diagnostic imaging department. They are introduced to Dr. Julio, the pediatric cardiologist who informs them that Parishad does indeed have a problem with her heart called an *atrial septal defect (ASD)*. He says that this is one of the most common types of congenital heart diseases and usually does not require surgery, but adds that Parishad will need to be admitted for more testing.

Within a short time, Parishad is admitted to the pediatric cardiac unit. Brandon Donnelly is the primary registered nurse caring for Parishad and her family. From his many years of experience working with families of sick children, Brandon believes that listening to their concerns and making sure that families are involved in care decisions is critical. During his assessment he is careful to share what he is doing with both Farzan and Golnaz, giving both the chance to ask questions and share their feelings. Brandon realizes that Golnaz feels as though she should have known something was wrong. She looks tearfully at Brandon and asks if she is a "bad mother." He does his best to reassure her that she did everything right in bringing her baby to the pediatrician. Golnaz also shares that breastfeeding has not being going as well as she had hoped. Since Parishad can be breastfed while in hospital, Brandon offers to contact one of the hospital's certified lactation consultants, to which Golnaz and Farzan agree gratefully.

The Nahmet family begins to settle into the unit as members of the health care team come in intermittently to assess Parishad, complete diagnostic tests, and explain what is happening. Several hours later, Ginny Calan arrives and introduces herself as a certified lactation consultant. During her assessment, she notes that the Nahmet family speaks English as a second language. While they are able to find creative ways to communicate about things such as breastfeeding and sleeping patterns, Ginny considers using a translator for important communications with this family. After completing her assessment of breastfeeding issues with Golnaz and her baby, Ginny concludes there is room for improvement with the latch, and does some preliminary teaching. She defers a longer teaching session until next morning, when she promises to return.

Ginny seeks out the family's primary nurse, Brandon. She confers with him about her recommendation that the Nahmets might benefit from a translator for her planned session in the morning. Brandon says he too had wondered if a translator would help to ensure that Golnaz and Farzan fully understood all the important information related to Parishad's health and treatment in order to participate in her care.

Ginny offers to make the arrangements for an official translator. Brandon is grateful when she also promises to contact the rest of the health care team (primary cardiologist, social worker, discharge planner) along with the family so that they can coordinate the best time for the translator to come. While this planning and orchestrating of persons and events is time-consuming, Brandon and Ginny know that everyone on the team and the Nahmet family will benefit from having an opportunity to ensure that effective communication takes place.

Learning Outcomes

After studying this chapter, you should be able to:

1. **Define key concepts related to professional roles and relationships, including professional identity, professionalization, role, role clarification, role conflict, role confusion, and role distance.**
2. **Describe how professional roles and relationships affect the capacity for interprofessional practice within a health care setting or situation.**
3. **Discuss the various roles that take place within a team context.**
4. **Summarize strategies for effective relationships.**
5. **Analyze the effects of relational communication and conflict within interprofessional practice situations.**

INTRODUCTION

THE OPENING VIGNETTE IN THIS CHAPTER REVEALS HOW PROFESSIONAL ROLES AND relationships are interdependent. In this chapter, we will explore the key concepts related to professional roles and relationships within interprofessional practice (IPP). We will also continue our focus on communication as we highlight the potential effect that positive, negative, or absent communication inevitably has on the capacity for IPP in any setting.

This chapter begins with a brief overview of relevant theory related to how people structure their identities and orient themselves within health care settings. Moving forward from that point, we will explore the impact of professional/patient roles on IPP. Understanding ourselves and others as individuals and within our professional (or patient) roles sets the stage for exploration of relationships that form between members of the IPP team, including patients. Key concepts such as power and authority and attitudes toward collaboration will be explored in terms of their impact on the quality of relationships formed. These concepts are central to the relationships dimension of the organizing framework that was described in Chapter 2.

After reading this chapter, you will have gained an understanding of key concepts with which you can analyze the relationships you encounter most in today's interprofessional health care environments. However, because many aspects of both role enactment and relationship formation focus on individuals, who they are, and how they interact with others, we invite you also to reflect at a personal level on how these concepts relate to you as an individual and as a health professional.

PEOPLE

IPP revolves around people. At its core, IPP demands that the people involved collaborate effectively and combine their efforts and skills toward setting and meeting goals. It therefore requires us to have a reasonable understanding of ourselves, of others with whom we work, and of those receiving care. The people involved in IPP are diverse, possessing different personal and professional identities, personality and communication traits, skills, and motivations for participating in or seeking health care. In the sections that follow, we will review briefly important concepts related to human beings that come into focus when we consider the roles we enact and how, within these roles, we form relationships in IPP.

Personality Traits The term **personality traits** refers to an individual's psychological makeup. Personality traits are the culmination of an individual's attitudes, values, beliefs, experiences, and behaviour (Myers & Anderson, 2008). Within IPP, personality traits play a significant role. Interprofessional team effectiveness and productivity are in part determined by a balanced mix of personality types (Choi & Pak, 2007), the lack of which can lead to negative dynamics that prevent productive discussions and timely and effective problem solving. An individual may possess any of numerous personality traits. Three of these (Machiavellianism, self-esteem trait, and self-monitoring trait) exert significant influence on the relationships and communication within the team and with patients (Myers & Anderson, 2008). *Machiavellianism* refers to an individual's tendency to believe that others with whom he or she is interpersonally linked are untrustworthy and able to be manipulated (Paulhus & Williams, 2002). *Self-esteem trait* denotes an individual's appraisal of his or her own self-worth (Robins & Paulhus, 2001). Finally, *self-monitoring trait* refers to an individual's tendency to pay attention to cues about the appropriateness of different forms of behaviour within his or her environment or situation (Bain, Baxter, & Ballantyne, 2007).

Self-Identity **Self-identity** may be thought of as the way an individual perceives, describes, and identifies himself or herself. The concept spans a number of fields of study, including psychology, sociology, and anthropology. Self-identity is a complex and dynamic entity that is responsive to our experiences and interactions with others and the environment (O'Hagan, 2001).

Erikson's *Life Stage Theory* (1968) is likely the best-known representation of the concept of self-identity. A main feature of Erikson's theory is the development of a conscious sense of self as the result of social interaction. Erikson referred to this sense of self as *ego identity*.

In the opening scenario of this chapter, Golnaz questions whether she is a bad mother because she did not realize immediately that there was something wrong with her baby. Under difficult circumstances such as this, it is possible that a person's self-identity as a "mother" may be challenged or disrupted by her child's illness. Conversely, the challenge of illness and loss related to health may propel the individual toward a greater and/or transformed sense of self (Golafshani, 2002). As depicted in the opening scenario, it is important for members of the IPP team to be aware of the impact of health-related situations on identity in order to support patients during this period of change and potential growth (Dugan, 2007).

Self-identity and how we conceptualize of ourselves as persons also influences both (a) our ability to engage in relationships with others and (b) how we function within teams (Thomas & Hynes, 2007). For example, one who perceives himself or herself to be team-oriented and a team leader is likely to exhibit behaviour that fits with that self-identity. The impact of this behaviour within the team is dependent upon factors such as other members' self-identities and their perceptions and expectations of the role of leader.

Professional Identity Similar to the concept of self-identity, **professional identity** is defined by three key elements: (a) a set of beliefs and attitudes a person holds about his or her profession, (b) an understanding of one's role and the boundaries between professions, and (c) a conception of how one should engage with others as members of an interprofessional team (Adams, Hean, Sturgis, & McLeod, 2006; Lingard, Reznick, DeVito, & Espin, 2002). Wackerhausen (2009) describes professional identity as occurring on both a micro level and a macro level. At the micro level are the qualities of individuals that qualify them to be designated as a particular type of professional. These are determined not only by education, but also by the behaviours exhibited by the individual, such as expectations of conduct, which are in keeping with the culture of the profession. The macro level refers to the public persona of a profession ascribed to an individual (e.g., how society views the profession of medicine translates into assumptions about an individual physician). The macro professional identity of an individual health professional is mostly external and determined by factors such as public perceptions, the views of other professions, economics, and technological and scientific advancements.

Professional identities may have a positive influence on work life in health care settings by creating expectations of interaction that embody the ideals of conduct. However, Wackerhausen (2009) holds that professional identities may also become barriers to collaboration. In interpersonal relationships with other professionals and patients, an individual's professional identity may act as a barrier that limits outlook on issues and situations. Professional identities may also lead to self-affirming behaviour that is counterproductive to building relationships for teamwork. Members of interprofessional teams can counteract any pitfalls associated with professional identity development by learning about others' professional identities and seeking out perspectives that differ from their own.

Values and Beliefs Values and beliefs are constructs that are closely linked. In this section we will explore briefly how values and beliefs influence IPP. In the broadest sense, a *value* is defined as a feeling about a person, thing, or situation/event (Myers & Anderson, 2008). Values can be thought of as enduring conceptions about a situation/behaviour/condition of life that is desirable at the personal or social level (Beebe & Masterson, 1997; Glen, 1999). Values form the underpinning of our perceptions of right and wrong and they are reflected in our beliefs, attitudes, and behaviours. Our beliefs structure our world and form the basis for how we respond to our environment and others. Beliefs accepted as important truths, and hence established and fundamental, are called *tenets*. In the health care professions, a set of tenets is often adopted by members as part of their education.

Individual values and beliefs are commonly thought of as unique, differing from person to person. However, some researchers and philosophers argue that a small group of values exists that is universal (Jahanbegloo, 2007; Rokeach, 1973). Recognizing our own personal values and beliefs is a necessary first step in being able to work collaboratively in such a way that healthy and harmonious negotiation will take place.

Professional Values Profession-specific values and beliefs can be enhancing or obstructive to the formation of interprofessional relationships. Professional orientations and value systems are instilled during the process of professionalization and further reinforced in practice. **Professionalization** is the process of assuming an occupational identity. It encompasses educational experiences and professional socialization, where values and norms common to one's profession are internalized and become a part of self-identity and behaviour (Adams et al., 2006; Hall, 2005). While professionals bring with them personal moral values formed from sources such as family and religion, the process of professionalization also contributes to the internalization of moral values (Glen, 1999).

The unique nature of professionalization may sometimes result in the development of differing professional value systems among the members of interprofessional teams.

Because value systems are often unwritten and sometimes unspoken, they may become virtually invisible in the context of interprofessional relationships. Yet at the same time, values and beliefs form the basis of the cognitive maps (Hall, 2005; Petrie, 1976) from which professionals practice. Therefore, it becomes important for health care professionals to understand each other's orientations and values, determining, for example, how they perceive clinical situations and approach teamwork.

In the opening vignette, Brandon and Ginny demonstrate the value they both place on effective communication and family-centred care through their desire to ensure that a translator is made available to the Nahmet family. Although they represent two different professions, it is important to recognize that these two members of the team share these same values. While not always the case, there are many times when professional values are shared by the various health professions. In these cases, they may act as a bridge when other types of conflict emerge.

As a first step to understanding the values and beliefs of another professional, we must clarify our own personal and professional value system. Helpful Tools 4.1 outlines a number of simple questions that focus on this objective. These questions may also be adapted to explore the values and belief of others.

Diversity In health care environments, the term **diversity** is used to refer to individual and collective differences based on culture, demographics (including gender and age), and cognitive factors (e.g., education preparation and learning styles). Patients may differ in terms of their ethnicity, gender, sexual orientation, educational preparation, age, and social status. Differences within interprofessional teams and between health care

Helpful Tools 4.1

Values Clarification Questions

Values clarification has many benefits, including helping you to rediscover the benefits and joys experienced in your health care practice. The following questions focus on identifying the values that underpin your practice and who you are as an individual.

1. Begin by creating an inventory of your personal values by answering the question: What do I value as an individual? Do not worry about how the values you identify are worded or if they fit with a particular definition or category of values.
2. Prioritize your list.
3. Next, create two other lists focusing on what you value as a health professional and what you think others (e.g., family, friend, society) expect for you/of you.
4. Review your list by considering if there are discrepancies between:
   a. what you value and how you behave,
   b. your personal values and your professional values, and
   c. what you expect of yourself and what you believe others expect of you as a professional.
5. Describe any discrepancies you are able to identify between your personal and professional values.

professionals and patients may have a positive or negative impact, depending upon the values of the people involved. Research findings, for example, have demonstrated that when patients perceived prejudice from health care professionals based on group identity differences, such as race, they were more likely to experience poorer health outcomes (Bird, Bogart, & Delahanty, 2004; Steffen, McNeilly, Anderson, & Sherwood, 2003). Integration of IPP models incorporating patient-centred care and collaborative care planning that values diversity has the potential to create much more positive experiences.

Within IPP, diversity is also an important consideration. A mix of professionals with various backgrounds is purported to enhance the function of a team in areas such as decision making. The concept of "value in diversity" has become commonplace in today's work environments (Neuliep, 2006). Diversity in interprofessional teams offers a greater range of knowledge, ability, life experiences, and perspectives, all of which afford a team more options and advantages in comparison to homogenous teams (Keyton, 1999; Shea-Lewis, 2002; Wachs, 2005).

Roles

A role is a set of expected behaviours and responsibilities enacted through both what we say and what we do (Myers & Anderson, 2008; Sampson & Marthas, 1990). The concept of a role is strongly linked to the notion of identity and can be thought of as positions (e.g., mother, child, nurse, doctor) that individuals take on and carry out. Roles, therefore, help us to develop both our self- and our professional identities. Roles may be ascribed, achieved, or assigned. *Ascribed* roles are based on intrinsic characteristics of the individual. For example, an individual is ascribed the role of child by virtue of being born. *Achieved* roles are acquired through our actions and are based on our interests, our accomplishments, and the activities in which we engage. Professional designations such as registered physiotherapist are examples of achieved roles. Lastly, an *assigned* role is one formally granted to an individual, for example by appointing him or her as chairperson or president of an organization.

Roles are significant in that they structure our relationships with others. They define and regulate the behaviour of individuals in the context of relationships, making it possible for us to know who people are, what we can expect from them in terms of behaviour and communication, and how we should respond to them in return (Sampson & Marthas, 1990).

Roles have particular significance in the formal relationships in interprofessional teams. Within this context, role enactment may contribute to the overall effectiveness and productivity of the team and the quality of outcomes. Professional roles play an important part in health care practice, not only from a theoretical perspective, as we often see described in literature focusing on sociological and psychological aspects of human interactions, but also from a practical perspective. In addition to the historical roots of our professional roles, formalization of these roles can be seen in various types of legislation, codes of conduct, and the standards of practice defined for health care professionals.

However, interprofessional teamwork is more complex than the merely cumulative effect of behaving consistently with individual and professional roles; it involves collaborative and cooperative interactions regulated by more fluid group roles.

The intersection of individual, professional, and group roles is complex and dynamic. When there is internal consistency and clarity of the values and expectations, the individual often feels competent in role enactment; but when this is lacking, *role conflict*, *role confusion*, or *role distance* may emerge.

Role conflict occurs when an individual experiences tension and has negative emotions that result from competing or conflicting sets of expectations and demands associated with a person's roles. **Role confusion**, which can occur among health care providers or in the relationship between providers and patients, generally involves a lack of understanding of roles or a failure to recognize the boundaries of roles or relationships. **Role distance** is separation or detachment between individuals and the roles they expect to occupy; they deny the conceptualized image implied by the role rather than the role itself and manifest behaviours such as indifference. All of these phenomena (role conflict, role confusion, role distance) challenge effective IPP and can lead to professional and personal stress and burnout.

Role of the Patient The role of the patient is a specific type of individual role. Buetow, Jutel, and Hoare (2009) suggest that the role of patients has changed significantly in recent history, converging with the role of the health care professional, to become the modern patient. The modern patient—compared to, say, the recipient of health care as recently as 25 years ago—is much more likely to be informed and actively involved in his or her care. Patients we meet today are much more aware of their rights and have greater capacity to both evaluate and utilize health services. These ideas are consistent with client- and family-centred care and with the focus of this text, IPP.

The role of the modern patient has important implications for health care providers. The modern patient–health professional relationship requires, among other things, more negotiation and shared decision making. The many benefits to this relationship include increased self-capacity and self-awareness for the patient, increased satisfaction with care felt by both patient and providers, and reduction in provider burnout (Buetow et al., 2009; Halbesleben, 2006). The drawbacks include the blurring of roles, which can lead to role conflict (see discussion above), discord, and poor quality of relationship.

Professional Roles and Role Clarification

Health care providers bring to their practice a lifetime of personal experiences that contribute to making them the people they are. However, they are required to function within the role requirements of their profession. Some of these requirements are informal, and relate to the professional values embedded within our collectives. For example, mutuality was identified as a key interpersonal value held by nurses providing care to patients with cancer (Coffey, 2006). Within the Canadian health care system, most of the members of the interprofessional team will belong to regulated professions. Under this type of structure, members of each of the health professions (e.g., physiotherapists, occupational therapists, respiratory therapists, physicians, dieticians) must be deemed by the provincial regulatory body for that profession to have met the requirements necessary in order to use the title (e.g., to refer to oneself as a registered dietician) and to maintain employment in that profession. Registration requirements generally include educational and practice components and demonstrating conduct consistent with the expectations for a member of the profession in question. It is important to keep in mind that these codes of conduct refer not only to how a professional behaves on the job, but also to how he or she behaves out in the world, recognizing that we are all ambassadors of our professions. In Chapter 9, we will further explore interprofessional health care regulation.

Currently, the use of competency frameworks in outlining professional roles and responsibilities is gaining widespread acceptance. One framework with real potential to impact IPP is the National Interprofessional Competency Framework, developed by the Canadian Interprofessional Health Collaborative (CIHC, 2010). (See Spotlight 4.1.)

Also incorporated into our professional roles are the expectations of practice based on our unique knowledge and skill set. When there is a lack of clarity related to our roles or to those of the other team members, role confusion may result and professionals may have difficulty knowing which role they should assume. It is essential that all members of the interprofessional team have a clear understanding of the roles of each member and are

Spotlight 4.1

National Interprofessional Competency Framework

The Canadian Interprofessional Health Collaborative (CIHC) comprises health organizations, researchers, educators, professionals, and students from across Canada. In 2008, with funding from Health Canada, a working group was formed to develop a national competency framework for interprofessional collaboration. This work began with a review of the literature related to competencies and a review of any frameworks in existence that related to interprofessional education and interprofessional collaboration. The final product, titled *A National Interprofessional Competency Framework*, consists of the following six competency domains and three key themes.

Competency Domains

- Collaborative Leadership
- Interprofessional Conflict Resolution
- Role Clarification
- Team Functioning
- Interprofessional Communication
- Patient/Client/Family/Community-Centred Care

Themes

- Context of Practice
- Level of Complexity
- Quality Improvement

Source: From *National Interprofessional Competency Framework*.

Helpful Tools 4.2

Role Clarification

The Canadian Interprofessional Health Collaborative (CIHC) (2010) National Interprofessional Competency Framework suggests the following activities and exercises that support health care professionals' role clarification:

- describing their own role and that of others
- recognizing and respecting the diversity of other health and social care roles, responsibilities, and competencies
- performing their own roles in a culturally respectful way
- communicating roles, knowledge, skills, and attitudes using appropriate language
- accessing others' skills and knowledge appropriately through consultation
- considering the roles of others in determining their own professional and interprofessional roles (p. 12)

able to clearly describe their own role and unique knowledge and skill. The CIHC framework identifies role clarification as one of the six competency domains. According to this framework, **role clarification** requires members of the interprofessional team to understand their roles and those of other professions, and use this knowledge to set and achieve appropriate goals. Role clarification requires that we identify not only what knowledge and skill is held uniquely by professions, but also what is shared. Through this process, we are able to determine which team member is most appropriate and most able to take responsibility for a given activity and context. For example, several members of a team might be able to provide teaching about a new medication to a patient (e.g., the pharmacist, the registered nurse, the physician, the nurse practitioner), but collaboratively determining in a specific situation which of these members will take leadership for this requires all members of the team to recognize and respect each other's role. Types of activities that demonstrate role clarification are included in Helpful Tools 4.2.

Roles in Teams

In addition to our understanding of the various individual roles that we take on, when involved in IPP we must also be aware of team roles. As teams are established and maintained, members take on roles related specifically to how the team itself functions. These may be chosen intentionally and members may be very conscious of their decision to take on a specific role (e.g., a member who values detail and takes pride in knowing exactly where and how to access policy information may often choose to be the information giver when this type of data is required). However, at times we also unknowingly take on team roles reflective of our own personality or values as they are experienced in the moment. For example, a member uncomfortable with conflict may repeatedly take on the role of harmonizer, trying to smooth ruffled feathers and keep the group working well together. In 1948, Benne and Heats identified three basic classifications of group/team roles in relation to their overall purpose, which continue to be commonly cited. Some roles focus on what was needed to accomplish a task (*task roles*). Others are focused on what is needed to maintain the group (*maintenance roles*). Finally, some are based on an individual's particular traits or orientations in the situation (*individual roles*). Within each of these categories, specific roles commonly enacted by group members have been identified. Table 4.1 highlights various team roles within this framework that may exist in IPP situations. In the opening vignette, we can identify Ginny (the certified lactation consultant) as an initiator when she raises the idea of providing a translator for the Nahmet family to ensure effective communication takes place.

When we are practising interprofessionally, it is important to focus not only on the outcomes of practice, but also on the overall functioning of the team. Understanding and applying the theory related to how individuals work together within a team and the roles that are at play is important to developing an awareness of team dynamics. This process also allows us to become more aware of pitfalls we may encounter working collaboratively.

Table 4.1 Roles in Teams

	Task Roles
Contributor/initiator	Proposes new ideas or alternative ways of approaching goal achievement and problem solving; helpful in moving the group into new areas for consideration and discovery.
Information seeker/giver	Requests clarification of moments, issues, and information provided by others, determines what information is needed, and searches for relevant information; provides accurate information and is seen as expert or authority on a particular subject.
Coordinator	Is involved in helping to organize and pull together ideas and themes to help move the group forward toward goals.
Evaluator	Critically evaluates ideas, proposals, and plans against standards; examines the appropriateness and practicalities of ideas and scrutinizes procedures for effectiveness.
	Maintenance Roles
Encourager	Provides praise and affirmation for the efforts of members; communicates acceptance and openness to others and their ideas; demonstrates warmth and promotes a positive team atmosphere.
Harmonizer	Mediates and tries to reconcile differences, conflicts, and disagreements within the team; goal is to reduce or diffuse tensions within the team and uses such tactics as humour and explanation.
Compromiser	Changes his or her position on issues or seeks a position between contending perspectives for the good of all members.

(*continued*)

Table 4.1 Roles in Teams (*Continued*)

	Individual Roles
Aggressor	Acts negatively and is hostile toward other members; may belittle, denigrate, and insult others' contributions and attack them personally in an effort to elevate his or her own status.
Recognition-seeker	Tries to get the attention of the team for him- or herself through boasting, flamboyance, or directing members away from team activities.
Dominator	Asserts authority over other members and manipulates others in an effort to control what happens within the team; may monopolize conversations and dictate to others how they should behave.
Help seeker	Uses the team to gain sympathy and personal accomplishment by sharing feelings of inadequacy and acting helpless.
Special-interest pleaser	Uses the interests of others (e.g., making suggestions of what others might like) in an attempt to avoid revealing his or her own feelings and opinions.
Self-confessor	Uses the team and its time to disclose personal feelings and share personal issues by disguising personal content in team-related issues and problems; aims to gain personal satisfaction or insight.
Disrupter	Uses team time and meetings as an opportunity to get away from work and have fun; distracts other members by engaging in other activities such as telling jokes and doing other, unrelated work.

Source: "Role in Teams" from Functional Roles of Group Members. Published by ICA Associates Inc., © 1948.

RELATIONSHIPS IN INTERPROFESSIONAL PRACTICE

While research examining the nature of relationships between health care professionals in general is just now coming into greater focus, for many decades the subcategory of nurse–doctor relationships has been a phenomenon of interest. In his seminal paper "The doctor–nurse game," Leonard Stein (1967) critiqued the relationship between nurses and physicians, which he described as an interprofessional game in which the dominant, typically male, doctor's clinical decision making was covertly guided by the seemingly passive, usually female, nurse. While even Stein would argue that we have since moved beyond this characterization (e.g., Stein, Watts, & Howell, 1990), relationships between members of the interprofessional team are not without their potential challenges. On the other hand, within the context of health care, the formation and maintenance of respectful, collegial, and supportive interprofessional relationships can be a solid foundation for rewarding practice that is much more likely to lead to desired patient outcomes.

Throughout this text, we have stressed not only the importance of IPP, but also the emerging evidence that the use of interprofessional teams results in high-quality, collaborative health care. The success of IPP is predicated on a host of relational dynamics, beyond just bringing people together, that result in functional and effective relationships between the members of interprofessional teams (D'Amour, Ferrada-Videla, San Martin-Rodriguez, &

Beaulieu, 2005). Keeping in mind that people and the relationships they form will always be at the centre of care, it's important to attend to the details of interprofessional relationships. These details enable us not only to focus on what is desirable within the relationship, but also to understand what we may be experiencing when things are not working.

In successful interprofessional relationships, health care professionals are able to maintain their specialized knowledge and skills, while also remaining open to the fluid nature of collaboration in which boundaries are not always clear. Interprofessional relationships require a sharing of professional, sometimes discipline-specific, knowledge and perspectives. They also thrive when sound relational communication skills are employed and when knowledge and application of group processes and skills takes place (Cohen & Bailey, 1997; Petrie, 1976). Kilgore and Langford (2009) argue that attaining high levels of mutual understanding among team members and demonstrating a willingness and preparedness to respond to the various needs of diverse patients requires overcoming barriers rooted in profession-specific and health care system issues. Reeves, Nelson, and Zwarenstein (2008) add that amid the current focus on IPP, there may yet be lessons to learn from the troubled relationship between nurses and physicians brought into focus by Stein in the 1960s and 1970s.

On the positive side, the trend toward more collaborative practice has enabled us to uncover many helpful strategies to support the development of healthy, positive relationships in IPP. Lindeke and Sieckert (2005) highlight three areas for development that promote positive relationships: (a) self-development strategies, (b) team-development strategies, and (c) communication-development strategies. While initially discussing nurse–physician relationships, the matrix of strategies these authors provide has applicability for all members of the interprofessional team. Table 4.2 provides an overview of these approaches.

Power and Authority IPP offers the potential for many very positive opportunities for collaboration, team-building, and relationship development. However, we would be remiss if we failed to acknowledge that traditional hierarchical health care structures have led to historical imbalances in power and authority among health care professions (San Martin-Rodriguez et al., 2005). The dynamics not only of our health care systems but also modern social systems in general have fostered gender and other stereotypes and disparities in social status. These can impact the relationships among health care professionals, creating power differences (Hall, 2005; San Martin-Rodriguez et al., 2005). Additionally, cultural and other forms of diversity play an influential role in establishing and maintaining the power imbalances that may impede the development of healthy professional relationships in health care settings and negatively impact health care (Burgess et al., 2010).

The concept of power distance has been discussed in relation to cultural diversity, but it has applicability to interprofessional relationships as well. **Power distance** refers to the degree to which those who are less powerful accept and expect power to be unequally distributed (Hofstede, 2001). It measures how individuals perceive power differences. Individuals from cultures with large power distances are more likely to accept hierarchal and paternalistic power relationships in workplace environments than those from cultures with small

Table 4.2 Strategies for Effective Relationships

Self-Development Strategies	
Develop emotional maturity.	Avoid perfectionist thinking; focus on constant improvement.
	Develop self-confidence that enables you to creatively address challenges, rather than taking an all-or-nothing approach.
	Focus on your own growth; become a lifelong learner; identify and employ best practices.
Understand the perspectives of others.	Create or capitalize on opportunities for interprofessional learning and interprofessional socialization.
	Avoid assumptions; take time and extend the effort to learn about each other's role.
Avoid compassion fatigue.	Employ self-renewal strategies.
	Consider lifestyle changes and self-care practices.
Team-Development Strategies	
Build the team.	Build trust.
	Create common ground through a patient focus.
Negotiate respectfully.	Try to balance power and authority.
	Define expectations for independent and collaborative tasks and make explicit expectations for joint interactions from the start.
Manage conflict wisely.	Don't avoid conflict; rather, strive for healthy conflict in which everyone is free to voice an idea.
	Focus on facts rather than opinions.
Avoid negative behaviours.	Encourage consistent, courageous, and deliberate leadership.
	Avoid the blame game and territorial issues.
	Speak frankly, but leave room for flexibility and open-mindedness.
Design facilities for collaboration.	Anticipate and negotiate for space requirements that support collaboration.

Table 4.2 Strategies for Effective Relationships (*Continued*)

Communication-Development Strategies	
Communicate effectively in emergencies.	Get your facts rights and prioritize, focusing on key data.
	Respond promptly and calmly.
	Follow up and debrief when the situation is calmer.
Use electronic communication thoughtfully.	Use an appropriate tone for professional electronic communication.
	Evaluate the content of messages and clarify any uncertainties before reacting.
	Be as concise as is possible and appropriate.

Source: Adapted from Lindeke, L. L., & Sieckert, A. M. (2005). Nurse–physician workplace collaboration. *The Online Journal of Issues in Nursing, 10*(1), manuscript 4.

power distances. The concept suggests that within teams where there is greater cultural diversity, there is a greater likelihood for communication challenges and other interpersonal problems. For example, in a health care environment with a strong hierarchal structure, a leader who perceives a large power distance may take offence when challenged by a team member who perceives a small power distance (Myers & Anderson, 2008). Research findings also indicate that power distance influences the level of comfort and engagement between patients and health care professionals (Gao, Burke, Somkin, & Pasick, 2009).

However, the complexity of power differences within IPP is underscored by the legitimate differences in legal authority that exist between health care professionals. Physicians, for example, are often the professional group with the greatest amount of authority (under health care legislation) to make decisions related to patient care. While equity between health care professionals is central to notions of collaboration and effective relationships in IPP, it would be naïve to fail to recognize that there are role differences that may impact relationship formation. Acknowledging that all members of the team are inherently important to ensuring quality health care is a necessary first step to finding ways to navigate around this common roadblock to collaboration. We revisit this topic in greater detail in Chapter 9.

RELATIONAL COMMUNICATION

Successful IPP is contingent on the development, maintenance, and management of the many relationships both among health care professionals and between health care professionals and patients. One key component in supporting these processes is relational communication, "the verbal and non-verbal messages [or communications] that create the social fabric of a [team] by promoting relationship between and among [team] members" (Keyton, 1999, p. 192). To this definition, Myers and Anderson (2008) add listening as a central activity, arguing that it is a communication skill that occurs before, during, and after member interactions.

Keyton (1999) holds that relational communication is the affective or expressive element of the communication that occurs within a team. The messages involved in relational communication create the climate that allows for task completion and goal attainment. These messages can be of either a positive or a negative quality and can affect either the entire team or just some individuals.

Interprofessional Communication

Interprofessional communication is identified as one of the six competency domains that form the National Interprofessional Competency Framework (CIHC, 2010). The competency statement specifically notes that "learners/practitioners from different professions communicate with each other in a collaborative, responsive and responsible manner" (p. 16). It involves both verbal (negotiating, consulting, interacting) and nonverbal (listening) modes. It also requires trust and respect.

Verbal and Nonverbal Communication There are multiple definitions for verbal and nonverbal communication within the literature. For our purposes, we will focus on the distinctions between the two concepts. **Verbal communication** is made up of the words and phrases we use to create meaning. **Nonverbal communication** (sometimes called *metacommunication*) refers to all other communication used to create meaning (Arnold & Boggs, 2011; Myers & Anderson, 2008; Sampson & Marthas, 1990). From a relationship perspective, verbal and nonverbal communication function to structure and organize our interactions, enabling us to establish and maintain relationships, convey relational messages, and form and manage our impressions of others and situations within the team and in the environment (Beebe & Masterson, 1997; Ketrow, 1999).

Effective verbal communication is a cornerstone not only of IPP, but of health care in general. Patients and our professional colleagues count on us to be able to communicate the most relevant information in a timely and appropriate manner. This entails using available communication strategies and technologies, maintaining confidentiality as appropriate while also ensuring full disclosure to all who may require the information. This seems like a tall order, but it is the very lynchpin of safe health care. Lindeke and Sieckert (2005) highlight the need for health care professionals working in interprofessional teams to be prepared to communicate in emergency situations. They cite Henry (2000) in creating a simple list of must-dos, including (a) getting the facts from informed sources, (b) keeping your perspective, (c) responding promptly, and (d) calmly sharing only what others need to know and ethically should know.

Two methods for interprofessional communication that are growing in popularity are referred to by the acronyms CARE and SBAR. CARE is a method for increasing assertiveness in communication; SBAR focuses on communication of patient information between members of the interprofessional team. Helpful Tools 4.3 provides a very brief overview of these techniques.

Nonverbal communication includes such behaviours as eye contact, body posture, facial expressions, and even seating arrangement in a team. It is important to note that most often nonverbal communication requires interpretation. We need to read between the lines, so to speak, to attribute a meaning to this type of communication.

Consider a conversation between Jane and Gary. Jane is sharing the details of her current work project with Gary, who listens but repeatedly checks the time on his watch. Jane finds herself speeding up her speech and leaving out details that she would otherwise have shared, interpreting Gary's actions to mean he is either impatient, late for an appointment, or bored. These may all be reasonable explanations, but it's important to keep in mind that there may be many other possible considerations. In this situation, Gary is actually checking the time because he has been assigned by the team to distract Jane and keep her occupied for as long as possible while they set up a surprise birthday celebration for her in the coffee room! In assuming she could read his nonverbal cues and trying to accommodate his wishes, Jane is actually working against the desired outcome. While this is a harmless example, it's easy to imagine how important clarification of nonverbal cues becomes when we consider professional communication within the context of health care. Table 4.3 provides an overview of some forms of nonverbal communication.

Helpful Tools 4.3

Interprofessional Communication Techniques

Use of communication techniques, such as CARE and SBAR, can help to ensure that communication between health care professionals is clear, efficient, and directed toward supporting quality patient care and outcomes.

- The acronym CARE (Smith, cited in Grover, 2005) is a simple assertiveness communication technique.
  - C—clarify the situation (e.g. problem or conflict).
  - A—articulate why the situation is a problem.
  - R—request a change in the behaviour or situation.
  - E—encourage this change thorough your actions.
- SBAR (situation–background–assessment–recommendation) is a standardized communication technique developed by Michael Leonard, Doug Bonacum, and Suzanne Graham at Kaiser Permanente of Colorado. The technique provides a framework for organizing basic information about patient care situations and can be used when communicating in situations such as reporting critical incidents or when making recommendations to other members of the health care team. Refer to the Additional Resources section at the end of this chapter for links to information about using SBAR.

Table 4.3 Sources of Nonverbal Communication

Communicative Attribute	Description
Personal appearance	Refers to how team members look; their clothing, body shape and measurements, general attractiveness. Personal appearance influences the perceptions and reactions of others.
Facial expression	Team members convey meaning through their faces. Facial expressions are culturally bound. In Western culture, facial expressions are used to communicate emotions such as anger, sadness, happiness, fear, disgust, and surprise.
Oculesics (eye behaviour)	Refers to eye movements and other eye behaviours. These include making eye contact, winking, staring, and blinking. Of these, eye contact is thought to be the most important.
Kinesics (body movements)	Refers to use of body movement such as a person's posture. Through these body movements, team members convey their emotional state, respond to ideas and issues, and send messages without verbally communicating them.
Proxemics	Refers to the use of space by members of the team and is divided into two types: distance and territory. Distance refers to the amount of physical space between members. Territory refers to ownership of space.
Vocalics (vocal cues)	Refers to the qualities of team members' voices, such as pitch, rate, volume, inflection, articulation, and pronunciation. Vocalics are very important to understanding the meaning of verbal communications.

Source: Based on Myers, S. A., & Anderson, C. M. (2008). *The fundamentals of small group communication*. Thousand Oaks, CA: Sage Publications.

Listening Listening is an important aspect of relational communication that occurs within interprofessional teams and between patients and health care professionals. Listening, sometimes referred to as a specific type of nonverbal communication, is integral to knowledge acquisition. Eighty-five percent of what we learn is through listening, and we spend about 45% of our day at it (Metcalfe, 2009). A common definition of **listening** is a dynamic process involving receiving, perceiving, and making sense of a message, the aim being to respond (Myers & Anderson, 2008). Burton (2002) refers to compassionate listening as withholding judgment and maintaining boundaries while hearing with the heart. Burton contends that when patients are not listened to or paid attention to, they are diminished. Stickley and Freshwater (2006) further add that listening involves use of all the senses, not just the ears.

It is important to stress the value of listening when communicating within the interprofessional team. Myers and Anderson (2008) describe five types of listening that are essential to relational development in health care teams:

- *Discriminative listening.* Refers to the ability to discriminate or distinguish stimuli from one another.
- *Appreciative listening.* Refers to the level of interest or desire to listen for reasons of enjoyment.
- *Empathic listening.* Refers to the willingness to listen to understand how another feels.
- *Comprehensive listening.* Refers to the desire to understand in order to learn and gain meaning.
- *Evaluative listening.* Refers to the need to evaluate information based on criteria.

Trust and Respect Trust and respect have been identified as key precursors to positive communication and effective work relationships among teams. Both are included in the CIHC National Interprofessional Competency Framework (2010). San Martin-Rodriguez and colleagues (2005) identify trust as a key element necessary for the development of collaborative interactions between health professionals. Trust involves the ability of one person or professional to rely on the truthfulness and integrity of another person or professional (van Servellen, cited in Grover, 2005). While trust can be either global (a general and open acceptance of individuals) or specific to an individual, in the context of IPP trust is often primarily dependent on competence and experience (San Martin-Rodriguez et al., 2005). Health care professionals who are judged as competent in their skills and knowledge and as having adequate experience are more likely to be trusted by others. Henneman, Lee, and Cohen (1995) note that building trust in someone requires time, patience, effort, and previous positive experiences with trusting someone.

While health care professionals identify a strong desire to be respected, they also may engage in professional behaviours that are interpreted as disrespectful by others (Casanova, Day & Dorpat, 2007; San Martin-Rodriguez et al., 2005). San Martin-Rodriguez and colleagues contend that a lack of understanding or appreciation for the contribution of other professionals is perceived as a major barrier to development of respect in collaborative interactions between health care professionals.

Conflict

Many of us have been socialized to avoid conflict as something negative. Wilmot and Hocker (2001) found that conflict often conjures in peoples' minds a variety of negative images, ranging from war to struggle. While the intensity of these images varies, all convey a perception of tension. Yet, not only is conflict natural in our daily lives, it might actually be considered an important and necessary aspect of them. **Conflict** in the context of IPP refers to the process that occurs when team members, because of the complex and interdependent nature of teams and their work, engage in a struggle rooted in a difference of beliefs, thoughts, attitudes, feelings, and/or behaviours (Cox, 2003). These differences may be either expressed (verbally or nonverbally) or perceived. Conflict is neither negative nor positive and is an unavoidable consequence of working in teams in health care environments.

While some professional socialization processes deal specifically with conflict, we often find that how health care professional groups tend to respond to conflict is transmitted through the attitudes of their educators and professional cultural norms (Lindeke & Block, 1998). In professions where historically conflict was perceived as negative, such as nursing, communication and relational patterns often developed with a goal of conflict avoidance (Baker, 1995; Hiemer, n.d.; Valentine, 1995). Instead, a more productive goal would be to identify areas of professional conflict, uncover the factors at play, and take appropriate action for healthy resolution. This sounds like a tall order, but it is essential to invest time and energy into creating positive relationships and the conditions wherein interprofessional teams can thrive.

The term **interpersonal conflict** refers to conflict that arises between two or more individuals (Cox, 2003). Cox distinguishes interpersonal conflict from **intergroup conflict**, which is defined as disagreement or difference between members of two or more groups or their representatives over authority, territory, or resources. Both forms of conflict involve factors and issues at the level of the individual, such as opposing personal values. However, an intergroup conflict will most often focus on issues at levels beyond the individual, such as professional territorialism. Interprofessional conflict can be a mix of both interpersonal and intergroup conflict. These conflicts often are rooted in differences in perceptions of team members' roles, level of accountability, or desired goals.

It's important to remember that when we avoid conflict at all costs, we may actually be putting our patients at risk. Having the freedom to disagree means we can engage in a process where alternative perspectives and options are discussed. This process is essential if we are to avoid groupthink, a situation that occurs when members of a group are so eager to get along that they avoid presenting alternative solutions (Lindeke & Sieckert, 2005). Instead of avoiding conflict, our goal is to find ways to identify conflict and manage it so that healthy discourse is encouraged. The CIHC National Interprofessional Competency Framework (2010, p. 17) uses the phrase "conflict positive" to promote the development of a set of agreements to assist with managing conflict. Specifically, these agreements should ensure that everyone is heard, including the patient, who is the expert in his or her own life and health experience. In ensuring that appropriate methods for dealing with conflict are applied, interprofessional teams create an atmosphere in which all members are comfortable engaging more fully in team processes. Chapter 6 will build on this discussion and discuss ways to resolve conflict.

IPP can be a tremendously rewarding approach to practice for health care professionals. Understanding not only our professional roles and how we enact them, but also the roles of the other team members, is critical to its success. As well, it's important to consider how we relate to other members of the team, the intersection of personal and professional values, and the potential for conflict and miscommunication, particularly in high-stress situations.

CONCLUSION

For IPP to be successful, understanding ourselves and the multiple personal and professional roles we take on is critical. Being aware of and demonstrating respect for differences among team members is central to the formation of positive IPP relationships. Communication is a key factor that promotes or inhibits relationships among health care professionals and between providers and patients. Effective interpersonal and interprofessional communication involves many modalities, including both verbal and nonverbal elements. Recognizing and responding to conflict when it occurs within the IPP team, rather than avoiding it at all costs, is an important skill for enhancing team functioning.

SUMMARY

- IPP demands that professionals collaborate effectively, requiring that we have a clear understanding of our professions, our roles, our competencies, and ourselves. It also requires that we develop an awareness of and respect for differing personal and professional values and diversity among health professionals and patients.
- Roles are behaviours enacted through what we say and what we do. Professional role enactment contributes to overall productivity of teams. However, the intersection of individual, professional, and group roles is complex and dynamic. When inconsistencies occur, role conflict may result.
- The success of IPP is predicated on a host of relational dynamics, beyond just bringing people together, that result in functional and effective relationships between members of interprofessional teams. In successful interprofessional relationships, health care professionals are able to maintain their specialized knowledge and skills, while remaining open to the fluid nature of collaboration in which boundaries are not always clear.
- Relational communication is a key component in supporting the development, maintenance, and management of relationships among health professionals and between professionals and patients. Effective interprofessional communication, including verbal and nonverbal modalities, is a cornerstone of successful professional collaboration. Trust and respect have been identified as two precursors to positive communication.
- Conflict is not inherently negative. In IPP, the goal is not to avoid conflict at all costs, but rather to recognize it and respond to it accordingly. In ensuring that appropriate methods for dealing with conflict are applied, interprofessional teams create an atmosphere in which all members are comfortable engaging more fully in team processes, likely leading to greater provider satisfaction and better patient health outcomes.

Key Terms

conflict
diversity
intergroup conflict
interpersonal conflict
interprofessional communication
listening
nonverbal communication
personality traits
power distance
professional identity
professionalization
role clarification
role conflict
role confusion
role distance
self-identity
verbal communication

Review Questions

1. Describe the relationship between personal values and professional values. How are personal and professional values acquired and transmitted?
2. Why is the concept of diversity important to consider in relation to both patients and the interprofessional team?
3. What are team roles and how do they relate to IPP?
4. Describe the three types of development strategies that can be used to promote positive interprofessional relationships.
5. How can interprofessional communication promote IPP?

Application Exercises

1. Consider your own health profession (or the one about which you are learning). How would you define that role? What sources of information can you use in seeking a definition for this professional role? Research the role of at least one other member of the IPP team. Compare and contrast these roles. What roles are common to both types of professionals and what roles are unique to each? Create a list of all the ways that you can envision that these two types of professionals might collaborate. If you work with or have the opportunity to study with individuals from the other professional roles you have chosen to learn about, engage them in discussion about what you have learned.
2. Watch a 30–60 minute episode of any type of health care–related drama currently on television (e.g., drama, soap opera, situation comedy, etc.). As you watch, make notes about the inter- and intraprofessional relationships portrayed. Identify any themes that emerge in relation to professional roles, values and beliefs, power and authority, and conflict. How realistically do you believe the television show portrays these relationships? If you could take on the role of consultant to this program, what changes would you suggest given your knowledge from this chapter?

Additional Resources

Websites

Institute for Healthcare Improvement SBAR Toolkit
www.ihi.org/IHI/Topics/PatientSafety/SafetyGeneral/Tools/SBARToolkit.htm

Guidelines

Registered Nurses Association of Ontario (RNAO) Healthy Work Environments Best Practice Guidelines
www.rnao.org

Online Videos

Toronto Rehab SBAR Videos
www.youtube.com/user/TheTorontoRehab/videos

Additional Readings

Bainbridge, L., Nasmith, L., Orchard, C., & Wood, V. (2010). Competencies for interprofessional collaboration. *Journal of Physical Therapy Education, 24*(1), 6–11.

Boaro, N., Fancott, C., Bakerm, G. R., Velji, K., & Andreoli, A. (2010). Using SBAR to improve communication in interprofessional teams. *Journal of Interprofessional Care, 24*(10), 111–114.

Burzotta, L., & Noble, H. (2011). The dimensions of interprofessional practice. *British Journal of Nursing, 20*(5), 310–315.

Wright, D., & Brajtman, S. (2011). Relational and embodied knowing: Nursing ethics within the interprofessional team. *Nursing Ethics, 18*(1), 20–30.

References

Adams, K., Hean, S., Sturgis, P., & McLeod, C. J. (2006). Investigating the factors influencing professional identity of first year health and social care students. *Learning in Health and Social Care, 5*(2), 55–68.

Arnold, E. C., & Boggs, K. U. (2011). *Interpersonal relationships: Professional communication skills for nurses* (6th ed.). St Louis, MI: Elsevier Saunders.

Bain, S. A., Baxter, J. S., & Ballantyne, K. (2007). Self-monitoring style and levels of interrogative suggestibility. *Personality and Individual Differences, 42*, 623–630.

Baker, K. M. (1995). Improving staff nurse conflict resolution skills. *Nursing Economics, 13*(5), 295–317.

Beebe, S. A., & Masterson, J. T. (1997). *Communication in small groups: Principles and practice* (5th ed.). New York, NY: Longman.

Benne, J. D., & Heats, P. (1948). Functional roles of group members. *Journal of Social Issues*, 4.

Bird, S. T., Bogart, L. M., & Delahanty, D. L. (2004). Health related correlates of perceived discrimination in HIV care. *AIDS Patient Care and STDs, 18*(1), 19–26.

Buetow, S., Jutel, A., & Hoare, K. (2009). Shrinking social space in the doctor–modern patient relationship: A review of forces for, and implications of, homologisation. *Patient Education and Counseling, 74*(1), 97–103.

Burgess, D. J., Warren, J., Phelan, S., Dovidio, J., & van Ryn, M. (2010). Stereotype threat and health disparities: What medical educators and future physicians need to know. *Journal of General Internal Medicine, 25*(S2): 169–177.

Burton, L. A. (2002). The medical patient: Compassionate listening and spirit-mind-body care of medical patients. In R. Gilbert (Ed.), *Health care and spirituality: Listening, assessing, caring* (pp. 163–178). Amityville, NY: Baywood Publishing Co.

Canadian Interprofessional Health Collaborative. (2010). *A national interprofessional competency framework*. Vancouver, BC: Author.

Casanova, J., Day, K., & Dorpat, D. (2007). Nurse–physician work relations and role expectations. *Journal of Nursing Administration, 37*(2), 68–70.

Choi, B. C., & Pak, A. W. (2007). Multidisciplinarity, interdisciplinarity, and transdisciplinarity in health research, services, education and policy: 2. Promotors, barriers, and strategies of enhancement. *Clinical and Investigative Medicine, 30*(6), E224–232.

Coffey, S. (2006). The nurse–patient relationship in cancer care as a shared covenant: A concept analysis. *Advances in Nursing Science, 29*(4), 308–323.

Cohen, S. G., & Bailey, D. E. (1997). What makes team work: Group effectiveness research from the shop floor to the executive suite. *Journal of Management, 23*, 239–290.

Cox, K. B. (2003). The effects of intrapersonal, intragroup, and intergroup conflict on team performance effectiveness and work satisfaction. *Nursing Administration Quarterly, 27*(2), 153–163.

D'Amour, D., Ferrada-Videla, M., San Martin-Rodriguez, L., & Beaulieu, M. D. (2005). The conceptual basis for interprofessional collaboration: Core concepts and theoretical frameworks. *Journal of Interprofessional Care, 19*(S1), 116–131.

Dugan, B. (2007). Loss of identity in disaster: How do you say goodbye to home? *Perspectives in Psychiatric Care, 43*(1), 41–6.

Erikson, E. H. (1968). *Identity, youth and crisis* (pp. 16–19). New York, NY: W. W. Norton and Co.

Gao, G., Burke, N., Somkin, C. P., & Pasick, R. (2009). Considering culture in physician–patient communication during colorectal cancer screening. *Qualitative Health Research, 19*(6), 778–89.

Glen, S. (1999). Educating for interprofessional collaboration: Teaching about values. *Nursing Ethics, 6*(3), 202–213.

Golafshani, N. (2002). Identity formation through second language learning: A journey through a narrative. *Electronic Magazine of Multicultural Education, 4*(1). Retrieved on March 1, 2010, from http://jonah.eastern.edu/emme/2002spring/golafshani.html

Grover, S. M. (2005). Shaping effective communication skills and therapeutic relationships at work: The foundation of collaboration. *AAOHN Journal, 53*(4), 177–182.

Halbesleben, J. R. B. (2006). Patient reciprocity and physician burnout: What do patients bring to the patient–physician relationship? *Health Services Management Research, 19*(4), 215–222.

Hall, P. (2005). Interprofessional teamwork: Professional cultures as barriers. *Journal of Interprofessional Care, 19(S1)*, 188–196.

Henneman, E. A., Lee, J. L., & Cohen, J. I. (1995). Collaboration: A concept analysis. *Journal of Advanced Nursing, 21*(1), 103–109.

Henry, R. (2000). *You'd better have a hose if you want to put out the fire*. Windsor, CA: Gollywobbler Productions.

Hiemer, A. (n.d.). Conflict resolution: Tools for nursing. *RN Journal*. Retrieved from http://www.rnjournal.com/journal_of_nursing/conflict-resolution-tools-for-nursing.htm

Hofstede, G. (2001). *Culture's consequences: Comparing values, behaviors, institutions, and organizations across nations* (2nd ed.). Thousand Oaks, CA: Sage Publications.

Jahanbegloo, R. (2007). *Conversations with Isaiah Berlin* (2nd ed.). London: Halban Publishers.

Ketrow, S. M. (1999). Nonverbal aspects of group communication. In L. R. Frey (Ed.), *The handbook of group communication theory & research* (pp. 258–287). Thousand Oaks, CA: Sage.

Keyton, J. (1999). Relational communication in groups. In L. R. Frey (Ed.), *The handbook of group communication theory & research* (pp. 192–222). Thousand Oaks, CA: Sage.

Kilgore, R. V., & Langford, R. W. (2009). Reducing the failure risk of interdisciplinary healthcare teams. *Critical Care Nurse Quarterly, 32*(2), 81–88.

Lindeke, L. L., & Block, D. (1998). Maintaining professional integrity in the midst of interdisciplinary collaboration. *Nursing Outlook, 45*(6), 213–218.

Lindeke, L. L., and Sieckert, A. M. (2005). Nurse–physician workplace collaboration. *OJIN: The Online Journal of Issues in Nursing, 1*(10), manuscript 4.

Lingard, L., Reznick, P., DeVito, I., & Espin, P. (2002). Forming professional identities on the health care team: Discursive constructions of the "other" in the operating room. *Medical Education, 36*(8), 728–734.

Metcalfe, S. (2009). *Cengage Advantage Books: Building a speech* (7th ed.). Boston, MA: Wadworth Publishing.

Myers, S. A., & Anderson, C. M. (2008). *The fundamentals of small group communication*. Thousand Oaks, CA: Sage Publications.

Neuliep, J. W. (2006). *Intercultural communication: A contextual approach* (4th ed.). Thousand Oaks, CA: Sage Publications.

O'Hagan, K. (2001). *Cultural competence in the caring professions*. London, UK: Jessica Kingsley.

Paulhus, D. L., & Williams, K. M. (2002). The dark triad of personality: Narcissism, Machiavellianism, and psychopathy. *Journal of Research in Personality, 36*(6), 556–563.

Petrie, H. G. (1976). Do you see what I see? The epistemology of interdisciplinary inquiry. *Journal of Aesthetic Education, 10*, 29–43.

Reeves, S., Nelson, S., & Zwarenstein, M. (2008). The doctor–nurse game in the age of interprofessional care: A view from Canada. *Nursing Inquiry, 15*(1), 1–2.

Robins, R. W., & Paulhus, D. L. (2001). The character of self-enhancers: Implications for organizations. In B. W. Roberts & R. Hogan (Eds.), *Personality psychology in the workplace* (pp. 193–222). Washington, DC: American Psychological Association.

Rokeach, M. (1973). *The nature of human values*. New York: Free Press.

Sampson, E. E., & Marthas, M. (1990). *Group process for the health professions* (3rd ed.). Albany, NY: Delmar Thompson Learning.

San Martin-Rodriguez, L., Beaulieu, M. D., D'Amour, D., & Ferrada-Videla, M. (2005). The determinants of successful collaboration: A review of theoretical and empirical studies. *Journal of Interprofessional Care, 19*(S1), 132–147.

Shea-Lewis, A. (2002). Workforce diversity in healthcare. *Journal of Nursing Administration, 32*(1), 6–7.

Steffen, P. R., McNeilly, M., Anderson, N., & Sherwood, A. (2003). Effects of perceived racism and anger inhibition on ambulatory blood pressure in African Americans. *Psychosomatic Medicine, 65*(5), 746–750.

Stein, L. (1967). The doctor–nurse game. *Archives of General Psychiatry, 16*, 699–703.
Stein, L., Watts, D., & Howell, T. (1990). The doctor–nurse game revisited. *New England Journal of Medicine, 322*, 546–549.
Stickley, T., & Freshwater, D. (2006). The art of listening in the therapeutic relationship. *Mental Health Practice, 9*(5), 12–28.
Thomas, M., & Hynes, C. (2007). The darker side of groups. *Journal of Nursing Management, 15*, 375–385.
Valentine, P. E. B. (1995). Management of conflict: Do nurses/women handle it differently? *Journal of Advanced Nursing, 22*(1), 142–149.
Wachs, J. E. (2005). Building the occupational health team: Keys to successful interdisciplinary collaboration. *AAOHN Journal, 53*(4), 166–171.
Wackerhausen, S. (2009). Collaboration, professional identity and reflection across boundaries. *Journal of Interprofessional Care, 23*(5), 455–473.
Wilmot, W. W., & Hocker, J. L. (2001). *Interpersonal conflict* (6th ed.). New York, NY: McGraw-Hill.

Chapter 5
Introduction to Collaboration

A pediatric diabetes team is engaged in a case review prior to the beginning of a busy clinic day. The endocrinologist, social worker, registered dietitian, and diabetes nurse educator are reviewing the clients scheduled for the day.

Debbie (social worker): I just met Melissa T. out in the hall on her way to clinic. She told me she's been thinking about letting her son Dylan participate in the summer camp program for youth with Type I diabetes. I am so pleased; she has been very reluctant to let him gain some independence. I think this is a big step for this family and especially for Dylan.

Joseph (endocrinologist): He's what, eight years old now? Remind me, who manages his blood glucose, diet, and insulin? Is it his mom exclusively or does Dylan play a role too?

Lana (diabetes nurse educator): Dylan just turned nine. His mom has been almost solely managing Dylan's diabetes. She's well organized, meticulous, and very particular about his care. Mary and I have been working with Dylan to help him understand his own care and talking to him about self-management. His mom has been reluctant, but Dylan is really eager to gain some control. He's told me he'd really like to go to camp. I think he's pretty much ready to go. What do you think, Mary?

Mary (registered dietitian): I agree, he's keen, but I don't think he's quite ready to take over his own care. The kids who go to camp need to be pretty independent and fully capable of caring for themselves. There's lots of support, of course, but Dylan's mom hasn't allowed him a lot of autonomy. I don't know that he's quite ready.

Joseph: Dylan's diabetes is pretty well controlled, I'm satisfied with the results of his blood work and his insulin routine. He's generally a pretty healthy active kid ... from my perspective he's a good candidate for the camp. Can we put a plan in place to get him and his mom ready? We have about two months.

Debbie (speaking to Joseph): I think that if you and I focus on supporting Dylan's mother, reassuring her that his diabetes is well under control, answering her questions, and helping her work through her concerns, she might be more agreeable to letting Dylan go.

Lana: Okay then, maybe Mary and I can focus on helping Dylan get ready. We can add a few extra sessions with him to support him to manage his own care. I can review with him his insulin administration and blood glucose monitoring technique and routine.

Mary: Two months, eh? Hmm ... well, it's definitely doable and would be beneficial for both Dylan and his mom. I can review his diet with him and maybe he can come to a few of the group sessions we run for kids, like the Healthy Eating Healthy Play group. He'd have an opportunity to interact with other kids who are veteran campers.

Lana: Great, I'll have a look at the clinic schedule over the next couple of months and see where we can fit in some extra appointments.

Debbie: I'll help Dylan's mother get started on the camp paperwork and other details. This decision is a big step and I anticipate the process may be tough for her. I'll keep an eye out for concerns that arise and may have to call on the team's support as we go forward. I'll let you know. Thanks, everyone.

After working together to support Dylan and his mother, Dylan attended summer camp for the first time. He returned to the clinic in the fall, proudly displaying the first-place ribbon he won in the canoe races.

Learning Outcomes

AFTER STUDYING THIS CHAPTER, YOU SHOULD BE ABLE TO:

1. **Define the concept of collaboration and describe its core elements.**
2. **Discuss the concept of collaboration in the context of practice.**
3. **Identify key barriers to collaboration in practice.**
4. **Apply strategies for successful collaboration within a team-based situation or activity.**

INTRODUCTION

AS DISCUSSED IN CHAPTER 1, COLLABORATION IS AN IMPORTANT ELEMENT OF INTERPROFESSIONAL practice (IPP). The requirement for health care teams to collaborate effectively in order to best serve the needs of patients appears as a foundational element of teamwork in virtually every professional discipline. Understanding how collaboration works, what supports collaboration, and what challenges interprofessional teams may experience in relation to practising collaboratively is essential if we hope to meet successful IPP outcomes, including improved patient care. The above vignette demonstrates a number of facets of the concept of collaboration in IPP. Faced with a complex patient issue, the pediatric diabetes team members interact with each other to clarify the issue and develop a plan to accomplish the goal that the family in the scenario had identified. As part of their planning, the team also makes provision for communication throughout the process. They demonstrate both a good understanding of the various roles within the team and respect for each other as professionals with divergent opinions.

Interprofessional collaboration is not a new concept in health care, having emerged in the literature during the 1970s and grown in prevalence over the past three decades. As early as 1978, the World Health Organization (WHO) identified interdisciplinary collaboration as essential to success with primary health care at a global level. As countries strive to improve both patient outcomes and health care systems, the expectation for collaboration to occur across health disciplines has become a worldwide imperative (Alberto & Herth, 2009). In Canada, this interest in collaborative practice has led to such initiatives as Interprofessional Education for Collaborative Patient-Centred Practice (IECPCP) and the Canadian Interprofessional Health Collaborative (CIHC), sponsored by Health Canada.

The focus of this chapter is to help readers understand the concept of collaboration and integrate it into their practice. It begins with a definition, followed by a review of the many facets of the concept and discussion of its application to practice environments.

DEFINING THE CONCEPT OF COLLABORATION

In this text we define collaboration as a process that requires relationships and interactions between health professionals, regardless of whether they perceive themselves to be part of a team or not. However, it should be noted that there is no universally accepted definition of the concept. There are varying definitions and a variety of ways to describe, explain, and demonstrate collaboration. Table 5.1 provides an overview of some of the

Table 5.1 Definitions of Collaboration

Author(s)	Definition of Collaboration
D'Amour et al. (2005)	"a complex, voluntary and dynamic process that occurs involving several skills" (p. 126).
Lindeke & Sieckert (2005)	"a complex process that requires intentional knowledge sharing and joint responsibility for patient care. Sometimes it occurs within long-term relationships between health professionals. Within long-term relationships, collaboration has a developmental trajectory that evolves over time as team members leave or join the group and/or organization structures change. On other occasions, collaboration between [health care professionals] may involve fleeting encounters in patient arenas" (para. 2).
Mattessich, Murray-Close, & Monsey (2001)	"a mutually beneficial relationship that is well-defined and entered into by more than one organization or individual to achieve mutual goals" (p. 24).
O'Daniel & Rosenstein (2008)	"health care professionals assuming complementary roles and cooperatively working together, sharing responsibility for problem-solving and making decisions to formulate and carry out plans for patient care"

definitions used in health care literature. Notwithstanding the differences, there are common themes to these definitions, including reference to the complexity involved in collaboration and the idea that collaboration has both process and relational components. As you will recall from Chapter 2, the organizing framework allows us to look at health care situations from the perspective of processes, relationships, tasks, and contextual factors. When considering the degree to which collaboration could or should be occurring, we must factor in not only the "how" of collaboration (processes), which we will discuss throughout this chapter, but also the "who" (relationships).

Core Elements of Collaboration

Although definitions of collaboration may vary, from a practical perspective it is helpful to consider what characteristics of the concept are overarching. A review of health care and social science literature reveals nine core elements seen as essential for its success: (a) problem-focused process(es), (b) cooperation, (c) interdependence, (d) shared ownership of goals, (e) action orientation, (f) non-hierarchical relationships, (g) shared accountability and responsibility, (h) communication, and (i) flexibility and adaptability. Each of these characteristics of collaboration is discussed below.

Problem-Focused Process(es) Collaboration is seen as a **problem-focused process(es)** (Canadian Health Services Research Foundation [CHSRF], 2006; Petri, 2010); that is, it involves the members of a team coming together to solve a problem or overcome an issue. There is also the sense that a solution derived through this process will be better, given the collective knowledge and wisdom of the team members, than one developed by any individual alone. Chapter 6 of this text discusses the problem-solving process in greater detail.

Cooperation Collaboration also requires **cooperation**, the action or process of professionals from various disciplines working jointly to achieve a common goal or produce an outcome. Cooperation requires energy and a commitment to working together with a focus on interdependence. It also requires reflecting upon your own professional views and perspectives as a part of the whole rather than as a stand-alone entity (Petri, 2010), "acknowledging and respecting other opinions and viewpoints while maintaining the willingness to change personal beliefs and perspectives" (Hall, 2005, p. 193). This can be difficult, especially if the work is not going well, as individual members of the team may feel that it would be easier to "just do it myself." Cooperation may be eroded by factors such as a lack of trust (Way, Jones, & Busing, 2000), the passing of time, the complexity of the context, the lack of measurable success of the plan, and the changing of patterns of interactions among individuals on the team (Gaboury, Bujold, Boon, & Moher, 2009).

Interdependence **Interdependence** "refers to the occurrence of and reliance on interactions among professionals whereby each is dependent on the other to accomplish his or her goals" (Bronstein, 2003, p. 299). Interdependence is based upon each professional understanding his or her own personal goals, but more importantly, also understanding the goals shared by the collaborating team. Inherent in interdependence is recognition of the value of other professionals' roles and trust in their abilities (Suter, Arndt, Arthur, Parboosingh, Taylor, & Deutschlander, 2009).

To support interdependence, both formal and informal processes develop. Formal processes may include meetings similar to the one depicted in the opening vignette, distribution of written communications, and presentations. Informal processes may include telephone conversations, hallway chats, or sharing ideas through email (Bronstein, 2003). These processes increase time spent together, which fosters an increase in trust in other members of the team and ultimately, interdependence.

Shared Ownership of Goals **Shared ownership of goals** means having mutual responsibility in all aspects of working to meet goals (Bronstein, 2003; CHSRF, 2006). There is an underlying sense of stewardship of the goal, and team members see that the benefits of the collaboration will be focused on the "other" (Axelsson & Axelsson, 2009). To foster a sense of shared ownership of goals when professionals, clients, and their families are involved in collaborative work, it is important to (a) have a clear understanding of the chosen goal, (b) ensure that the goal is external to the team members, (c) frequently check back to see that the team continues to have a mutually shared goal, and (d) ensure that the decisions made, and the plans created, remain true to this goal (Bronstein, 2003).

Action Orientation Collaboration has an action orientation, with a sense of movement toward an outcome. The problem-solving and goal-attainment elements inherent in the definitions of collaboration suggest that it involves a change in the status quo. This change is directed toward quality improvement, and so a key outcome is the creation of a plan for action. Collaboration does not simply involve circular discussion about what is but rather includes plans for what could be.

Non-Hierarchical Relationships Health care has traditionally involved professional relationships that were hierarchical in nature (Hall, 2005). For example, historically physicians have directed nurses' work, managers or team leaders have directed staff members, and administrative personnel have been directed by more senior executives. Collaboration requires a shift to **non-hierarchical relationships**, which are based upon each member having an equal say or equivalent level of power within the team. This involves moving away from control over work by a superior profession to a partnership in which each member's voice carries the same weight and is equally respected by the team (Axelsson & Axelsson, 2009). Each member of a team has a variety of skills, knowledge, and abilities that must be acknowledged as unique, and of equal value and importance. The power within the team must be shared. In non-hierarchical relationships each member is empowered to share his or her knowledge and take an equal role in decision making (Orchard, 2010). This structure implies an underlying respect for each team member and trust in others. It also requires that team members understand their own scope of practice and be prepared to demonstrate leadership and contribute their thoughts and opinions. They must have confidence in themselves and a willingness to speak up.

Shared Accountability and Responsibility One aspect of a non-hierarchical approach within a team is the need to assume shared accountability and responsibility for both the decisions made and the outcome of the work accomplished (Bronstein, 2003; Petri, 2010). In traditional models of health care practice, decision making was discipline-specific, and errors were seen as partly due to the decision maker's lack of skill. An example might be a decision to discharge an elderly woman home. Without the information gathered through a social work or occupational therapy assessment, indicating that the patient would be safe on her own, this decision may have been a poor one; but responsibility would have rested solely with the professional responsible for the discharge. Another stance typical of practice in the past was that the individual wasn't responsible for the outcome of a decision because he or she had just done what he or she was told to do. For example, a nurse might disown responsibility for the outcome of an intervention on the basis that she was just following the doctor's order. When employing a practice approach based in collaboration, team members share accountability for the decisions, the plan of action, and the outcomes (Lindeke & Sieckert, 2005; Way, Jones, & Busing, 2000). In Chapter 9 of this text we discuss this notion of shared accountability and responsibility in more detail.

Communication Another key element of collaboration is communication, which is not surprising given how central communication is to IPP. As discussed in Chapters 3 and 4, communication is a complex phenomenon that requires a specific set of circumstances in order to achieve the desired outcome, be it transmission of information, exchange of ideas, or, as discussed in Chapter 6, negotiation toward resolution of complex challenges. In a true collaboration, team members will undertake open, honest communication. They must be prepared to both agree and disagree in a manner that is clear, professional, and focused on the task at hand. They must understand the terminology and language used within the interactions, and be able to articulate their perspectives and challenge others' perspectives in a way that is not judgmental or personalized. In addition, they must be prepared to listen to feedback objectively and adapt their thinking.

This is easier said than done. Sometimes professionals become entrenched in their way of managing patient care. Routines become established and decisions automatic. For many, the first reaction to a challenge is defensiveness. Imagine a scenario in which an expert clinician is challenged by a novice practitioner in a team meeting about a proposed plan of care. The challenge may come in a less-than-tactful manner ("Are you kidding? That's just wrong") and the clinician may react negatively in a verbal manner that is judgmental ("What, you think you know more than I do?"). Both statements may be open and honest. But the result of this communication is detrimental to the process of collaboration. Skilled, professional communication is essential for success in collaboration (O'Daniel & Rosenstein, 2008; Suter et al., 2009).

Flexibility and Adaptability Given the cooperative, give-and-take nature of collaboration, two related core elements are flexibility and adaptability. During collaboration, team members must be prepared to make concessions in their own thinking and their own plans. Creating opportunities for teams, as a whole, to be together and make decisions requires team members who are prepared to compromise and committed to joint decision making. The defined scope of practice for each of the health-related disciplines describes professional responsibilities that seem to overlap. Collaboration requires team members who know and understand the scope of practice of the other team members as well as their own, and who do not create silos of practice but rather opportunities for collaboration (Bronstein, 2003). A willingness to understand the scope of practice of others, an ability to adapt one's own professional orientation to new contexts, and the flexibility to do so quickly are all essential to collaborative IPP (Bronstein, 2003; Hall, 2005).

Now that we have gained a better understanding of the key features that constitute collaboration within IPP, let us return to the opening vignette involving the pediatric diabetes team. This situation allows us to consider in greater depth how the members of an interprofessional team can exemplify collaborative IPP. In this scenario, the team is faced with the challenge of supporting a reluctant mom in her decision to send her son Dylan to the summer camp program for youth with Type I diabetes in a relatively short period of time. Accomplishing this goal requires collaboration to ensure that both Dylan and his mother are ready to experience success with this initiative. The team cooperates with the patient and his family, partnering with them to develop a plan. Team members are all busy and have had individual professional goals for Dylan, but join forces to work toward this shared goal. Their collaborative work is action-oriented; they spend a minimal amount of time focusing on where Dylan and his mom are currently in this journey, electing instead to focus on where they need to be when camp begins. Each team member expresses his or her opinion openly and professionally. These opinions differ at the outset of the discussion. When the registered dietitian expresses her opinion that Dylan is not ready for this type of venture, they discuss options and put in place a plan to move him toward readiness. This plan involves cooperation and coordination between the registered dietitian and the nurse. They both commit to reworking their scheduled visits in order to accommodate Dylan's learning needs. The team relies upon the expertise of the social worker to manage mom's preparation. They also rely on the physician to monitor the medical management of Dylan's diabetes. Each team member shares the accountability for his or her role in the plan and they all also share in the success of achieving the joint goal.

Indicators of Effective Collaboration

It is important to consider what kind of indicators we can examine to determine if effective collaborative team practice is occurring. One feature to look for is the level of respect demonstrated among team members (San Martin-Rodriguez, Beaulieu, D'Amour,

& Ferrada-Videla, 2005). Teams that are collaborating effectively demonstrate increased respect among members (CHSRF, 2006). Another indicator of collaboration is a clarity of roles within the team (San Martin-Rodriguez et al., 2005); that is, members demonstrate an understanding of their own role and that of others (CHSRF). Effective management of conflict also indicates a high level of collaboration (San Martin-Rodriguez et al., 2005). Additionally, there is a collective desire to meet the needs of patients by working together, and collectively take accountability for the plan as well as the outcomes (CHSRF).

COLLABORATION IN PRACTICE

How does the theoretical information discussed in the above section translate into the everyday work of health care? As with many concepts, successful collaboration can be envisioned on a continuum. Many teams, such as the one in the opening vignette, function at a very high level of collaboration. Others struggle and may be less successful, but manage to establish and maintain a quasi-collaborative way of practice that adequately meets the needs of the patient and satisfies the team. Finally, some teams function with very few indicators of effective collaboration; patient care occurs within a hierarchical structure in which interaction between members is minimal.

Imagine that the relationships in the team of the opening vignette were hierarchical, with little collaboration happening. How might the meeting depicted be different? It is likely that the interaction would be minimal. There might be a dominant team member with decision-making authority who sets the agenda. In such a situation, other members might provide reports on their activities, but their opinions would be neither sought nor shared. The dominant member would determine the plan of care for Dylan, and each member would carry out his or her assigned responsibility. Although the desired result of sending Dylan to camp might be realized, team members may come away frustrated with the process and feeling as though things were beyond their control.

The complex nature of health care means that there will be variations in the level of success of collaborative efforts. Health care issues and team memberships change. As well, even when they appear to be facing the same circumstances, patients have individual needs and desires related to their care. For successful collaboration, health care professionals need to be aware of the intricacies of IPP and continuously develop their collaboration skills. In addition, each experience of collaboration, positive or negative, should provide an opportunity to critically reflect upon the core elements and outcomes in the situation. This reflective process promotes individual and team learning. Collaborative skills may also be developed through formalized educational and practice-based programs and other opportunities. Learning collaborative skills is a key aspect of interprofessional education (IPE) initiatives (see Chapter 8). Spotlight 5.1 provides an example of an effective program focusing on collaboration for professionals in practice.

Spotlight 5.1

Effective Collaboration in Action: Palliative Care and Collaborative Practice Mentorship Program

Purpose of the Program

- To build collaborative relationships between interprofessional primary health care teams and experts in palliative care
- To increase palliative care knowledge among the primary care providers
- To improve symptom management for patients (pain, nausea, etc.)
- To improve patient and family satisfaction with palliative care

Participants

- A mentor dyad (palliative care physician and palliative care advanced practice nurse) and a mentee dyad (nurse practitioner and family practice physician)

Program

- Mentor pairs are drawn from universities with palliative care expertise and are provided with a one-day workshop addressing the concepts of collaborative practice and mentoring.
- Mentees are provided with a two-day workshop using the Learning Essential Approaches for Palliative and End of Life Care (LEAP) and an extra 2.5-hour collaborative practice module.
- Mentor-mentee pairs then have a minimum of eight weeks of interactions including videoconferences, shadowing opportunities, or modalities of choice.

Evaluation

- Key results include (a) increased knowledge related to palliative care, (b) improvements in collaborative efforts, and (3) increased confidence in areas such as communication, collaboration, assisting, supporting, and providing guidance to patients and families with issues related to end-of-life experiences (Cancer Care Ontario, 2012).

For more information visit www.cancercare.on.ca.

CHALLENGES TO EFFECTIVE COLLABORATION

Given the complex and chaotic nature of work environments in health care, the development of collaboration within a team can take time. Teams may also be faced with a number of barriers, some of which will be specific to their practice environments and contexts. Practitioners and teams that take a proactive stance toward the development of effective collaboration position themselves for success. To this end, it may be advantageous for teams to anticipate, consider, and brainstorm solutions to barriers that they may encounter as they work toward collaboration. A small team project can provide an opportunity to examine issues and barriers, and positive reinforcement for the team's efforts.

Common Barriers to Effective Collaboration

As a learner or professional involved in IPP, it is important to understand the possible challenges that will impact your ability and that of others to engage in collaboration. Gaining knowledge of these potential issues and challenges is a first step toward overcoming them and strengthening collaboration. Within the literature, several barriers to successful collaboration related to professional perspectives, practice approaches, the practice environment, and the context of the situation have been identified:

- *Professional climate*. A very traditional hierarchy within an organization or a health care culture steeped in isolated ways (silos) of practice can make true collaborations more difficult. The "rules" within an organization can also lead to patterns of behaviour that support *monodisciplinary* decision making (Elissen, van Raak, & Paulus, 2011).
- *Territorial professional stance*. Historically, socialization within professional schools has been monodisciplinary in nature. Although IPE is being integrated into professional education, "silo making" persists (Orchard, 2010). As a result, health care professionals might not look to other professionals and might take a stance that prevents them from collaborating to resolve shared problems.
- *Loss of focus*. This occurs when professionals or their interests, rather than the patient, become the focus of practice activities. In situations in which collaboration is established for the wrong reasons, outcomes tend to be negative (Axelsson & Axelsson, 2009).
- *Poor communication skills*. Quality improvement and risk management literature is clear on the fact that many adverse events have poor communication as one of the key causative factors (O'Daniel & Rosenstein, 2009; Suter et al., 2009). It may also lead to misunderstandings, negative emotions, and interpersonal conflicts.
- *Time*. Health care environments are chaotic, and often there appears to be little or no time to focus on activities other than direct patient care. Collaboration takes more time; for example, shared decision making requires more time than reaching a decision independently.

Table 5.2 outlines strategies that might be implemented by IPP teams and individual members to overcome these barriers.

Table 5.2 Strategies to Overcome Barriers to Effective Collaboration

Barrier	Strategies to Overcome It
Professional climate	■ When possible and appropriate, include representation from various levels within the organization in collaborative efforts. Avoid discouraging the participation of others because you question their added value to the initiative. ■ Plan for small steps and small wins; begin with a core team and add members as the successes increase. ■ Be open and receptive to listening to feedback, and involve the biggest naysayers—those who overtly question the value of the collaboration. ■ Celebrate and share successes; provide praise and encouragement.

Table 5.2 Strategies to Overcome Barriers to Effective Collaboration (*Continued*)	
Barrier	**Strategies to Overcome It**
Territorial professional stance	■ Don't allow the members to fall into individualized professional stances. ■ Enter into collaboration with a stance of "un-knowing" (Bronstein, 2003). ■ Demonstrate a thirst for knowledge in the way you ask questions and how you approach learning. ■ Consciously give yourself and others encouragement and praise. Review successes, clarify goals, and consider the addition of resources. ■ Practise effective conflict management (see Chapter 6). ■ Take the time to recognize similarities and differences and give consideration to who is the best person to "do the work" in a given situation and time.
Loss of focus	■ Involve the patient in collaborative efforts whenever possible. ■ Ensure that patient care goals are external to the team. ■ Continuously review and revise goals and assess whether the collaboration is effective and meeting the intended purpose.
Poor communication skills	■ Listen when others speak rather than focusing on how you will respond. Seek as much clarification as possible in order to understand what is being communicated. ■ Approach concerns regarding the tone or intention of communication using a conflict management approach. Consider giving others the benefit of the doubt and ask for clarification if you don't understand. ■ Take a deep breath and avoid reacting immediately to communication that you may find unsettling. Take some time to consider how best to respond. ■ Ensure your communication conveys respect, particularly when offering constructive feedback. ■ Do not selectively share opinions with different people in order to gain support for your own perspective.
Time	■ Recognize the workloads of those on your team. ■ Properly resource the team to promote effective use of time. ■ Offline discussions should be avoided. If they are necessary, relevant details should be reported back to the team. ■ Ensure that meeting and team activities are the focus by developing clear agendas and timelines.

OPPORTUNITIES FOR SUCCESS

It would be very helpful if all collaborations began with the elements, skills, and circumstances necessary for their success. It would also be beneficial if we could hand-pick our collaborators on the basis of their level of competence in collaboration. The reality of many practice environments is that they are not ideally suited to collaboration. Therefore, it is important for health professionals to actively cultivate environments that facilitate successful and effective collaboration. Table 5.3 outlines some relevant strategies to this end.

Table 5.3 Strategies for Successful Collaboration

Strategy	Description
Up-front preparation	■ Mentally prepare yourself for collaboration by deciding at the outset that you are prepared to fully participate. ■ Have a compelling reason to collaborate. The more you are invested in the process, the more likely you are to work to ensure that it is successful. ■ Imagine potential barriers and think through possible solutions or responses.
Set the stage	■ Support democratic processes that give consideration to all members when planning the activities involved in collaboration (e.g., when setting meeting times). ■ Establish norms and assumptions that will underpin collaboration such as a commitment to engaging in ways that reflect an egalitarian power structure. These norms and assumptions are most effective if they are documented and shared with others. ■ Understand your own role and consider your own strengths and weaknesses. Enter into collaboration prepared to learn and to support the learning of others. ■ Agree on guiding principles for interactions, then hold yourself and other members accountable to them. ■ Have a clear understanding of the goals of collaboration and ensure that others have the same level of clarity. Keep goals focused on the needs of the patient; however, be mindful of the secondary gains for those involved in the collaboration. ■ Foster trust for yourself and others. For example, follow through on tasks you agree to complete, maintain confidentiality, and support any decision agreed upon.
Plan for action	■ Clarify who is taking an action forward, such as identifying who will follow up on test results or interview the family member of a patient. ■ Decide on the structure of communication, how success and outcomes of the collaboration will be measured, what approaches will be used to address conflict, and when the collaborative effort will terminate.
Evaluation	■ Engage in formative and summative evaluation of the collaborative effort and the intended purpose (see Chapter 10). ■ Debrief the findings of the evaluation, celebrating the positive results and reflecting upon where improvements are needed on the basis of the findings. ■ Engage in reflection at both the individual and the team levels. Individual reflection is a powerful tool, and team reflection, although it takes more effort, may provide even greater insight. ■ Discuss what learning has taken place during the process, both team learning and individual learning.

It is worth noting that these strategies are not intended solely for either the designated or the informal leaders within the practice environment. Rather, they are strategies that should be considered by all professionals engaged in IPP. Healthy collaboration involves participation by all members of the team (Bronstein, 2003). Any member can and should take a leadership role when he or she is the most appropriate expert or has the most knowledge of the issue under consideration (see Chapter 7 for a detailed discussion of leadership for IPP).

BUILDING FOR SUSTAINABILITY

A collaborative culture cannot be built overnight. However, a series of small collaborations resulting in quick gains (e.g., a small project that can be accomplished with relative ease and minimal effort by the team but that has positive results) can help begin the process. Persistence and perseverance by those involved in IPP at all levels will go a long way to germinating interprofessional collaboration within an organization. Being inclusive and inviting participation serves as a method of succession planning. People involved in successful collaborations are more likely to want to continue interacting in this manner.

One of the challenges faced by organizations, even those that have traditionally practised in a collaborative manner, is the ability to sustain not only individual but also organization-level collaborations. As members involved come and go, changes to the mix of personalities and skills within a team and/or organization can impact interactive processes or derail the work altogether. For example, collaborative teams that rely on one strong leader may be destabilized when that leader moves on. It is important that the members of the team be vigilant against possible threats to sustainability.

One strategy to promote the sustainability of collaboration in IPP is to "take the pulse" of the team on a periodic basis, using activities such as a "check-in." In this way, the team creates an opportunity for members to raise issues within or related to the team, revisit the goals or vision for the work, and use the desired outcomes as touchstones for continuing the collaboration and reaffirming commitments. Helpful Tools 5.1 provides an example of such an exercise. The notion of a check-in can be broadened to the level of the organization as part of the overall evaluation of IPP implementation (see Chapter 10).

Another strategy is to elicit the feedback of an objective outsider, asking that person to describe what he or she observes and to interpret the team's or the organization's goal(s), the work already under way, the role of the team members, and the successes that have been achieved. Within an organization, the outside-observer role might be formalized through the use of an external consultant hired to review the organization or a specific project. Informally, within IPP teams, colleagues external to the team or even sometimes a student involved in a health care learning experience might fulfill this role. For example, imagine that the pediatric diabetes team in the opening vignette includes an early childhood education (ECE) student member who has completed an IPP course in her program of study. That person might share her knowledge about collaborative teams and provide informal feedback based on her observations of the team's collaborative efforts.

Helpful Tools 5.1

Be a Collaborator: Behaviour Checklist

- Helps the team establish long-term goals and clarify current objectives or tasks
- Helps the team see how their work fits with the entire organization
- Encourages the team to set shared goals
- Regularly reminds the team of the need to revisit their goals and action plan
- Pitches in to help out other team members who need assistance
- Works hard to achieve team goals and to complete the current tasks even though he/she may not agree with them
- Demonstrates respect for team members by listening attentively to their opinions
- Gives his/her opinion in a professional, clear and concise manner, whether it matches with the general consensus or not
- Considers other points of view and alters practice when appropriate

Source: Excerpt "Collaborator: A Checklist of Behaviors" from *Team Players and Teamwork: New strategies for developing successful collaboration* by Parker, G.M. Published by John Wiley & Sons, © 2007.

If collaboration is to be sustained, it must be adequately supported. Professionals in leadership roles should consider providing adequate resources to support collaborative efforts within an organization. Often a new project begins with resources and enthusiasm and as time passes and new projects are on the horizon, older work gets overlooked and under-resourced. As noted earlier in this chapter, collaboration, in contrast to independent work, takes time, is more labour-intensive, and requires ongoing support. However, the investment is well worth the effort. Collaborative practice in interprofessional teams supports positive outcomes for patients, such as improved quality of care and patient satisfaction, and increased satisfaction and feelings of well-being for providers (D'Amour & Oandasan, 2005).

Health care is practised by a wide variety of professionals in a multitude of dynamic, ever-changing contexts. To develop and sustain collaboration among the varied professionals within such a system requires strategies that can handle such an environment. One important strategy is to develop tools to foster professional growth and support collaboration, such as frameworks, project plans, and guidelines. These provide a template or starting point, and also incorporate the evidence upon which new processes are built and provide a measuring stick for success.

One such evidence-informed tool is outlined in Helpful Tools 5.2. The Registered Nurses' Association of Ontario Best Practice Guideline (BPG) entitled *Collaborative Practice Among Nursing Teams* (2006) has many recommendations for individuals, the organization, and the system to consider in building and sustaining a collaborative and healthy work environment. Although this BPG is written with nurses in mind, many of the core elements are transferrable to other health care professions.

Helpful Tools 5.2

RNAO Health Work Environments Best Practices

The *RNAO Best Practice Guideline* provides recommendations organized into individual/team, organizational, and external/systems.

Example: Individual/Team Recommendation

1.1 Nurses develop knowledge about values and behaviours that support teamwork and the impact of teamwork on patient/client safety and patient/client outcomes. As such nurses:

- Inform themselves about the attributes of supportive teams
- Articulate their belief in the value of teamwork
- Demonstrate their willingness to work effectively with others

Example: Organizational Recommendation

2.3 Organizations support systems and processes that promote team functioning and continuity of patient/client care.

Example: External/System Recommendation

5.1 Accreditation bodies of health services organizations include evidence-based standards and criteria on effective teamwork as part of their standards.

Source: Excerpt from "RNAO Best Practice Guideline" from *Collaborative practice among nursing teams.* Published by Registered Nurses' Association of Ontario, © 2006.

CONCLUSION

Collaboration is increasingly being recognized as a core element of IPP. It is important that health care professionals understand how it works, what supports it, and what challenges interprofessional teams may experience in relation to practising collaboratively. The role effective collaboration plays in positive patient outcomes raises the urgency of developing teams that practise in a collaborative manner.

SUMMARY

- Collaboration is a process that requires relationships and interactions between health professionals, regardless of whether they perceive themselves to be part of a team or not.
- The core elements of collaboration are (a) problem-focused process(es), (b) cooperation, (c) interdependence, (d) shared ownership of goals, (e) action orientation, (f) non-hierarchical relationships, (g) shared accountability and responsibility, (h) communication, and (i) flexibility and adaptability.

- Challenges to collaboration include hierarchical environments, a territorial professional stance, poor communication skills, time, and loss of focus.
- The responsibility for supporting collaboration in health care rests with each individual practitioner, not only those in formal leadership roles. Additionally, for collaboration to be successful at the level of direct practice, it must also exist and be supported throughout the various levels of an organization.
- Collaboration does not occur overnight, but rather requires continuous effort. However, the benefits of developing and sustaining collaboration within and between health care teams far outweigh any challenges.

Key Terms

cooperation
interdependence
non-hierarchical relationships
problem-focused process(es)
shared ownership of goals

Review Questions

1. Describe the core elements of collaboration.
2. Identify two of the key barriers to success for collaborative work. What strategies might overcome these barriers?
3. What kinds of strategies can be put in place at the level of the (a) individual team member, (b) team, and (c) organization to enhance the potential for successful collaboration in IPP teams?

Application Exercises

1. At your next team or group meeting, observe the actions, behaviours, and outcomes related to the gathering. Consider the following questions in the light of your own contributions and those of other members:
   - Do I see evidence that members understand their own and others' roles and responsibilities on this team?
   - How would I answer if I were asked: What is the goal of working together on this team? Do the goals support patient-centred care? Are any of the goals professional-centred?
   - Can I recognize any or all of the elements of collaboration in this work? Could it be described as collaboration? If so, why? If not, why not?
   - What, if any, are the barriers to collaboration in the team? What strategies might I (or the team) initiate to improve collaboration?

Additional Resources

Websites and Electronic Documents

RNOA Best Practice Guideline: Collaborative Practice Among Nursing Teams
www.rnao.org

Exemplary Care: Registered Nurses and Licensed Practical Nurses Working Together, Association of Registered Nurses of Prince Edward Island
http://www.arnpei.ca/images/pdf/RNsandLPNsWorkingTogether.pdf

Nova Scotia's New Collaborative Care Model
www.gov.ns.ca/health/MOCINS

Nursing in Collaborative Environments, Registered Psychiatric Nurses Association of Saskatchewan, Saskatchewan Association of Licensed Practical Nurses and Saskatchewan Registered Nurses Association
http://www.health.gov.sk.ca/nursing-collaborative-environments

Working Together: A Framework for the Registered Nurse and Licensed Practical Nurse, Nurses Association of New Brunswick
http://www.nanb.nb.ca/PDF/Working_Together_Final.pdf

References

Alberto, J., Herth, K. (2009). Interprofessional collaboration within faculty roles: Teaching, service, and research. *Online Journal of Issues in Nursing, 14*(2).

Axelsson, S. B., & Axelsson, R. (2009). From territoriality to altruism in interprofessional collaboration and leadership. *Journal of Interprofessional Care, 23*(4), 320–330.

Bronstein, L. (2003). A model for interdisciplinary collaboration. *Social Work, 48*(3), 297–306.

Canadian Health Services Research Foundation (CHSRF). (2006). *Teamwork in healthcare: Promoting effective teamwork in healthcare in Canada*. Ottawa, ON: Author.

Cancer Care Ontario. (2012). *Palliative care and collaborative practice mentorship program*. Retrieved from https://www.cancercare.on.ca/about/programs/otherinitiatives/palcare

D'Amour, D., Ferrada-Videla, M., San Martin-Rodriguez, L. S., & Beaulieu, M. D. (2005). The conceptual basis for interprofessional collaboration: Core concepts and theoretical frameworks. *Journal of Interprofessional Care, 19*(S1), 116–131.

D'Amour, D., & Oandasan, I. (2005). Interprofessionality as the field of interprofessional practice and interprofessional education: An emerging concept. *Journal of Interprofessional Care, 19*(S1), 8–10.

Elissen, A. M. J., van Raak, A. J. A., & Paulus, A. T. G. (2011). Can we make sense of multidisciplinary co-operation in primary care by considering routines and rules? *Health and Social Care in the Community, 19*(1), 33–42.

Gaboury, I., Bujold, M., Boon, H., & Moher, D. (2009). Interprofessional collaboration within Canadian integrative healthcare clinics: Key components. *Social Science & Medicine, 69*, 707–715.

Hall, P. (2005). Interprofessional teamwork: Professional cultures as barriers. *Journal of Interprofessional Care, 19*(S1), 188–196.

Lindeke, L. L., & Sieckert, A. M. (2005). Nurse–physician workplace collaboration. *Online Journal of Issues in Nursing, 10*(1), Retrieved from http://www.nursingworld.org/MainMenuCategories/ANAMarketplace/ANAPeriodicals/OJIN/TableofContents/Volume102005/No1Jan05/tpc26_416011.html

Mattessich, P. W., Murray-Close, M., & Monsey, B. R. (2001). *Collaboration: What makes it work?* (2nd ed.). Saint Paul, MN: Amherst H. Wilder Foundation.

O'Daniel, M., & Rosenstein, A. H. (2008). Chapter 33. Professional communication and team collaboration. In R. G. Hughes (Ed.), *Patient safety and quality: A handbook for nurses*. Retrieved from http://www.ahrq.gov/qual/nurseshdbk/docs/O'DanielM_TWC.pdf

Orchard, C. A. (2010). Persistent isolationist or collaborator? The nurse's role in interprofessional collaborative practice. *Journal of Nursing Management, 18*, 248–257.

Parker, G. M. (2007). *Team players and teamwork: New strategies for developing successful collaboration*. San Francisco, CA: Jossey-Bass.

Petri, L. (2010). Concept analysis of interdisciplinary collaboration. *Nursing Forum, 45*(2), 73–82.

Registered Nurses' Association of Ontario (RNAO). (2006). *Collaborative practice among nursing teams*. Toronto: Author.

San Martin-Rodriguez, L., Beaulieu, M. D., D'Amour, D., & Ferrada-Videla, M. (2005). The determinants of successful collaboration: A review of theoretical and empirical studies. *Journal of Interprofessional Care, 19*(S1), 132–147.

Suter, E., Arndt, J., Arthur, N., Parboosingh, J., Taylor, E., & Deutschlander, S. (2009). Role understanding and effective communication as core competencies for collaborative practice. *Journal of Interprofessional Care 23*(1), 41–51.

Way, D., Jones, L., & Busing, N. (2000). *Implementation strategies: Collaboration in primary care—family doctors & nurse practitioners delivering shared care*. Discussion paper written for Ontario College of Family Physicians. Retrieved from http://www.eicp.ca/en/toolkit/hhr/ocfp-paper-handout.pdf

World Health Organization (WHO). (1978). Declaration of Alma-Ata. Retrieved from http://www.euro.who.int/__data/assets/pdf_file/0003/98301/E68395.pdf

Chapter 6

Problem Solving, Conflict Resolution, and Negotiation

Mrs. Wang is a 69-year-old Chinese female who lives independently in a highrise condominium apartment. She is an active member of her community and volunteers with other seniors and young children. Mrs. Wang has a history of depression with psychosis that was first diagnosed shortly after she immigrated to North America 20 years ago. With the help and support of a team of health care professionals, Mrs. Wang has been able to maintain good health and has had very few hospitalizations in the past. However, since recently being diagnosed with Type II diabetes, Mrs. Wang has been hospitalized on several occasions for exacerbations of depression and poor blood sugar control. Three days ago, she was found semiconscious in her home by her daughter, Man Yee. After being treated for her diabetic emergency and stabilized, Mrs. Wang is now currently admitted to the psychiatric unit of her local hospital.

The interprofessional team caring for Mrs. Wang is concerned about her recent pattern of admissions and suggests that there may be a need to explore any underlying problems.

INITIAL PATIENT INTERVIEW

As a first step to uncovering the problem, a meeting is arranged between Mrs. Wang; her daughter, Man Yee; her primary nurse, Phil; and her inpatient psychiatrist, Dr. Bali. After introductions and an opportunity to get (re)acquainted, Phil asks Mrs. Wang to share her understanding of what has been happening and the circumstances that led to her admission. Mrs. Wang provides a detailed description of her activities post-discharge from her previous admission. She reports she stopped taking her insulin injections because she felt they were affecting her chi. Asked to clarify, Man Yee explains that *chi* is the flow of energy in a person's body and that her mother believes her insulin injections, in combination with the other medication she is taking (Glyburide, Olanzapine, and Benztropine), reduces her energy to the point where she cannot participate in the activities about which she cares. Mrs. Wang emphatically agrees with her daughter's explanation of the situation.

During the interview, Dr. Bali assesses Mrs. Wang's judgment and finds no issues. Mrs. Wang also does not report any changes in her own mental status or any symptoms of either depression or psychosis. Before the meeting ends, she expresses a wish for the team to help her to feel better and get her energy back.

Team Meeting #1

Later the same day, the interprofessional team members involved in Mrs. Wang's care meet to discuss her situation. The team's agenda for the meeting is to identify the issues involved in Mrs. Wang's situation and clarify the problem. The team would also like to generate possible solutions to the problem. Dr. Bali and Phil begin by presenting the information they gathered from their interview with Mrs. Wang and her daughter. During discussion, Cora, a medical resident working with Dr. Bali, proposes that Mrs. Wang's noncompliance may be due to her psychiatric diagnosis and symptoms she is experiencing. She adds that it is not uncommon for patients to misrepresent their experiences out of fear that they will be kept in hospital under provincial mental health legislation. Phil responds strongly to Cora's hypothesis and challenges her interpretation of the problem in this situation. Phil asserts that there is no evidence to suggest that Mrs. Wang is not competent and indicates his discomfort with the label "noncompliant." Sensing tension and disagreement here, Dr. Bali quickly interjects and changes the topic. He suggests that the team continue to gather information about Mrs. Wang's situation. The team spends the remainder of their meeting revisiting their decision making about Mrs. Wang's medication regimen only. They also identify tasks for each member to follow up on and report back to the team at the next meeting.

Team Meeting #2

At the next team meeting, individual members share the information they have gathered. Together, they identify what the problems are in Mrs. Wang's situation and articulate that their goal is to identify possible interventions that will stabilize Mrs. Wang's blood glucose, without significantly compromising or impinging upon her energy level and ability to function. They also plan next steps, which include sharing their perceptions of the problem with Mrs. Wang and collaborating with her in the development of a plan to meet her health needs.

Learning Outcomes

AFTER STUDYING THIS CHAPTER, YOU SHOULD BE ABLE TO:

1. **Define problem solving and describe various models for this fundamental group process.**
2. **Summarize the phases involved in the problem-solving process.**
3. **Discuss conflict resolution within the context of problem solving in IPP.**
4. **Describe the benefits of negotiation a problem-solving tool.**

INTRODUCTION

AS THE ABOVE VIGNETTE ILLUSTRATES, MEMBERS OF INTERPROFESSIONAL TEAMS ENGAGE IN the process of problem solving on a regular basis. McClam and Woodside (1994) comment on the central and vital nature of problem solving in health care environments. They note that all human living essentially is a series of problems, and members of the "helping" professions are ultimately in the business of problem solving.

The most common problems encountered by interprofessional health care teams involve patients and their reasons for seeking care (e.g., health care dilemmas, life situations, lack of resources). Other problems encountered may directly involve the interprofessional team, such as conflicts and workload issues. While problem solving and other related processes in health care, such as decision making and negotiation, can and do occur at the individual level, they are often better addressed in an interprofessional team context. In most situations, an interprofessional team brings to these processes multiple skills, differing viewpoints, and varied knowledge that results in more creative and better solutions.

The ability to effectively resolve problems and the approaches used to resolve them can vary greatly from individual to individual and team to team. Some individuals may simply be more adept at solving problems than others. In general, effective problem solving comes by way of learning and through the application of what we learn.

Within the literature, there is considerable support for the use of systematic, structured approaches to problem solving. Wildman and Warner (2003) stress that while we all engage in problem solving in the course of our work lives, we often do so without structure and full understanding of the processes involved. Yet we use these processes to make vital decisions and generate solutions that have an impact on patients, ourselves, and the broader organizational systems in which we work. In health care environments, spontaneous and/or random approaches to problem solving, with little skill or thought, may lead to negative health outcomes and put patients and even care providers at risk. The use of systematic approaches/strategies for problem solving offers the most effective way for interprofessional teams to address problems and find solutions.

Our goal in this chapter is to help you begin to develop a systematic approach toward problem solving and engage in other, related processes as members of interprofessional teams. To that end, we will begin with a discussion of problem solving and examine different aspects of it. We then examine problem solving in the context of conflict and conflict resolution, considering how negotiation can facilitate the process. On the way, we will reflect on Mrs. Wang's situation, while we present tools and ideas to help you to think critically about these ideas and practise your problem solving skills. The organizing framework, presented in Chapter 2, will be used as an example to highlight how a structured approach to problem solving may be applied. While problem solving itself is a process, the focus of a problem that the interprofessional team encounters may be related to a process, a relationship, a task, or contextual factors.

PROBLEM SOLVING

Problem solving is defined as the invention of an alternative solution to a problem that is different from any existing solution (Adams & Galanes, 2006; Frey, 1997; Maier, 1958). It is a structured and complex process consisting of a set of activities designed to analyze a problem systematically and generate, implement, and evaluate solution(s). The process of problem solving is common to both work and non-work environments (Robertson, 2001). At all levels within a health care system, individuals and teams will invariably experience varied work-related problems. These problems may range from minor issues, such as why a patient's intravenous infusion pump is sounding an alarm, to more significant issues, such as are described in the opening vignette.

Whether a problem is minor or major, Wildman and Warner (2003) emphasize the importance of professionals, individually and as part of interprofessional teams, developing competence in solving problems. Problem-solving competence involves the ability "to identify and understand the type of problem, issue, or challenge that [teams and individuals] face, decide on an appropriate strategy or process to help solve it, and be able to apply the chosen process efficiently and effectively" (Wildman & Warner, 2003, p. 1). In this section, we introduce knowledge and tools to assist in the development of problem-solving competency within the context of interprofessional practice (IPP).

Patients and Problem Solving

As we have noted, interprofessional teams are centrally involved in collaborating with patients to find solutions to their health-related problems. Patients seek help from health care professionals because they encounter problems they cannot solve alone and/or do not have the resources to solve. Patients' problems may be emotionally, psychologically, physiologically, or interpersonally/socially related and, not uncommonly, may include several of these components. Patients may also experience problems either directly or indirectly. For example, in the opening vignette, Mrs. Wang's daughter is indirectly being affected by her mother's problem.

Problem solving with patients requires the interprofessional team to establish and build a therapeutic relationship with the patient. Interprofessional team members must demonstrate respect for patients by getting to know them and their situation and by demonstrating a valuing of their perspectives as legitimate and important.

Throughout the problem-solving process, mutual learning and respect are essential elements of the collaborative effort between the interprofessional team and the patient (McClam & Woodside, 1994). It is important for interprofessional teams to keep in mind that although patients may seek help to problem-solve, their level of motivation with respect to problem solving may range from highly motivated to resistant. Patients are experts in their own health experience and their problems. They may, however, lack a clear understanding of the problem-solving process and the skills and resources to find effective solutions to their problems. Similarly, interprofessional teams are often experts in problem solving, but may lack knowledge about the patients they are seeking to help. Therefore, if the process is to be effective, both parties must work to establish a relationship that involves teaching/learning, genuine respect, and a willingness to collaborate.

The Problem-Solving Process

Many models have been proposed that outline the steps of the problem-solving process (see Table 6.1). Features common to these models are:

- problem solving is seen as a learned process,
- problem solving consists of identifiable stages understood to be directional in some way,
- it is acknowledged that problem solving is not always a linear process,

Table 6.1 Problem-Solving Models

Model	Steps
Austin, Kopp, and Smith (1986)	1. Clarify the problem and obtain information.
	2. Set goals.
	3. Generate alternative solutions.
	4. Plan and organize for action.
	5. Evaluate progress.
	6. Follow up on action.
Egan (1990)	1. Explore and clarify the problem.
	2. Set goals.
	3. Develop and execute strategies.
Mandell and Schram (1985)	1. Gather data.
	2. Identify the problem.
	3. Plan.
	4. Implement.
	5. Evaluate.
Levi (2001)	1. Recognize and define the problem.
	2. Analyze problem.
	3. Generate alternative solutions.
	4. Choose from solutions.
	5. Implement solution(s).
	6. Evaluate outcomes of implementation.

- although the number of stages varies, all models identify a problem situation, seek to resolve it, develop potential solutions, and judge those solutions,
- the stages of problem solving may overlap and do not always occur discretely, and
- a relationship between problem solving and decision making exists.

It is important to stress that problem solving and decision making are distinct but related processes. The two are all too commonly equated, resulting in failure to fully discover possible solutions prior to determining the most appropriate course of action. **Decision making** is defined as the selection of an alternative from an existing set of options when no externally correct alternatives exist (Myers & Anderson, 2008). We might think of decision making as the mechanism(s) that individuals and teams use to make choices and judgments. Problem solving and decision making are related in that decision making is a part of the problem-solving process. In the course of solving a problem, decision making can occur at different points, called *decision points*.

Over time, interprofessional teams develop their own unique strategies for problem solving. Which strategy is used is influenced by factors such as the team's development, other team processes (e.g., norms and communication), and the organizational system in which the team in situated. However, there is clear consensus that health care teams should adopt structured and consistent methods to resolve problems (e.g., Elwyn, Koppel, Greenhalgh, & Macfarlane, 2001; Forsyth, 2006; Thompson, 2004). Levi (2001) summarizes the value of using a problem-solving model, noting that it optimizes a team's ability to make good decisions and generate solutions to problems.

Table 6.1 identifies the steps of a variety of models/approaches that interprofessional teams might use. It is easy to identify common elements in the models. The value of these structured approaches depends on factors such as the development of the team, context, other team processes, and the type of problem encountered (Levi, 2001). Structured models/approaches are generally more useful in addressing complex and unstructured problems (VanGundy, 1981).

In this text, we present a model of problem solving described by McClam and Woodside (1994). It organizes the process into three phases: problem identification, decision making, and problem resolution. This model offers a number of advantages for interprofessional teams: (a) it is comprehensive and incorporates key concepts related to problem solving found within the literature; (b) it is intended for professionals working in the human services; (c) it reflects principles of an interprofessional approach; and (d) it is patient-centred.

This model is also highly consistent with the PRT framework described in Chapter 2. As a reminder, the **process dimension** of the organizing framework describes the "how" of engaging in IPP, including such elements as (a) actions, (b) progression or change over time, and (c) outcomes or results. Processes are dynamic and often multidimensional. The **relationship dimension** includes variables related to the interpersonal realm of health care practice—the "who" of the IPP process. It also includes elements associated with the relationships that exist, such as communication styles, methods, and approaches;

leadership and membership styles; and relational dynamics and conflict. This dimension often poses the greatest challenge for professionals engaging in IPP. The **task dimension** is the "what" of the IPP approach. Variables found within this dimension include actions, behaviours, and desired outcomes. It is often within this dimension that the goals for patient care become illuminated. The three core dimensions (process, relationship, and task) share a reciprocal relationship with a number of **contextual factors**, unique to each situation or problem (for an overview, please refer to Chapter 2, Figure 2.2). Clearly determining along which dimension a problem exists allows an interprofessional team (or individual health care provider) to be more cognizant of the kinds of subtle elements that may be impacting a situation.

Returning to McClam and Woodside's (1994) model of problem solving, the three phases provide users with a method for working through relatively simple to highly complex situations. The first phase, *problem identification*, consists of collaboration between those involved in the problem, gaining an understanding of expectations, and identifying the problem. *Decision making*, the second phase, consists of selecting goals, generating alternatives/options, and making decisions. *Problem resolution*, the third and last phase, involves the activities of planning, taking action, and final evaluation of actions, outcomes, and of the process itself. Each of these phases will be discussed in greater detail in the sections that follow.

Problem Identification Phase In his classic work, Duncker (1945) defined a **problem** as a situation in which an individual or team

> has a goal but does not know how this goal is to be reached. Whenever [the individual or team] cannot go from the given situation to the desired situation simply by action, then there is recourse to thinking .... Such thinking has the task of devising some action which may mediate between the existing and the desired situation. (p. 1)†

More simply: "you have a problem when you are required to act but you don't know what to do" (Robertson, 2001, p. 3).

Problems come in different types, sizes, and complexities (Wildman & Warner, 2003). Simple problems are those that are clearly defined, are straightforward to solve, and require less information to understand and address. Complex problems are often multidimensional many uncertain and changing variables; they are also information-intensive and may be hard to evaluate.

It cannot be overstated how important it is for interprofessional teams to be able to identify, frame, understand, and analyze problems properly. Problem identification is a critical first step in the problem-solving process. Yet this stage is often rushed or even skipped (Levi, 2001). Failure to properly identify a problem or misconstruing a situation as a problem can result in time wasted by taking action that does not address an actual problem, while one persists. It may also lead to errors and poor decisions about the real problem.

A key step in problem identification is developing an understanding of the expectations of those involved in the problem situation. Expectations, whether those of a patient or the team, shape both problem identification and resolution. Gaining an understanding

†Source: Excerpt from *Psychological Monographs*, On Problem-Solving, Volume 58, Issue 5, by Karl Duncker. Published by The American Psychological Association, © 1945.

of a patient's expectations serves many purposes, including (a) clarifying the patient's understanding of what is happening, (b) clarifying and providing some indication of the direction of the problem-solving process, and (c) clarifying the level of commitment of clients and how their expectations factor into the problem. In the opening vignette, Phil and Dr. Bali assess Mrs. Wang's expectations by asking her to explain her understanding of how the medication she is taking affects her energy level and what she would like to see happen. Through the responses of Mrs. Wang and her daughter, they gain a better understanding of what she perceives to be happening and an indication of the direction required for a collaborative resolution.

The final step of the problem identification phase is, of course, identifying the problem. This means developing a problem statement and analyzing and evaluating it. The best approach here is a systematic method, which increases the likelihood that the statement accurately reflects a given situation and has not been misunderstood. A general structured approach to problem identification is outlined in Helpful Tools 6.1.

Helpful Tools 6.1

General Problem Identification Process

1. **State the problem(s).** Provide a detailed and specific description of the problem based on the following questions. If the problem seems complex, develop several statements for all of the problems identified.
   a. What is happening or not happening? What makes it a problem?
   b. Where, how, and to whom is it happening?
   c. What is at stake?
   d. Who owns the problem?
   e. Does the statement reflect a problem or a desired outcome or solution?
2. **Check assumptions.** What assumptions are being made related to this problem and are they true/accurate? (*Note:* If these assumptions are not accurate, reconsider whether a problem exists or revise the problem statement.)
3. **Verify that a real problem exists.** What would happen if nothing were done about this problem? (*Note:* If the answer is "nothing," reconsider whether a problem exists and repeat steps 1 and 2.)
4. **Identify relevant and supporting information and data.** What information, documentation, and data are relevant to this problem? Is this information accurate?
5. **Verify understanding of the problem.** Do all team members agree with the understanding of the problem that has been articulated? (*Note:* If an agreement cannot be reached, consider other possible interpretations of the facts identified.)
6. **Prioritize the problem.** If there are several problem statements, which take precedence? Is there one that is overarching and would impact or resolve other identified problems?

Let us apply the general structure in Helpful Tools 6.1 to identify and clarify the problem with which Mrs. Wang and the interprofessional team are faced in the opening vignette. We can see that there is a lack of clarity about the focus of the problem. Here it is important to recognize that in a given situation, a problem may be multifaceted or there may be several related problems. The key to clearly articulating the problem is to try to identify all possible problems. Once that is accomplished, it is important to either (a) determine the main problem under which the other problems fall or (b) decide which problem is the most important. Below is an example of one of a number of problems that the interprofessional team in the opening vignette might identify using steps 1 to 4 of the problem identification process.

1. **State and provide description of the problem:** Mrs. Wang's blood glucose is not in good control because she is not taking her prescribed medication.
   - Mrs. Wang reports she stopped self-injecting her insulin following discharge from the hospital and was admitted because she had a diabetic crisis.
   - Mrs. Wang's belief is that the medication negatively affects her chi and, as a result, she chose to stop injecting her insulin.
   - Mrs. Wang's daughter is concerned about her mother's situation and health.
   - Mrs. Wang, her family, and the interprofessional team own the problem.
2. **Check assumptions:** Mrs. Wang has chosen to stop taking her medication. This is a reasonable assumption based on the assessment of Mrs. Wang's ability to make judgments. The alternative would be that she is being denied her insulin or someone has forced her to stop taking it.
3. **Verify that a problem exists:** There are consequences if the identified problem is not addressed, the most serious of which is that Mrs. Wang will continue to experience diabetic crises, putting her life at risk.
4. **Gather supporting information:** Hospital records, diagnostic tests, and Mrs. Wang's statements to the interprofessional team provide supporting information.

At this point we would also suggest that you consider along which dimension of the PRT framework the problem exists for the team. Is the issue related to a specific health care process that must be addressed? Does it deal with relationships? Or is it about a specific task? In this case, we can easily see that the problem does not relate to either a basic health care delivery process or interprofessional or interpersonal relationships. Returning to the vignette and the summarized details above, we see that the issue of Mrs. Wang not taking her insulin falls under the category of *task*: it relates to the "what" of a health care situation.

As we move to the decision-making phase of McClam and Woodside's (1994) model of problem solving, we will keep in mind that our priority focus is on the accomplishment of a task, while the other dimensions of process and relationship may be relevant in terms of exacerbating the problem or finding solutions.

Decision-Making Phase The decision-making phase comprises three steps—goal setting, generating alternatives, and decision making—each of which takes place in sequence.

Goal Setting The next step after a problem has been defined, analyzed, and understood is to set goals. A **goal** is a statement of intention that indicates where the client/team wants to be in the end of the problem-solving process. Quite simply, it describes the intended or desired outcome. As the first step of the decision-making phase, goal setting establishes the direction for both the team and the patient and guides the remaining parts of the problem-solving process. They also provide the structure for evaluating the end result.

For goals to be effective, they must be clear, unambiguous, and reachable (see Helpful Tools 6.2). Well-constructed goals increase the likelihood of solving problems successfully (Dixon & Glover, 1984). They increase awareness of the possible consequences and assist interprofessional teams and patients to identify ideal and viable solutions. In the opening vignette, there is a clear difference between the goal articulated by Mrs. Wang and the goals of the team. Mrs. Wang's stated goal is to "feel better and get her energy back." The team's underlying goal might be to "identify interventions that will stabilize Mrs. Wang's blood glucose without significantly compromising or impinging upon her level of energy and ability to function." These two goals are generally focused in the same direction, which is to help Mrs. Wang improve her quality of life. However, Mrs. Wang's goal is open to multiple interpretations, as there are many ways to define "feeling better";

Helpful Tools 6.2

Tips for Goal Setting

1. **Identify observable behaviours and actions.** E.g., "My goal is to run a race."
2. **Describe criteria that would indicate that the goal has been successfully reached.** E.g., "My goal is to run a marathon."
3. **Specify conditions for evaluation.** E.g., "My goal is to run a marathon this coming autumn."
4. **Be realistic.** E.g., "I want to enter a marathon this autumn and complete it" is a more realistic goal for a person who has no experience with long-distance running than "I want to enter a marathon next week and win the race."
5. **Develop sub-goals for the main goal.** Sub-goals act as the steps to be taken toward the main goal. They make the overall goal more manageable and easier to attain. For example, joining a running group to gain support and mentorship, beginning by running short distances such as 2–5K and increasing the distance each week by a certain amount, etc.

her statement does not give any indication of behaviours required to achieve the result. The team's goal is clearer and unambiguous, and indicates measurable outcomes.

Generating Alternatives After setting clear goals, the next step of the decision-making phase is to generate alternative solutions to the problem(s) identified. In this step, the interprofessional team collaborates with the patient(s) to generate as many different alternatives as possible to meet the goals that have been set and resolve the problem situation. It is important to keep in mind that the alternatives generated should directly address the goals.

As a rule, patients should be involved as much as possible when problems directly or indirectly relate to them. The level of a patient's involvement in this step will be determined by many factors, including both capacity and willingness to participate.

Generating alternatives requires critical and creative thinking. Critical thinking is a complex cognitive activity that incorporates a number of skills, such as the ability to apply knowledge and assemble information and resources. The skills involved in critical thinking are used to produce new ideas or knowledge in new forms. An interprofessional team that uses critical thinking throughout the problem-solving process is more likely to generate relevant and congruent solutions that will be successful in addressing problem situations (McClam & Woodside, 1994).

Creative thinking leads to alternatives that are imaginative and innovative. Interprofessional teams that think creatively demonstrate flexibility and originality. They are able to reimagine resources and generate novel uses and adaptations. Creative thinking allows a team to look beyond the conventional boundaries of a problem situation and the standard solutions and to consider other ideas, including those of the patient.

One of the most common strategies that teams use to generate alternatives is *brainstorming* (see Helpful Tools 6.3). Brainstorming relies on creative thinking and involves team members spontaneously sharing ideas or solutions to the problem being examined. In brainstorming, the ideas generated often "spin off" other ideas. The aim of this method is to generate ideas and not evaluate them. It centres on quantity of ideas, and teams should expect that some ideas generated may be of low quality. Ideas that are unethical, offensive, and inappropriate are unacceptable in any circumstances and should be avoided (Myers & Anderson, 2008).

Helpful Tools 6.3

Brainstorming Steps

1. Reframe problem statements into a challenge to stimulate ideas.
2. Set a time limit for the brainstorming session (e.g., 30 minutes). Larger teams will require more time.
3. Identify a team member who will facilitate the process and record ideas and alternatives.
4. Develop rules that the team agrees to abide by (e.g., members should encourage creativity; no negative and derogatory ideas; no evaluation of ideas).
5. Start by sharing or shouting out ideas and solutions to the problem.
6. Following the session, review, analyze, and make decisions about the options using a structured process.

Making Decisions The final step of this phase, decision making, involves careful analysis of the alternatives generated, then making a choice. The analysis is a crucial task that must be completed first, to prevent a wrong choice and subsequent mistakes.

Making decisions as an interprofessional team is generally more complicated than as an individual. However, all teams manage to develop some method for combining individual inputs into a single team decision (Forsyth, 2006). These methods, called *social decision schema*, are mostly implicit. However, Peniwali (2007) suggests that successful analysis and decision making requires explicit and deliberate methods. Some common explicit social decision schemes, described below, are delegation, statistical aggregation, voting, consensus, and random choice (Forsyth).

- *Delegation*—Decision making is left to one individual member or a subsection of the team. Delegated decision makers may or may not seek consultation with other members of the team when making decisions. Delegation may be the default method of decision making in interprofessional teams with hierarchical and autocratic structures. Factors such as workload and scope of practice may also lead a team to delegate decision making.
- *Statistical aggregation*—Individual team member decisions are averaged to yield a team decision. Ranking and averaging alternatives is an example of statistical aggregation. Statistical aggregation is least appropriate for decision making related to client problems, which are often complex. However, statistical aggregation is efficient and saves time.
- *Voting*—Team members vote to indicate their preferences from among the various alternatives generated. A choice is made on the basis of that alternative favoured by the majority (usually meaning 50% or more).
- *Consensus*—The team discusses alternatives until it reaches unanimous agreement without voting. Decision making based on consensus requires the most time, but it leads to greater commitment to the decision. Consensus is the preferred method of reaching a decision in teams, particularly in problem situations that require sensitive judgment. However, the method may not be possible in all situations.
- *Random choice*—A team abandons reasoned approaches and leaves final decisions to chance (e.g., flipping a coin).

Brockner and Wiesenfeld (1996) note that a method of decision making, implicit or explicit, is most likely to be successful and accepted as fair if:

- it is applied in a consistent and impartial manner on the basis of accurate information,
- it offers the opportunity to evaluate the decision and correct it prior to its implementation,
- it best represents the interests of patients and other parties,
- it involves the patient and other parties (if applicable), and
- it is in keeping with professional standards of practice and ethics.

With regard to the opening vignette, the most favourable approach for the team to use—considering factors such as the complexity of Mrs. Wang's problem situation and the level of involvement of members in the problem-solving process—would likely be the consensus method.

Problem Resolution Phase The last phase of the problem-solving process, problem resolution, begins once a decision has been made about which of the strategies previously generated is most likely to meet the goals set and resolve the problem. This phase consists of planning for implementation, taking action, and a final evaluation. As in the previous phases, ongoing collaboration between the interprofessional team and the patient is important if problem resolution is to be achieved.

Planning for Implementation The steps involved in planning for implementation may be varied. They generally include a review and evaluation of the processes leading to this step, assessing readiness for change and addressing any related issues, and developing a plan of action.

A review and evaluation of the preceding steps is intended to help avoid costly mistakes and to ensure that details and important information are not missed. A review should include assessment of the perceptions of the problem and the level of satisfaction with the choices made. This review may reveal that the identified problem has changed because the circumstances or the environment has changed. In such a case, the problem that was identified no longer fits and fails to represent the situation accurately. This step also allows the client and/or the interprofessional team the opportunity to assess whether the solution should be implemented or whether to terminate the problem-solving process.

The implementation plan is an action plan that outlines the exact steps necessary to resolve the identified problem. The plan puts into operation the chosen strategy. It will generally include a sequence of specific activities to be enacted, including their timing and who will be taking the action. It must incorporate the goals set in the previous phase of problem solving.

Change is an important concept at this juncture. Most solutions generated to resolve a problem involve some form of change, usually in behaviour (Egan, 2007). We know from theory, research, and even personal experience that while change is a fact of human life, it may often be associated with feelings of fear and confusion. In problem situations, this phenomenon is heightened and may result in resistance to planning and taking action (McClam & Woodside, 1994). It is important that teams possess the skills to manage change effectively. This includes the ability to assess their own and patients' preparedness for change and the willingness to incorporate ways to address change-related issues into the overall resolution plan. Having a systematic and clearly articulated plan for action is one way to help dispel fears and resistance to proposed changes.

A number of structured approaches are available to help interprofessional teams effectively accomplish planning for implementation. The most common are linear models that identify the tasks or actions to be taken in a particular order and attach a time frame to each action. These approaches also consider constraints and barriers that might be encountered. Alternatively, nonlinear models may be appropriate when problems are complex or require several tasks to be completed concurrently. Most health care–related problems, due to their complexity and time-sensitivity, necessitate nonlinear approaches. These are harder to organize, and present challenges with follow-through. They also require a higher level of problem-solving competence. Leadership (see Chapter 7) is critical when using nonlinear models to plan and structure the resolution of a problem.

Taking Action Taking action involves carrying out the steps of the plan that has been developed. In problem-solving situations involving patients, this step is characterized by significantly more participation by the patient. Often, there is a reversal of roles as the patient assumes more responsibility and carries out the plan with support from the team.

Let's reconsider Mrs. Wang's problem situation. Suppose that she, her daughter, and the interprofessional team work together to devise a plan that involves changes to her medications and the addition of non-pharmaceutical interventions, such as frequent contact with an outpatient nurse, a visiting pharmacist, or perhaps some type of outreach support person. The goals of this plan would be to minimize the side effects of her medication, gain better control of her blood glucose, better manage her symptoms, and maintain a good-to-high level of activity. The majority of the actions associated with these goals, such as adhering to the new medication regimen, would be carried out by Mrs. Wang, with support from the team. The team's supportive role may include providing information and resources to manage symptoms, monitoring her progress, and helping her develop a support network and address barriers should they arise. The team, along with Mrs. Wang, may also engage in data collection and information gathering, which would be helpful when evaluating the outcome of the process.

Final Evaluation In the ideal problem-solving process, the action taken to resolve a problem eventually ends and final evaluation begins. In reality, problem solving is more iterative and resembles a feedback loop or system. Robertson (2001) notes that often when teams problem-solve, make decisions, and act on these decisions, additional problems arise that require further problem solving. Thus, the findings of the final evaluation step act as inputs that feed back into the process. For example, in the case of Mrs. Wang, the barriers or issues she might experience as she and the team carry out their plan may initiate a new problem-solving process.

Although evaluation is the final step, you will have noticed that it also occurs throughout the process at different points. This type of ongoing evaluation is referred to a *formative evaluation*. Formative evaluation provides feedback about the effectiveness of particular steps as the problem-solving process progresses. For example, at several points in the problem identification and decision-making phases we have outlined, activities are evaluated in an effort to ensure accuracy and avoid mistakes.

Evaluation that occurs at the end of the problem-solving process is referred to as *summative evaluation*. Summative evaluation focuses on the entire process and is used to assess the outcomes as well as determine how effectively the process was enacted. A number of methods can be used to conduct a summative evaluation; however, whichever is used, the evaluation should broadly address whether goals were met and whether the parties involved are satisfied with the outcomes.

Pitfalls of Team Problem Solving As we noted previously, members of interprofessional health care teams are not strangers to the processes of problem solving. Much of the work and the care teams provide involves some fundamental level of problem solving. However, many of us are generally more familiar with problem solving on our own or with patients rather than in teams. Although problem solving at the team level has many advantages, it is also complex and challenging. There are a number of potentially devastating pitfalls. Here is a brief overview of the most common ones and ways to avoid them:

- *Cognitive limitations and differences in style*—Cognitive pattern styles and biases, team norms, and the communication structure within a team play a role in the team's ability to engage in the phases of problem solving (Levi, 2001). Differences in cognitive style may lead to disputes and disagreements. Additionally, differences in professional orientation may make it more difficult to agree upon which approaches to use and to reach consensus. Lastly, the cognitive work demanded by complex problems may at times be too taxing for members, leading to behaviour such as social loafing and absenteeism (Forsyth, 2006). To avoid this pitfall, teams should break complex problems down into sub-problems and take the time to clearly define each problem using a systematic approach.
- *Resistance*—Resistance to use of formal problem solving, whether by some or all the members, can stall resolution of problems. Reasons for such resistance include the perception that formal procedures will hinder team progress and feelings of awkwardness with these processes (Poole, 1991). To overcome this, Myers and Anderson (2008) suggest that team members consider the many benefits afforded by these procedures, such as the time and energy they save.
- *Inadequate discussion*—Effective discussion is integral to problem solving. Without it, teams cannot make accurate problem statements and they rush through problem solving, making mistakes along the way. Inadequate and ineffective discussions are characterized by poor communication and inappropriate behaviours. They may be the result of team members lacking the needed interpersonal and communication skills. Poor communication skills include poor listening, use of jargon, and poor nonverbal behaviour. Inappropriate behaviours may often be egocentric, including conduct such as dominating, sidetracking discussions, and use of tactics such as procrastination. Attention to communication within a team and committing to developing and improving interpersonal skills can help teams foster effective discussion.
- *Polarization*—Polarization is the tendency for a team to respond to a problem situation and the decision making involved in a more extreme way than members of the team would respond individually (Forsyth, 2006). It occurs as a result of many common social and team processes, such as normative pressure, social decision schema, and social comparison. Polarization can lead to mistakes and missteps in the problem-solving process, for example by fostering a "one-track mind" and fixation on certain ideas. However, it may also offer some benefits, such as when teams rapidly support and take up new ideas and innovations. To avoid problems associated with

polarization, teams should develop awareness and understanding of the concept and watch out for it during problem-solving activities.

- *Groupthink*—Groupthink is a term coined by researcher and scholar Irving Janis (1982), who defined it as "a mode of thinking that people engage in when they are deeply involved in a cohesive [team], when the members strivings for unanimity override their motivation to realistically appraise alternative courses of action" (p. 9). It represents a distortion in the thinking/reasoning of a team, which renders them incapable of making rational decisions and prone to mistakes. Indicators of groupthink in teams are closed-mindedness, overvaluing and exalting the team, and pressure toward uniformity. There might also be any of a number of contributing factors, an important one being leadership style (see discussion of leadership styles in Chapter 7). To avoid groupthink, teams should (a) work to maintain an environment of open inquiry and communication, (b) take every opportunity to correct misunderstandings, misinterpretations, and biases, and (c) use structured procedures such as those discussed in this chapter.

CONFLICT RESOLUTION

In Chapter 4, we introduced the concept of a conflict. *Conflict* is defined as the process that occurs when team members, because of the complex and interdependent nature of teams, engage in a struggle rooted in a difference of beliefs, thoughts, attitudes, feelings, and/or behaviours. A maxim of conflict is that it is inevitable in teams. Teams bring together people with different preferences and motivations that may pull them in different, sometimes opposing, directions. They also might create a social dilemma for members, who often have to choose between focusing on outcomes that might serve them best as individuals and team outcomes. This type of situation may lead to competition rather than cooperation in interprofessional teams. Team members' professional orientations, and other factors such as power and status structures existing in the health care system, may create tension and underpin disagreements.

Conflicts in teams often progress through stages, beginning with an initial conflict period and then escalating beyond the initial disunion. The escalation may be characterized by splits within a team and behaviours such as arguing and public displays of emotion (Forsyth, 2006). It's not hard to see why processes to address conflict when working in teams, as can arise with IPP, are essential. **Conflict resolution** refers to a range of methods that may be used to address conflict, whether at the interpersonal level, between different groups or teams, or even between countries, in such a way that an acceptable solution may be found.

Conflict in Problem Solving

Conflict can occur at any point during the processes in which an interprofessional team is engaged. Not only may it be the cause of a problem, but it may also arise in the course of problem solving itself. Conflict may emerge during the problem identification phase, or when decisions are being made about how to resolve a problem. Members of an interprofessional team, for example, may disagree with one another's analyses of a problem situation. In the opening vignette to this chapter, we see that this is the case between Phil, Mrs. Wang's primary RN, and Cora, the psychiatric resident.

In the decision-making phase of problem solving, a team may also experience conflict over which procedure or method to use to make decisions (Forsyth, 2006). Many of these conflicts can be avoided or addressed by predetermining the procedures and methods that will be used for problem solving. Among more formal interprofessional health care teams, such as those constructed for higher level committees, procedural rules of order are often adopted to regulate behaviour and discussion. For teams working collaboratively to provide patient care, having a clear sense of team members' roles and responsibilities, how information is communicated, how decisions are made and by whom, and how dissent is expressed may be critical to smooth team functioning around decision making.

Resolving Conflicts

Whether a conflict becomes a problem for an interprofessional team most often depends on how the conflict is addressed. Conflicts that are not addressed will often eventually subside. However, the likelihood that they will reemerge or become a problem is high. The most appropriate way for a team to address conflicts that escalate is to confront them, and work through them in a systematic manner. Doing so potentiates the team's development and may become a source of valuable learning and information. The ability to address conflict is so crucial to effective IPP that is has been identified as one of the six domains of the National Interprofessional Competency Framework developed by the Canadian Interprofessional Health Collaborative (CIHC, 2010) (see Spotlight 6.1).

In general, all of us draw upon one or more of a global set of basic conflict resolution tactics. Five of the conflict resolution tactics most commonly described in the literature are presented in Table 6.2 (e.g., Forsyth, 2006; Masters, 2005; Myers & Anderson, 2008). Within teams, these tactics may be used with varying results. Cooperation, however, is the strategy most likely to lead to adequate resolution of conflict within teams and tends to yield the best results.

Confronting conflicts and resolving them appropriately and productively in interprofessional teams requires knowledge and skills. These skills can be learned and practised. Good conflict resolution involves a deliberate and planned process. Basic steps that are essential to conflict resolution include:

- creating an appropriate atmosphere (appropriate timing, location, opening well),
- clarification of perceptions (thought and attitude processes are explored with effective listening),
- identifying "real" issue and shared needs,
- generating options,

- developing doable action plan and implement it (requires consensus), and
- evaluating outcomes of actions and the resolution process.

Smith (2001) also asserts that prior to initiating steps to resolve a conflict, there should be a pre-resolution period in which members of a team engage in self-reflection to address their emotional responses to the conflict. Helpful Tools 6.4 provides a useful conflict resolution technique that can be applied to most situations.

Table 6.2 Common Conflict Resolution Tactics

Tactic	Description
Competing/fighting	This tactic involves requiring or forcing others to accept one's point of view. Those who use this approach have a win–lose perspective and are often results-oriented, self-confident, assertive, and focused primarily on the bottom line and maximizing their own outcomes. Under extreme circumstances, aggressiveness and domination may be used to "win."
Avoiding	This tactic involves inaction as a means of addressing conflicts. Traditionally, avoidance has been viewed in health care environments as necessary to organizational functioning (Masters, 2005). This tactic is characterized by passivity and withdrawal from the situation or passing responsibility onto other team members. Users of this style may also fail to show adequate concern or make an honest attempt to find a solution to a problem. Although it is not preferable, avoidance can be appropriate in situations in which there is a need to delay resolution, provide time for reflection, and reduce tension. It may also be the only option available to someone who does not have control over a situation.
Collaborating/cooperating	This tactic reflects a desire to find creative solutions that are acceptable to all parties involved in a conflict. Collaborating or cooperating requires open and honest communication and consideration of the outcomes for all involved. This tactic engages the process of problem solving.
Accommodating/yielding	This tactic involves sacrificing one's own concerns and giving in to the demands or perspectives of others. Sometimes this behaviour is motivated by a desire to maintain relationships and unity with other members of a team; sometimes, individuals or teams may use this tactic because they realize there is an error in their position. Accommodating or yielding can therefore represent either superficial or genuine agreement (Forsyth, 2006).
Compromising	This tactic requires the user to take a mid-range perspective. Compromising involves finding solutions to conflict that only partially satisfy those involved. Members may split the difference between positions and engage in give-and-take tradeoffs. Compromise may be acceptable in conflicts that are not critical and/or when a quick solution is desired. Using this style often involves negotiation (Masters, 2005).

Spotlight 6.1

CIHC National Interprofessional Competency Framework: Interprofessional Conflict Resolution Domain

The Canadian Interprofessional Health Collaborative (CIHC) National Interprofessional Competency Framework, as described in Chapter 4, articulates competencies grouped into six domains that are necessary for effective interprofessional collaborative practice. The interprofessional conflict resolution domain describes the values, attitudes, and behaviours necessary for members of interprofessional teams to engage positively and constructively in conflict resolution. These values and behaviours include:

- recognizing that conflict may occur in the course of providing care and that it can potentially be beneficial to the care process,
- identifying sources of potential conflict and developing knowledge of strategies and approaches to resolving conflict,
- fostering a safe and open environment to share diverse perspective and opinions, and
- establishing structures and processes to facilitate the process of conflict resolution.

Source: Canadian Interprofessional Health Collaborative(CIHC). (2010). *A national interprofessional competency framework* (pp. 17-18). Vancouver, BC: Author.

Helpful Tools 6.4

The Two-Challenge Rule

The "two-challenge rule," originally developed by human-factors experts for the aviation industry, is an excellent conversational technique professionals can use in practice, particularly in conflict situations in which patient safety is a concern. The technique takes an advocacy–inquiry stance "characterized by public testing of conclusions and reasoning, inquiry into alternative points of view, and seeking to enhance free and informed choice" (Pian-Smith et al., 2009, p. 85). Thus, the technique allows the user to be assertive without being confrontational and non-collaborative.

The two-challenge rule involves open questioning, using (a) an advocacy statement describing the user's opinion or position on this issue ("I notice that ... I learned it should ...") followed by (b) an inquiry question that reflects a genuine curiosity and invites the other person to share thoughts and ideas ("Can you clarify your view?" (Pian-Smith et al., 2009). If no answer or an unclear response is provided, the user applies the format again with a different statement and question that conveys the concern. Again, if there is no response or the answer is nonsensical, the user is empowered to take action that ensures the safety of the patient or resolution to the problem.

Spotlight 6.2

Mental Health Conflict Simulation for First Responders

Use of technology and creative mechanisms to simulate conflict and conflict resolution approaches is an emerging area of research and innovation that may have great impact on the ability of health care providers to practise and develop these important skill sets.

As a result of a unique collaboration between the University of Ontario Institute of Technology, Durham Regional Police Services, and Ontario Shores Centre for Mental Health Sciences, four simulations were developed with interactive videos and an adaptive learning system that puts police in realistic simulated situations and gives them opportunities to respond to them and also receive detailed feedback.

The simulations, developed within a Flash framework, have a self-contained library with additional learning resources and are based on actual police experiences involving persons presumed to have a mental illness. The purpose of these learning objects is to promote a better understanding of some of the challenges individuals with a mental illness experience and facilitate the ability of frontline officers to respond to specific situations using the most appropriate therapeutic communication strategies.

The knowledge and skills these interactive learning objects are targeting have a broad applicability that extends beyond policing to include members of other helping professions, staff working in mental health facilities, and faculty and students in related programs in postsecondary educational institutions.

The simulations may be viewed at http://cirt.uoit.ca/LOs/mainMenu.

The similarities you may have noted between the above steps and those of the problem-solving process we have discussed are not surprising, given how closely related problems and conflicts are. When a resolution process fails or does not result in a satisfying outcome, a team may use a specific strategy, such as negotiation, to bring about resolution. Spotlight 6.2 summarizes a unique simulated learning tool focusing on conflict resolution and problem solving related to situations in which first responders are interacting with individuals with acute mental illness.

NEGOTIATION: A PROBLEM-SOLVING TOOL

Negotiation is "a reciprocal communication process whereby two or more parties to a dispute examine specific issues, explain their positions, and exchange offers and counter-offers to reach agreement or achieve mutually beneficial outcomes" (Forsyth, 2006, p. 435). As we noted in the above discussion, negotiation is most consistent with the conflict resolution tactic of compromise. It sometimes involves a formal process, such as when a specific health care union or professional organization negotiates an employment contract with the hospital employer. Alternatively, it may involve little more than on-the-spot bargaining with an interprofessional team colleague about a minor issue related to who will be responsible for an element of patient care. Sampson and Marthas (1990) highlight the importance of negotiation in health care environments, noting that it may be a central feature of team-based practice in organizational environments with rigid structures in which power and control are centralized and resources may be limited.

Negotiation involves a set of skills and knowledge of particular interventions and tactics. Learning these skills and ways of intervening in conflict situations can be a valuable asset in an interprofessional team. Health care professionals who develop negotiation skills can play a pivotal role in bringing about resolution to conflicts at critical junctures. Negotiation skills are also an asset when partnering and collaborating with patients.

Approaches to Negotiation

Fisher and Ury (1981) describe three classic approaches that individuals use to negotiate in problem or conflict situations: soft negotiation, hard negotiation, and principled negotiation.

Soft negotiation is a gentle style most often motivated by the desire to maintain relationships. Soft negotiators will often disclose their bottom line and are willing to make agreements that are not always in their best interests. Soft negotiators may use avoidance as a tactic and will change their position on an issue and make concessions in an effort to promote interpersonal harmony.

By contrast, the goal in *hard negotiation* is victory. Hard negotiators have a tendency to perceive others as adversaries, demand that concessions be made, and use competitive tactics such as influence.

In interprofessional teams, the ideal approach to conflict and settlement of issues is through *principled negotiation*. The focus of principled negotiation is to sidestep positional bargaining where one or another position is taken. This approach instead focuses on the problem and trying to reach an outcome that is amicable and efficient for all involved. It is akin to the problem solving approach we have outlined in this chapter, which seeks to invent options that optimize outcomes for all parties. Principled negotiators will employ objective criteria to generate many options from which to choose (Lens, 2004). The maxim "Be soft on people and hard on the problem" best sums up this approach.

Sampson and Marthas (1990) identify three levels of focus we should keep in mind during the process of negotiation: individual factors, contextual factors, and substantive factors. An awareness and application of these considerations during negotiation will help to build negotiation and conflict resolution skills.

Individually focused factors refer to an individual's or a team's collective negotiation style and cognitive factors. Cognitive factors lead to a tendency to bias situations or issues in our favour and can make negotiation difficult. Reflection is an important tool here, as it is important to cultivate an awareness of the ways in which we orient ourselves with respect to our thinking and reasoning about a conflict or problem.

Contextual factors refer to the climate and conditions of the negotiation process. Our aim in negotiating with an awareness of contextual factors is to attempt to alter the climate and conditions, such that we positively influence the process and facilitate resolution of the problem or conflict. Activities we can engage in include opening and maintaining channels of communication, diffusing negative feelings or perceptions, maintaining a focus on the issue, using a structured agenda, and establishing fair procedures early in the process.

Substantive factors are issues that impact and influence negotiation. In a substantive focus, these are directly addressed in an effort to bridge gaps between the parties and precipitate resolution. Actions that can be taken include addressing and directly discussing rivalries and constituents, making parties aware of the tradeoffs and concessions early in the process, identifying areas of overlap and agreement and exploring areas of possible compromise, acknowledging power issues, and taking into account the impact of the resolution on the continued relationships between team members or teams.

Leadership in Problem Solving and Conflict Resolution

Leadership will be explored in depth in Chapter 7. However, it is important to note the connection between leadership and positive outcomes in relation to problem solving. Whether formal or informal, appointed or shared, leadership can be used to assist the processes of problem solving, conflict management, and negotiation. Leaders can use their communication skills and knowledge of both group process and team development to support the problem-solving process. In brainstorming, for example, a leader may take on the facilitator role, organizing the processes and monitoring the steps and criteria the team has identified. Leaders can also apply various techniques and skills such as providing feedback and effective listening to help a team and patients resolve conflict.

A leader can positively influence conflict resolution and negotiation by focusing on the contextual and substantive factors we discussed in the previous section. As a mediator, a leader should attempt to modify the contextual factors in favour of an amicable resolution. In the opening vignette for this chapter, for example, Dr. Bali acts as an informal mediator and responds to the disagreement between Cora and Phil using an avoidance style. He is quick to change the subject and ignore the initial conflict. Although this strategy may be effective in the moment, it leaves the issues that Cora and Phil are struggling with unaddressed and increases the potential that they might emerge and escalate later in the process of problem solving. It is therefore important for a leader to gain an awareness of his or her style of conflict resolution and monitor for any negative influence it may have.

IPP gives health care providers the opportunity to work collaboratively to find positive and creative solutions to health care situations. But although it can lead to better patient outcomes and provider satisfaction, it is not without challenges. Understanding how to engage in problem-solving processes, related both to patient care and to team processes, is essential. Additionally, developing good skills related to conflict resolution and negotiation not only will enhance your practice, but may significantly impact the functioning of the entire interprofessional team.

CONCLUSION

Developing competency in problem solving is critical for effective IPP. Each of the three problem-solving phases, (a) problem identification, (b) decision making, and (c) problem resolution, includes multiple progressive steps. Problem solving often involves key elements of the related processes of conflict resolution, negotiation, and leadership. Developing a robust skill set around these required competencies supports IPP and team functioning. It also increases team member facility in addressing problems impacting the three IPP dimensions (relationship, process, and task) or contextual factors of the PRT organizing framework described in this text.

SUMMARY

- Problem solving is a common and vital team-level process. To practise IPP effectively, interprofessional team members must develop competency in problem solving.
- Problem solving is defined as the invention of an alternative solution to a problem different from any previously existing one. The majority of problems encountered by interprofessional teams are patient-related. To successfully help patients to resolve these problems, teams must develop collaborative teaching and learning relationships and involve patients in the problem-solving process.
- All teams develop unique approaches to solving problems. Regardless of the method used, problem solving is most effective when structured and guided by principles.
- The process of problem solving consists of three overlapping and interconnected phases: problem identification, decision making, and problem resolution. Each phase involves several progressive steps.
- Problem solving and decision making are related but distinct processes. Decision making is defined as the selection of an alternative from an existing set of options, when no externally correct alternative exists. Decision making is a part of problem solving and can occur at different points during the process.
- Conflict resolution, negotiation, and leadership are processes closely related to problem solving. Conflict resolution is a form of problem solving in which the problem encountered is a conflict. When resolving conflicts, teams will use one or more of the basic tactics: competing, avoidance, collaborating, accommodating, and compromise. The most effective but time-consuming tactic is collaborating.
- Negotiation is a tool that can be used in problem solving and to resolve conflicts. It is defined as a reciprocal communication process whereby two or more parties to

a dispute examine specific issues, explain their positions, and exchange offers and counteroffers to reach agreement or achieve mutually beneficial outcomes. It is most often associated with the conflict resolution tactic of compromising.

- During problem solving and negotiation, a leader can act as a facilitator of the process. During negotiation, the leader may mediate discussion and use negotiation and problem-solving skills to help individuals come to amicable solutions.

Key Terms

conflict resolution
contextual factors
decision making
goal
negotiation
problem
problem solving
process dimension
relationship dimension
task dimension

Review Questions

1. What are the advantages and disadvantages to using problem-solving methods and procedures?
2. Groupthink is often considered a negative phenomenon in teams. Can you think of any benefits or advantages of groupthink in a team?
3. Of the conflict resolution tactics reviewed, which do you think you use most often when you are in teams and groups? Why do you think you use this tactic?

Application Exercises

The following activities are intended to sharpen your ability to identify problems, clearly articulate them, and generate alternatives to resolve them.

1. Find a newspaper article about a health care–related issue. Identify as many problems as you think there may be. Who do you think owns the problem and why? Are the problems that you identify the same as those identified by others in the story, such as the author? How would you collect additional information to support your assessment of the problem (identify the methods you would use)?
2. Review Mrs. Wang's situation in the opening vignette. Write a problem statement for Mrs. Wang based on the information available to you.
3. Use Helpful Tools 6.1 to identify and analyze a problem you are experiencing in the workplace, at school, and/or at home. Using the tips for brainstorming, try to generate as many possible solutions as you can think. What criteria might you use to decide which solutions are best?

References

Adams, K., & Galanes, G. J. (2006). *Communicating in groups: Applications and skills* (6th ed.). Boston, MA: McGraw-Hill.

Austin, M. J., Kopp, J., & Smith, P. L. (1986). *Delivering human services*. New York, NY: Longman.

Brockner, J., & Wiesenfeld, B. M. (1996). An integrative framework for explaining reactions to decisions: Interactive effects of outcomes and procedures. *Psychological Bulletin, 120*, 189–208.

Canadian Interprofessional Health Collaborative (CIHC). (2010). *A national interprofessional competency framework*. Vancouver, BC: Author.

Dixon, D. N., & Glover, J. A. (1984). *Counseling: A problem-solving approach*. New York, NY: Wiley.

Duncker, K. (1945). On problem-solving. *Psychological Monographs, 58*(270).

Egan, G. (1990). *The skilled helper: A systematic approach to effective helping* (4th ed.). Pacific Grove, CA: Brooks/Cole Publishing Company.

Egan, G. (2007). *The skilled helper: A problem-management and opportunity-development approach to helping* (8th ed.). Pacific Grove, CA: Brooks/Cole Publishing Company.

Elwyn, G., Koppel, S., Greenhalgh, T., & Macfarlane, F. (2001). *Groups: A guide to small group work in healthcare, management, education and research*. Abingdon, UK: Radcliffe Medical Press.

Fisher, R., & Ury, W. (1981). *Getting to YES: Negotiating agreement without giving in*. Boston, MA: Houghton Mifflin.

Forsyth, D. R. (2006). *Group dynamics* (4th ed.). Belmont, CA: Thomson/Wadsworth.

Frey, L. R. (1997). Individuals in group. In L. R. Frey & J. K. Barge (Eds.), *Managing group life: Communicating in decision-making groups* (pp. 52–79). Boston, MA: Houghton Mifflin.

Janis, I. L. (1982). *Groupthink. Psychological studies of policy decisions and fiascos* (2nd ed.). Boston, MA: Houghton Mifflin.

Lens, V. (2004). Principled negotiation: A new tool for case advocacy. *Social Work, 49*(3), 506–513.

Levi, D. (2001). *Group dynamics for teams*. Thousand Oaks, CA: Sage Publications.

Maier, N. R. F. (1958). *The appraisal interview; objectives, methods and skills*. New York, NY: Wiley.

Mandell, B., & Schram, B. (1985). *Human services: Introduction and intervention*. New York, NY: John Wiley & Sons.

Masters, K. (Ed.). (2005). *Role development in professional nursing practice*. Sudbury, MA: Jones and Bartlett.

McClam, T., & Woodside, M. (1994). *Problem-solving in the helping professions*. Pacific Grove, CA: Brooks/Cole Publishing Company.

Myers, S. A., & Anderson, C. M. (2008). *The fundamentals of small group communication*. Thousand Oaks, CA: Sage Publications.

Peniwali, K. (2007). Criteria for evaluating group decision-making methods. *Mathematical and Computer Modeling, 46*(7–8), 935–947.

Pian-Smith, M. C., Simon, R., Minehart, R. D., Podraza, M., Rudolph, J., Walzer, T., & Raemer, D. (2009). Teaching residents the two-challenge rule: A simulation-based approach to improve education and patient safety. *Simulation in Healthcare, 4*(2), 84–91.

Poole, M. S. (1991). Procedures for managing meetings: Social and technological innovation. In R. A. Swenson & B. O. Knapp (Eds.). *Innovative meeting management* (pp. 53–109). Austin, TX: 3M Meeting Management Institute.

Robertson, I. S. (2001). *Problem-solving*. Hove, UK: Psychology Press.

Sampson, E. E., & Marthas, M. (1990). *Group process for the health professions.* (3rd ed.). Albany, NY: Delmar Thompson Learning.
Smith, S. B. (2001). Resolving conflict realistically in today's health care environments. *Journal of Psychological Nursing & Mental Health Services, 39*(11), 36–45.
Thompson, L. L. (2004). *Making the team: A guide for managers* (2nd ed.). Upper Saddle River, NJ: Pearson Prentice Hall.
VanGundy, A. (1981). *Techniques of structured problem-solving.* New York, NY: Van Nostrand Reinhold.
Wildman, P., & Warner, J. (2003). *Problem-solving & decision-making toolbox: 32 fully reproducible, ready-to-use tools to help you build your know-how to solve problems, be more creative and make better decisions* [electronic resource]. Amherst, MA: HRD Press.

Chapter 7
Leadership

It's 6:13 a.m. on a snowy March day. Anna Maria, a registered practical nurse (RPN), is making rounds to check on her patients admitted to the general surgical unit at a local community hospital. As she walks into room 403, she immediately notes something amiss. Turning on the light, she assesses at a glance that her patient, Mr. Foutier, is not breathing. She cannot palpate a pulse. Without delay, Anna Maria presses the code button and initiates cardiopulmonary resuscitation (CPR).

The events in room 403 mobilize the interprofessional team in a rapid response. Anna Maria's nursing colleagues on the unit immediately race to the scene. As they arrive, a seamless transition is made from one-person to two-person CPR, and Hannah, one of the registered nurses on the unit, begins documentation. Simultaneously, the hospital operator calls a "Code Blue" over the hospital intercom, indicating the location of the event. Within minutes, the respiratory therapist (RT), physician on call, phlebotomist, and orderly all arrive. Each is aware of both his or her own responsibilities and those of the other members of the team. Anna Maria informs the team in a few short sentences that Mr. Foutier is one-day postoperative for a bowel resection secondary to carcinoma. He has a history of atrial fibrillation and insulin-dependent diabetes.

Carmenzita, the RT, moves to the head of the bed and with a nod being all the required communication between herself and Dr. Lee, intubates the patient and begins manually bagging Mr. Foutier. At the same time, several of the nurses in the room are connecting the patient to a cardiac monitor, starting a second intravenous line, rapidly checking blood glucose levels by doing a capillary glucose test, and ensuring that the physical space in the room is able to accommodate these activities by sliding furniture out of the way. Helene, the unit clerk, brings Mr. Foutier's chart into the room along with requisitions for blood tests just as Myuri, the phlebotomist, prepares to draw blood. She checks with Dr. Lee, the leader of this resuscitative effort, about any specific laboratory tests he wishes and Dr. Lee asks one of the nurses to confirm if Mr. Foutier is taking any medications that require levels to be drawn. Doug, the orderly, had taken over CPR to give Anna Maria a break from the physical exertion, and begins mentally preparing to transport the blood specimens to the lab by asking who will be take over CPR. Meanwhile, Dr. Lee begins ordering first-line medications to be administered intravenously.

It has been only eight minutes since Anna Maria walked into Mr. Foutier's room, and yet the work accomplished by the team represents years of experience and extremely high levels of expertise. However, what is most central to whether this event unfolds in a chaotic fashion or whether the activities of the team seem synchronized and orderly is the ability of team members to work interprofessionally, to understand their roles, and to respond to the variable need to be either a leader or a follower.

Learning Outcomes

AFTER STUDYING THIS CHAPTER, YOU SHOULD BE ABLE TO:

1. **Define leadership and shared leadership.**
2. **Compare and contrast different perspectives and theories about leadership.**
3. **Describe five key elements common to leadership (vision, communication skills, change, stewardship, developing and renewing others).**
4. **Discuss the emerging notion of the quantum leadership paradigm.**
5. **Critically analyze the role of interprofessional leadership in health care.**

INTRODUCTION

IN THIS CHAPTER, WE WILL FOCUS ON LEADERSHIP FOR INTERPROFESSIONAL PRACTICE (IPP). Leadership is considered an essential component of professional practice (Collins-Nakai, 2006; Galuska, 2012), and central to effective IPP (e.g., Martin & Rogers, 2004; Ross, O'Tuathail, & Stubberfield, 2005; Registered Nurses' Association of Ontario [RNAO], 2013). Leadership might be thought of as the "glue" that holds together the other important elements of IPP that we have explored thus far. For example, as we discussed in Chapter 6, leadership plays an important role in group processes, such as problem solving and conflict resolution.

The importance of leadership is clearly demonstrated in the opening vignette involving cardiopulmonary resuscitation (CPR). In the scenario, key aspects of IPP such as collaboration, teamwork, and problem solving are brought to bear, facilitated by the leadership of a designated team member, in an effort to resuscitate the patient. Although the process illustrated in the scenario and in many real-life situations may seem effortless, leadership of interprofessional teams is complex and fluid, involving a number of interwoven processes and actions, as well as the sharing of power and expertise.

Leadership within IPP teams is also not without its challenges (Reeves, MacMillan, & van Soeren, 2010). At a very basic level, effective leadership in interprofessional situations requires a clear definition that is well understood and respected by all members of the interprofessional team (Øvretveit, 1990). Having this common definition and understanding, as simple as it may sound, is often extremely challenging given barriers such as professional socialization, professional boundaries and the protection of these boundaries through both conscious and unconscious actions, and the division of work among health care professionals (Evetts, 1999; Reeves et al., 2010).

IPP and the leadership to drive teamwork is more than getting along and/or being nice to one another. Moving from merely congenial relationship to strong working partnerships that lead to optimal patient outcomes requires substantive and sustained efforts that include power redistribution and shared clinical decision making (Grinspun, 2007). Key factors that can facilitate teamwork include having champions who can drive such a change, role clarity, trust, respect, valuing and being valued within the teamwork setting, and cultural readiness within the workplace (Clements, Dault, & Priest, 2007).

Our goal in this chapter is to assist readers to develop knowledge and understanding of leadership so that they can begin to develop and apply the necessary leadership competencies to IPP. This chapter is divided into two main sections. The first section deals with definitions of leadership and discusses key elements and approaches necessary to both understand and enact leadership. The second section explores more specifically health care leadership in the context of IPP.

DEFINING LEADERSHIP

Leadership is a difficult concept to define (Grossman & Valiga, 2009; Willumsen, 2006). This task is made even more arduous by the ever-changing health care environment and the increasing complexity of care that patients require. Scan the literature on leadership and it becomes abundantly evident that there are a multitude of definitions, theories, and research studies attempting to describe the nature of leadership and the characteristics that define it as a concept. This large and diverse body of knowledge led Bennis and Nanus (1985), several decades ago, to declare that there was a lack of consensus regarding what is meant by leadership. Nevertheless, Grossman and Valiga (2009) suggest there is emerging clarity with respect to what constitutes true leadership and how to distinguish it from other, related concepts such as management.

At a broad level, Redfern (2008) defines **leadership** simply as the ability to influence others. Bass (1990) recommends that a working definition of leadership incorporate ideas such as individual characteristics, the ability to influence behaviour, team goals, team processes, and contextual factors. Forsyth (2006, p. 376) proposes that leadership is "the process by which an individual[s] guides a [team] in their pursuits, often by organizing, directing, coordinating, supporting and motivating their efforts." This definition is applicable to IPP, as it is conceived at the team level and reflects a number of integral processes and actions. Yuki's (2002, p. 7) definition is even more germane to IPP: "the process of influencing others to understand and agree about what needs to be done and how it can be done effectively, and the process of facilitating individual and collective efforts to accomplish the shared objectives." This incorporates the features suggested by Bass and emphasizes that leadership is process-oriented and requires the collective efforts of all members. Galuska (2012, p. 333) states that "oversight for high-quality care, systems improvement, collaboration, communication, teamwork, conflict resolution, advocacy, and policy influence" are key competencies of leadership, and considers these critical in all practice settings and in policy.

As highlighted by the above definitions, leadership is both important and necessary to interprofessional team functioning (Myers & Anderson, 2008). However, what it resembles and how it is enacted within a team vary greatly depending on a multitude of factors. For example, organizational structures and processes may dictate what leadership looks like within a team. Organizational policies and procedures, communication and other processes, team development, and the characteristics and professional orientations of members may all play a role in determining how leadership is both conceptualized and enacted within a team.

The process of leadership has many characteristics, which have been described broadly within the literature. Leadership is reciprocal, transactional, transformational, adaptive, and cooperative (Forsyth, 2006). Reciprocity in leadership processes refers to the idea that not only do leaders influence the members of a team, but but also they are influenced by them in turn. Thus the style of leadership that exists in a team will foster corresponding membership or followership styles. In the same way, membership style may set the tone for the type of leadership style that emerges within a team as it develops. Leadership is both a transactional and a transformational process. As a transactional process, leaders and members of a team cooperate to accomplish goals. They exchange their knowledge and skills, time, and other assets for mutual benefit. As a transformational process, leadership brings about individual and collective shifts within teams, such as those associated with changes in values and beliefs. These changes may occur as a result of the support and motivation that leaders encourage in the team environment (Bass, 1990; Grossman & Valiga, 2009). Leadership is an adaptive process that requires cooperative interactions. Ideally, the process of leadership should help teams to move from goal setting to goal attainment by fostering cooperative relationships and through exerting influence in legitimate and empowering ways.

Forms of Leadership

Leadership often takes two main forms within a health care team: (a) shared leadership in which multiple team members formally or informally rotate through leadership activities and (b) leadership roles occupied by individuals who are either appointed or elected. Each of these forms is associated with a particular paradigm-based approach to leadership.

Appointed or elected leaders are associated with an individually focused, traditional approach based on personal traits. An appointed leader is someone chosen to lead a team, and the role may be an aspect of a person's job description. For example, commonly appointed leadership roles in health care might include shift leader or supervisor, program coordinator or director, clinical educator, and various other levels of administrators. An appointed leader is generally charged with the task of directing the team or group.

An elected leader is someone chosen by his or her team to lead the team, usually through either discussion and consensus or voting. The IPP team in the opening vignette provides an example. This structure, which exists in some health care environments that support collaborative practice models, is most often determined by status and hierarchy, which are dictated by implicit and explicit status characteristics and the related power distribution (Grinspun, 2007, 2010). This arrangement is often further reinforced by factors such as organizational structure and legislated scope of practice. This may be most suitable in particular circumstance (e.g., Dr. Lee is the designated leader during CPR because of her regulated scope of practice enabling her to diagnose and prescribe). As we discuss below, it is important to keep in mind that effective leadership in IPP has less to do with holding a particular title or status position than with possessing and being able to utilize appropriate knowledge and skills.

Shared leadership is "a dynamic, interactive influence process among individuals in groups for which the objective is to lead one another to the achievement of group or organizational goals or both. This influence process often involves peer, or lateral, influence and at other times involves upward or downward hierarchical influence" (Pearce & Conger, 2003, p. 1). Shared leadership can be viewed from two perspectives. The first centres on the notion of member competence and frames leadership as a flexible process. It involves a member of a team assuming the role of leader, based on his or her level of competence within the context, in order to help the team accomplish a particular task. From this perspective, leadership is functional and the leader does not have to encompass all the skills necessary to lead the team in all situations. This notion of shared leadership, whereby more than one team member can assume the role of leader, is captured by Yuki's (2002) definition. Referring back to the interprofessional team in the opening vignette, it is conceivable that, depending on a number of factors such as the complexity and expertise required during the cardiopulmonary emergency, facility protocols, and availability of team members, the RT or clinical nurse specialist on the team could also take on the role of team leader. In reality, however, this typically happens only in the absence of a physician.

The other view of shared leadership posits that leadership is a set of behaviours that can be exhibited by any team member at any time. Leadership behaviours include encouragement, assisting the team to become organized, and helping to build consensus during problem solving and conflict resolution. Leadership is conceptualized as both flexible and fluid, with leadership responsibilities and opportunities moving throughout the team from member to member. If we consider the interprofessional team in the opening vignette from this perspective, it is conceivable that at different times during CPR intervention, various team members exhibit leadership behaviours. These behaviours would collectively demonstrate the leadership of the team in providing the best-quality care for the patient.

The view of shared leadership as a set of behaviours should not be confused with leadership focused on task completion. Cummings et al. (2010) refer to this form of leadership as *dissonance leadership*, which they note does not achieve optimal outcomes for work environments. Instead, their comprehensive review points to a trend in outcomes patterns that supports the conclusion that "relationship or people focused leadership practices contribute to improving outcomes for ... work environments and for productivity and effectiveness of healthcare organizations" (p. 378).

Leadership Theory

The drive to understand leadership has resulted in a number of theories that attempt to explain leadership or introduce concepts that focus on the various aspects of leadership. Table 7.1

Table 7.1 Leadership Theories

Theory	Features
Great Man Theory	■ Popular early theory that posits history has been most profoundly influenced by great men who have brought about change. ■ Focuses on charisma, insight, intellect, or desire for personal gain that leads individuals to become influential.
Trait theories	■ Emerged in response to the limitations of "great man" leadership; trait theories, however, share similarities with the Great Man Theory. ■ Assume leadership comes from the inherent trait(s) an individual possesses. ■ Attempt to identify characteristics that distinguish leaders from other people. ■ A key limitation is that these theories cannot explain why people with leadership traits are not leaders.
Situational leadership theories	■ Propose that leaders take action to do what is needed when the time is right. ■ A key limitation is that these theories do not account for the important role of followers.
Behaviour theories	■ Theories based on the counterargument that leaders are "made, not born." ■ Focus is on leadership action and behaviours. ■ Leadership is constructed as behaviour that can be learned through teaching and role modelling.
Leader–member exchange theory	■ Leadership occurs when effective relationships develop between leaders and followers, which results in growing influence (Uhl-Bien, 2006). ■ Leader and followers gain the benefit that relationships offer. Participation and contribution of followers are sought; however, not a true sharing of leadership. The balance of power in the relationship is held by the designated leader.
Transactional leadership	■ Focus is on the relationship between a leader and followers within a hierarchal context. ■ Leader and followers engage in a mutually beneficial, contractual relationship in which the leader provides rewards in exchange for commitments and/or loyalty from the followers. ■ Commonly used in business and health care settings.
Transformational leadership	■ Focus is on the relationship between a leader and followers that is beyond a system of reward and punishment. ■ Leader and followers work together toward reaching long-term goals that are values- and principles-based. ■ Leader's role is to motivate and inspire followers and facilitate fulfillment of their potential, which also enhances the performance of the group.
Quantum leadership paradigm	■ "defines leadership as an interactional field where leader–follower relationship is the asset" (Erçetin & Kamaci, 2008, p. 865).

summarizes a number of theories that have been proposed over the years. The vast majority of these can be categorized into three broad groups: the traditional leadership perspective, the functional or style leadership perspective, and the situational leadership perspective.

Traditional Leadership Perspective The **traditional leadership** perspective focuses on the notion that leadership is innate and inherent to an individual; the "Great Man Theory" (see Table 7.1) is the archetype of this view.

The traditional leadership perspective holds that a leader is born and embodies certain characteristics or traits that make him/her a leader. Considerable research has focused on this notion in an effort to identify the specific traits of "born leaders". A significant amount of this research has focused on personality traits (Myers & Anderson, 2008). Within this research, contradictions to the perspective have emerged, leading scholars to consider factors not related to personal traits. Problems noted include phenomena such as the lack of stability in one's leadership ability when teams undergo a change in membership, in the prevailing context in which the team is functioning, in the overall situation, and in the specific task at hand. Additionally, the characteristics of a leadership personality have been difficult to pinpoint (Sampson & Marthas, 1990).

Functional or Style Leadership Perspective The **functional or style leadership** perspective focuses on how leaders lead. It is concerned with the level of the functional capacity of the individual occupying the role of leader and the style of leadership he or she uses. The functional or style leadership approach shifts focus from a list of personality traits to the skill sets of the individual and the functions, actions, and behaviours that he or she engages in to assist and guide a team. The leadership capacity of an individual is determined by the extent to which he or she can successfully help the team to meet its goals and objectives.

The different styles that leaders use to lead a team have been described extensively within the literature. Many are familiar with the work of Kurt Lewin and his colleagues (1939), who conducted research on three basic styles (autocratic, democratic, and laissez-faire). The main characteristics of these are summarized in Table 7.2.

Myers and Anderson (2008) remind us that all these styles may have their merits, given different situations and the context and configuration of an interprofessional team. Although a democratic style leads to the most satisfaction, an autocratic style might be required if a team desires expediency (Foels, Driskell, Mullen, & Salas, 2000; Sampson & Marthas, 1990). For example, in an emergency situation in which time is of the utmost importance, such as the cardiorespiratory resuscitation depicted in the opening vignette, an authoritative and decisive style is often necessary. However, in such situations there is usually an implicit understanding and agreement by those involved that this style is warranted.

Situational Leadership Perspective The **situational leadership** perspective focuses on the notion that the situation in which a team is operating influences, if not determines, leadership behaviour. This approach to leadership is less concerned with traits or the functional capacity of any one individual. Instead, attention shifts to the contributive, cumulative ability and capacity of the team. This approach posits that effective leadership requires different strategies at different times in the life of a team (Myers & Anderson, 2008).

Table 7.2 The Three Basic Leadership Styles

Style	Characteristics
Autocratic	■ Leader-centred; puts individual needs above team needs. ■ Authoritative; secretive. ■ Uses dominating approach to influence the team. ■ Fosters defensive team climate and conflict. ■ Tendency to use conflict for personal gain.
Democratic	■ Member-centred; inclusive of all members. ■ Emphasizes utilization of the resources available to the team. ■ Encourages supportive team climate. ■ Mediates conflict for amicable resolutions that benefit the team.
Laissez-faire	■ Uses a non-centred, non-directive style. ■ Non-committed and somewhat removed from the team. ■ Allows the team to drift and leaves outcomes to chance. ■ Avoids conflict.

Source: Based on Sampson, E. E., & Marthas, M. (1990). *Group process for the health professions* (3rd ed.). Albany, NY: Delmar Thompson Learning.

Contemporary Leadership Perspectives The leadership theories belonging to the perspectives described thus far have been critiqued as leader-centric and unidirectional, lacking in their ability to incorporate the relational aspects of leaderships and failing to acknowledge followers. In recent decades, more **contemporary leadership** theories have been proposed that promote the notion of leadership as a social process of influence that involves relational interactions between leaders and followers. This transition toward relationship-based leadership theory is marked by the introduction of Burns' (1978) *transforming leadership* theory (Goertzen, 2013). Transforming leadership occurs when "one or more persons engage with each other in such a way that leaders and followers raise one another to higher levels of motivation and morality" (p. 20). Burns' theory frames leadership as a moral process of engagement based on shared motives, values, and beliefs between the leader and followers. In this dynamic, followers define their needs, and the leader, guided by moral and ethical principles, works to recognize the needs and motives and elevate them to the collective level at which they can be worked on. Several contemporary leadership theories have been built upon Burns' work, the most notable of which is transformational leadership theory (see Table 7.1).

Other popular relationship-based leadership theories and views include relational leadership theory (Uhl-Bien, 2006) and authentic leadership theory. **Relational leadership theory** is defined as "a social influence process through which emergent conditions (i.e., evolving social order) and change (i.e., new values, attitudes, approaches, behaviours, ideologies, etc.) are constructed and produced" (Uhl-Bien, 2006, p. 668). This perspective aims to transcend hierarchy by emphasizing that leadership can happen in any direction.

Luthans and Avolio (2003, p. 243) define **authentic leadership** as "a process that draws from both positive psychological capacities and a highly developed organizational context, which results in both greater self-awareness and self-regulated positive behaviour on the part of leaders and associates, fostering positive self-development." Although authentic leadership overlaps with elements of other leadership theories, Wong and Cummings (2009) hold that the "in-depth focus [of authentic leadership] on leader and follower self-awareness/regulation, positive psychological capital, the moderating role of organizational climate, and sound propositions that link model constructs contribute to the assessment that authentic leadership is both a new theoretical perspective and a return to timeless, genuine, and basic leadership attributes and processes core to several leadership theories" (p. 534).

The evolution of leadership theory from traditional to contemporary approaches demonstrates two key trends in how we understand leadership. There is distinct movement away from thinking of leadership as a set of innate and/or inherent traits only a few people possess. Additionally, there is movement toward a more nuanced approach to leadership that is complex and multifaceted, involving elements that include individual characteristics, relationships, and interactions between people working together and the situation at hand. Grossman and Valiga (2009) summarize this emerging perspective, noting that leadership "can be learned. It is deliberate. It is not necessarily tied to a position of authority. A leadership role is something each one of us has the potential to fulfill" (p. 3). This perspective and the contemporary theories associated with it, such as shared leadership, align well with IPP.

Elements of Leadership

As the discussion reviewing various leadership perspectives demonstrates, leadership is complex and multidimensional. Fortunately, some common and fundamental elements have been identified. With this knowledge, we can begin to engage in a discussion about how these ideas apply to leadership in health care practice in general, and the kind of leadership that may be best aligned with IPP. Authors Grossman and Valiga (2009) have identified five elements common to the literature about leadership: vision, communication skills, change, stewardship, and developing and renewing others. This list should be seen not as exhaustive, but rather as a general overview of elements suitable for our discussion here. It is also important to remember that although these elements are unique, they are interrelated and interdependent.

Vision Having a vision or *visioning* refers to the ability to see what the future may bring. Rogers and Reynolds (2003) define **vision** similarly, noting that it is "a picture of the results you want to create, an ideal sense of what is possible, a statement of destination" (p. 71). Visioning is identified by many experts as a fundamental aspect of leadership (e.g., Kouses & Posner, 1995; Rogers & Reynolds, 2003; Thornberry, 2006). Whether leadership occurs at the individual or the team level, it is important to be able to conceive of and articulate possibilities that might not occur to others. Within the literature, visioning is often discussed at higher levels, such as creating a vision for an organization as part of a strategic planning exercise. While individual health care practitioners, such as social workers, physiotherapists, and pharmacists, may be involved at this level, it is important to remember that goals central to IPP, such as improved patient outcomes, represent a shared vision. In working with patients to develop goals related to their specific health care or when collaborating within the interprofessional team to develop goals that articulate new and innovative ways to provide care, IPP teams are engaging in shared visioning.

Envisioning possibilities for brighter futures at any level requires hard work, creativity, imagination, and commitment. It also takes critical thinking skills and the ability to assess current situations and forecast how they can be made different. With all these elements needing to come together, it is not surprising that visioning can be challenging for team leadership (e.g., Hall, Weaver, Handfield-Jones, & Bouvette, 2008). It can bring a team together and spur personal and team development; however, creating and bringing a shared vision to fruition is time-consuming and requires that other key elements of leadership be brought to bear, such as strong communication skills and the ability and desire to really listen to all perspectives.

Communication Skills As we have noted previously, effective communication is central to IPP. A number of the elements involved in IPP, such as teamwork, collaboration, and problem solving, rely on effective communication. It is no surprise then that communication is a key element of leadership (Grossman & Valiga, 2009).

Effective communication is essential to other elements of leadership. Visioning, for example, involves more than just having a great idea; it includes being able to share that idea in such a way that it is meaningful to others and relevant to the situation at hand. Effective communication skills enable others to take ownership of or feel included in new ideas about future possibilities.

A key communication skill, which we reviewed in Chapter 4, is listening (Metcalfe, 2009). Within a team environment, listening to the ideas of other team members is essential to creating and actualizing a shared vision and related goals. Consider what would happen if the members of the team in the opening vignette did not communicate well and, in particular, were not listening effectively to information, ideas, and instructions. In such a scenario, costly mistakes would likely be made, and contribute to a poor outcome. Although ineffective communication skills do not always have such high-stakes implications in team-related health care situations, this example illustrates that without strong communication skills, attainment of common goals is put at risk.

The communication skills of members of a health care team can vary, with only some receiving formalized training and practice to develop these skills during their professional education and others learning on the job and through personal experience (Duffy, Gordon, Whelan, Cole-Kelly, & Frankel, 2004; Hall & Weaver, 2001). However, effective communication skills are requisite for all team members in IPP, the more so if leadership is to be shared among the members. Such skills can be acquired and improved through learning and practice, and it is the responsibility of all team members to reinforce and encourage effective communication.

Change **Change**, a consistent theme of health care practice, is the process of making or becoming different. This simple definition belies the fact that it is a complex process that has been written about and studied extensively (Porter-O'Grady, 2003). Our understanding of change in health care environments is largely informed by research and theories derived from the field of organizational studies. There are number of ways to view and categorize it. Within the context of health care practice and IPP, team change is often categorized as either emergent or planned. *Emergent change* unfolds in an unplanned and seemingly spontaneous way. It is influenced by internal and external factors out of the control of any one individual, team, or organization. *Planned change* is a deliberate process that is consciously thought out and executed.

In the opening vignette of this chapter, both emergent and planned change processes are illustrated. The cardiac arrest Mr. Foutier experienced is an emergent change; it unfolded spontaneously and to a great extent was precipitated by factors and individual characteristics that despite the efforts of the patient (e.g., changes to diet and lifestyle, following medication protocols) and the team (e.g., patient plan of care and recommendations, support) could not be controlled or mitigated fully. The team's actions in response to the crisis are an example of a planned change. In health care environments, such as hospitals, responses to cardiac arrests follow a process that is structured by guidelines and based on algorithms that outline the steps for bringing about a change in the patient's status. Additionally, the vignette illustrates that while it may be useful to categorize change theoretically, it is important to understand change in the moment as a dynamic, nonlinear process having some elements of uncertainty and unpredictability.

According to the definition of the concept, IPP teams are engaged in change whenever involved in activities such as seeking to improve care, planning and working toward a goal related to their patients or the health care system, and responding to emerging situations. Leadership in IPP, therefore, must involve understanding and manage change. This requires that IPP team members develop their ability to assess change, plan where possible, and cultivate a culture that embraces and supports change and the challenges it brings (Buck & McPherson, 2006).

Stewardship The concept of **stewardship** entails the notion of duty and responsibility to others, as opposed to focusing solely on oneself. "Stewardship represents primarily an act of trust, whereby people ... entrust a leader with certain obligations and duties to fulfill and perform on their behalf .... [It] involves placing oneself in service of ideas and ideals and to others who are committed to their fulfillment (Sergiovanni, 2007, p. 59). A sense of service to others is inherent in this element of leadership (Grossman & Valiga, 2009; Sergiovanni, 2007). Stewardship is aligned with the definition of leadership proposed by Yuki (2002) and emerging perspectives that espouse a "leader among leaders" philosophy, fostering the notion of collective responsibility for achieving new goals.

Within an IPP team, effective leadership requires that all professionals have a sense of stewardship. This must apply not only to their relationships with the patients for whom they care directly, but also to those with other professionals with whom they interact and the environment in which they practise. For example, if a health care provider is to be leader who demonstrates stewardship, he or she must work toward change and improvement that has the potential to benefit patients, staff, and the organization.

Developing and Renewing Others Leadership involves helping others to develop their own capacities. It also involves assisting them to maintain their effort and commitment toward making a common vision become a reality. **Developing and renewing others** may involve conscious efforts, such as mentoring, or behaviours that indirectly influence others, such as role modelling (Grossman & Valiga, 2009). Developing and renewing others and stewardship are closely related elements of leadership. To develop and renew others, IPP team members must possess a sense of stewardship and be committed to helping other members to develop leadership and other IPP-related skill sets, such as effective communication and problem solving. Also, the literature demonstrates that administrators in health organizations and settings play a critical role in enabling or blocking the development of leadership skills for effective professional and team-based practice (Galuska, 2012; Grinspun, 2010). Similarly, the role of organizational culture also proves critical for leadership growth or stagnation (Galuska, 2012; Grinspun, 2007, 2010; Shirey, 2009).

Leadership in Problem Solving and Conflict Resolution

Whether formal or informal, appointed or shared, leadership can be used to assist the processes central to the functioning of IPP teams, such as problem solving, conflict management, and negotiation (see Chapter 6). Leaders are able to use their communication skills and knowledge of both group processes and team development to support the problem-solving process. In brainstorming, for example, a leader may take on the facilitator role, organizing the processes and monitoring the steps/criteria that the team has identified. Leaders may also apply various techniques and skills, such as providing feedback and utilizing effective listening, in order to help a team and/or patients resolve conflict.

A leader is in the position to positively influence conflict resolution and negotiation by focusing on the contextual and substantive factors we discussed in the previous section. A leader may act as a mediator in the process of negotiation, seeking an amicable solution (Sampson & Marthas, 1990). The role of a mediator is to maintain a neutral stance while acting as a link between parties in conflict. The conflict resolution style of a leader is central to his or her ability to mediate a conflict situation. The style of the leader can influence and bias the process of negotiation and conflict resolution. It is therefore important for a leader to gain an awareness of his or her style of conflict resolution and monitor for any negative influence it may have on the negotiation process.

Leadership and Followership

We cannot discuss leadership without mentioning the concept of followership. The two concepts, although separate, are very interdependent. Further, within a conceptualization of leadership as a shared process among people (or within a team) who are interacting, it becomes virtually impossible to view leadership and followership as distinct. A number of experts in the field of leadership studies have noted that both leaders and followers are important in the process of accomplishing something new; leaders need followers and followers are essential if change is to occur (Bennis, 2006; Campbell & Kinion, 1993; Goffee & Jones, 2006). **Followership**, as the term suggests, is the act of following a leader and involves many of same attributes that are associated with leadership. The roles of leader and follower both involve effective communication skills, visioning, and other elements traditionally ascribed to effective leadership (see discussion below). With such overlap in attributes and characteristics, it is not surprising that within the literature there is a sense of duality when discussing leadership and followership. Followers and leaders should possess the ability to interchange roles as needed and depending on the situation (Campbell & Kinion, 1993; Grossman & Valiga, 2009; Sullivan, 1998). The notion of a leader/follower has particular application to health care professionals who endeavour to work collaboratively. In IPP, team members must be able to dynamically shift from leading when appropriate and/or necessary to stepping aside at other times in order to allow other members to lead. This fluid leadership/followership exchange is something that should happen both willingly and with the commitment to both lead and follow with integrity.

Understanding leadership and one's own leadership capacity is a developmental and iterative process. The ideas related to leadership discussed in this section offer a foundation from which to build an understanding of leadership and to continue to develop a personal leadership approach. In the next section of this chapter, we discuss how these foundational ideas are applied specifically to leadership for IPP.

NEW LEADERSHIP PARADIGM FOR NEW HEALTH CARE

Over the past several decades, there has been much discussion about the chaotic nature of health care systems and the inadequacy of the Newtonian scientific approach that has been applied to respond to the constant changes experienced in these systems (McCallin, 2003; Plsek & Greenhalgh, 2001; Sharp & Priesmeyer, 1995). The scientific approach encourages linear thinking, with a focus on predicting and controlling human systems and behaviours. The influence of this approach is evident in many aspects of health care practice. For example, when providing care, health care teams tend to break problems down into smaller parts, parcelling out these sub-problems to individual professionals on the basis of an assumed accordance between the practitioner's expertise and the nature of the problem. These sub-problems are then addressed by means of rational reasoning and linear problem solving (Plsek & Greenhalgh, 2001). As we discussed in Chapter 6, this approach fails us when, as is often the case, problems are complex, involving unpredictable and unknown variables.

Leadership within the Newtonian scientific paradigm focuses on managing and adapting to change through goal setting, gaining the commitment of others to achieve goals, and decreasing uncertainty (Malloch & Porter-O'Grady, 2009). Newtonian leadership emphasizes a top-down management and control style, which is in keeping with traditional theories and approaches to leadership (Grossman & Valiga, 2009).

The Newtonian scientific paradigm is now seen as increasingly ill suited to address the growing complexity of patient care within a constantly changing health care system. This has led to a search for approaches better aligned with the realities in today's world. Within the literature, many authors have suggested we look to new science, a set of theoretical constructs that include chaos theory and quantum physics, for solutions. These constructs are seen as an appropriate theoretical toolkit for understanding and engaging within health care systems characterized by pacesetting changes, such as system restructuring and redesigns, cost containment strategies, and technological advancements (Grossman & Valiga, 2009; Porter-O'Grady & Malloch, 2007; Sharp & Priesmeyer, 1995; Vicenzi, White, & Begun, 1997; Wheatley, 2006).

The notion of chaos in health care may at first suggest a less than positive picture. However, it is actually a useful tool to both understand the current situation within health care and to consider how leadership within that context can be different. The term **chaos** refers to behaviours so unpredictable that they appear to be random and disorganized (Vicenzi et al., 1997). In health care, as in other systems, the tendency is to respond to unpredictable changes by bracing against the uncertainty (Erçetin & Kamaci, 2008). Burns (2002) highlights, however, that chaos is actually a complex pattern within a system that, despite defying prediction, is not random but determined by the conditions involved in the situation. In many ways, this definition characterizes what we observe in our everyday world today and in health care systems as well. For example, consider the situation in the opening vignette. Anyone involved in similar emergency situations can attest to the informal and seemingly unpredictable nature of events as they unfold. Typically, it may seem virtually impossible to predict the outcomes of the various behaviours being observed. Yet, considered together, these behaviours demonstrate an organized pattern that relates back to the conditions and elements involved in the situation (Burns, 2002).

The application of chaos theory to health care practice and environments represents a radically new and potentially very powerful tool for understanding and dealing with our health care system at all levels. By thinking about, visualizing, and managing patient and health care problems dynamically and nonlinearly, professionals, teams, and organizations can open the door for creative and innovative solutions. Practising and participating in this manner requires professionals to shift their thinking about the environment they work in and how they lead.

The Quantum Leadership Paradigm

Wheatley (2006) argues that if "new science" approaches are to be applied to how we view and manage health care systems, then the same lens should be used in our approach to leadership in this context. To this end, quantum science has become useful in developing a new leadership paradigm that corresponds with the new science view of health care systems

Table 7.3 Leadership Assumptions of Quantum Physics

Assumption	Description
Leadership is an interaction field.	Both leaders and followers participate fully in leadership. Leaders and followers create common ground where they perceive themselves to be working together for a shared vision of future possibilities.
Leadership cannot be structured and estimated.	Leadership requires that we take risks, not knowing or being able to determine for certain the outcome of our actions. Rather than leading to hopelessness, this awareness allows us to create practice that is fluid, with many potential action alternatives rather than hard-and-fast rules.
Discontinuity of leadership is fact.	Leadership is not continuous, and the inevitable turnover in leadership roles is something we should embrace as natural and desirable, rather than something to be avoided. Because leaders are guides, not supervisors, they learn alongside followers and role transition can be fluid.
Impact of leadership depends on interaction.	Leaders can influence followers by force only to a certain extent. Interactions that extend beyond authority and are based in mutual trust, respect, and attachment have a much more potent impact.

Source: Ercetin, S. S., & Kamaci, M. D. (2008). Quantum leadership paradigm. *World Applied Sciences Journal, 3*(6), 865–868.

(see Table 7.3). Malloch and Porter-O'Grady (2009) summarize **quantum science** as a paradigm that views the world around us as a complex grouping of adaptive systems. Quantum science is concerned with understanding complex and intersecting relationships. It "looks at change; how it works, what it means ... [and is] actively interested in adaptation, integration, interaction ... and the continuous dynamics of movement" (Malloch & Porter-O'Grady, 2009, p. 2).

Within the quantum science perspective, there is the recognition that while individuals are important, their collective relationship to a system (e.g., health care system) is more critical. The leadership paradigm the follows from this perspective privileges the interactional relationship between leaders and followers as the foundation for effective leadership (Erçetin & Kamaci, 2008; Malloch & Porter-O'Grady, 2009). The basic tenet of this paradigm is that leadership occurs through an interactional field between followers and leaders that cannot be structured or predicted. Leadership within this context must look for global patterns rather than try to predict what will happen and how to avoid it. It involves working to develop and support skills and alternative actions that will ready individuals for change and foster innovative responses to organizational chaos (Erçetin & Kamaci, 2008).

The quantum leadership paradigm aligns well with contemporary views of leadership discussed in this chapter, emphasizing shared leadership, a leader–follower dualism, the notion that "leadership can be performed by different people at different periods and the call for leadership to support interaction styles that potential goal attainment" (Erçetin & Kamaci, 2008, p. 687). Within this paradigm, leaders and followers do not perceive themselves as different from each other. They both contribute to and are expected to work toward shared goals and address challenges within the system in which they work.

A perspective parallel to quantum leadership is that of *whole system change* (Edwards et al., 2011), which builds on the interdisciplinary field of ecosystems management (Gunderson & Holling, 2002). Whole system change can be defined as "the uneven, nested cycles of adaptation that evolves within closely coupled, complex socio-ecological systems over time" (Edwards et al., 2007, p. 2). The whole system change perspective has a focus on changing and developing what is happening within a human system (e.g., team, organization, community) as a whole and not just components or processes. Engaging systems holistically allows for what is most salient and important at the individual and the collective level. It enables successful promotion of desired changes that are comprehensive.

The complementary nature of quantum leadership and whole system change in scaling up interprofessional teamwork is worth exploring. Quantum leadership launches leaders and followers into a more fluid and unstructured path, creating a shared vision of the possible. In a complementary way, whole system change can insert this new form of leadership into the multiple elements and complex relationships at the system levels.

LEADERSHIP FOR INTERPROFESSIONAL PRACTICE

As we discussed in Chapter 1, the complexity of health care and health care systems today have been key drivers of the movement toward IPP. As an alternative approach to traditional service delivery, IPP emphasizes elements such as teamwork and cooperation that necessitate a radically different perspective on leadership in health care. The following sections focus specifically on leadership concepts and practices as they relate to IPP.

Approaches to Leadership in Interprofessional Practice

Leadership within health care systems has historically been rooted in military and traditional understandings of leadership (McCallin, 2003). McCallin notes that "it is unlikely that models [such as these] that have not worked in the past will be any better in an era of far-reaching social reform where culture is changing and people must learn to think and act differently in a rapidly changing context. This means that ... [interprofessional teams] cannot rely on past models of leadership to facilitate ... team development [and IPP goals]" (p. 366). Leadership for IPP must be responsive to change and aligned with the values of IPP, such as shared accountability for outcomes and key elements of IPP including cooperation, teamwork, problem solving, and negotiation. By a number of accounts (see, e.g., McCallin, 2003; Marquis & Huston, 2009), the forms of leadership most likely to meet these requirements are shared and authentic leadership. Recall that we defined shared leadership as a perspective wherein the various members of a team share responsibility for the team processes and outcomes, while taking on formal and informal leadership roles depending upon the situation. Authentic leadership further enriches a person's effectiveness by his or her working with others to build optimism and confidence, promoting inclusiveness, and fostering transparent relationships that advance commitment (Avolio & Gardner, 2005). Building on this theory, Laschinger and Smith's study found that "new graduates' perceptions of the quality of interprofessional care were related to a combination of higher authentic leadership and structural empowerment" (2013, p. 27).

Although shared leadership provides a broad framework for leadership enactment in IPP, it does not specifically reflect the context within which IPP occurs. In this regard, the new science leadership paradigm may be an even more useful framework. This paradigm incorporates the features of shared leadership and situates leadership within the realities of the current health care environment. The new science paradigm's understanding of the environment directs those involved in IPP to orient themselves differently in relationship to each other and the ongoing changes they experience in their work environments. From this perspective, all members of the IPP health care team must work to understand that "chaos is a good thing because it is what makes us evolve and grow.... [Professionals] will need to be willing to make educated guesses, use their intuition, and be comfortable with uncertainty and ambiguity" (Grossman & Valiga, 2009, p. 116). The new science approach to leadership also acknowledges in a very real way the discontinuity of leadership. It challenges each leader-member of an IPP team to share his or her talents when appropriate and to recognize when others' abilities are better suited to accomplish team goals. Erçetin and Kamaci conclude that when teams manage to share leadership power, the "result of such sharing is the use of everyone's potential, the enrichment of the views and actions, [and] the adoption and administration of decisions made in easier and more effective ways" (2008, p. 867).

Interprofessional Leadership Within the IPP literature, growing attention has been given to the subject of interprofessional or collaborative leadership, specifically to shared leadership, relationship-based leadership, and new science leadership approaches. For example, Shelton and Darling (2001) used basic quantum physics principles and new science leadership paradigm assumptions to develop their quantum skills model. Additionally, Wirrmann and Carlson (2005) apply this model to primary care team practice to suggest new ways leadership in this context can be viewed. They argue that shared leadership in public health (and other areas of practice) requires practitioners to think and act in new ways, which can be achieved through developing "quantum skills." Spotlight 7.1 provides, in a real-world example, a summary of the results of a study exploring the interprofessional role requirements of leadership in relation to discharge planning in a neonatal intensive care unit.

Interprofessional Leadership Competencies and Guidelines We have previously described the CIHC (2010) National Interprofessional Competency Framework, which identifies six competency domains for IPP. According to this framework, collaborative leadership supports a process of shared decision making and leadership, but it also

Spotlight 7.1

Collaborative Leadership: Who Should Lead Discharge Planning Teams?

Collaborative leadership is defined as health care professionals understanding and applying leadership principles that support a collaborative model (CIHC, 2010). Evidence collected from key informant interviews, conducted as part of a case study examining the role of interprofessional collaboration on the discharge planning process in a neonatal intensive care unit, demonstrated the need for a discharge planning team leader.

The role of the discharge planning team leader should be both task-oriented (ensure sure the team is on track with the discharge process) and relationship-oriented (facilitate communication among the discharge planning team members), with equal emphasis on both. A team leader is needed to delegate the discharge-planning task among the different professionals involved in an infant's care. As well, a leader can make sure everyone has an opportunity to communicate ideas, opinions, or concerns. He or she is responsible for coordination of this information, which can then be shared with the physician responsible for the discharge decision.

Source: Manogaran & Gamble, 2011.

assumes that the individual maintains accountability for his or her actions and responsibilities, as defined by one's professional scope of practice (CIHC, 2010). As described within this chapter, collaborative leadership allows for the selection of a leader within a given context depending on the nature of the situation. Whether enacting the role of leader or follower, all members of the interprofessional team are accountable for the processes selected to achieve outcomes. Types of activities that support collaborative leadership are included in Helpful Tools 7.1.

Another helpful tool to support the development of interprofessional leadership is the Registered Nurses' Association of Ontario's (RNAO) evidence-based healthy work environment best practice guideline (PBG) *Developing and Sustaining Interprofessional Health Care: Optimizing Patient, Organizational and Systems Outcomes* (2013). The BPG addresses a gap in the available literature by providing a repository of the best available evidence specific to IPP. It prominently features recommendations for supporting leadership development at the individual, the organizational, and the systems levels (see Additional Resources at the end of this chapter).

Leadership Development Effective team members are capable of leading, following, and perhaps most importantly alternately transitioning between the two states. In order to navigate these various roles, individual practitioners must be aware of their own personal traits and professional values. They must also be able to assess their personal skill sets in relation to key leadership activities, including elements such as creating a shared vision, effective communication, supporting change, stewardship, and developing others. One's own individual capacity for leadership is less about a fixed, innate potential than it is about personal and professional development that requires commitment and ongoing work.

Helpful Tools 7.1

Activities to Support Interprofessional Leadership

The Canadian Interprofessional Health Collaborative's (CIHC) (2010) National Interprofessional Competency Framework suggests the following activities related to leadership that support a collaborative practice model:

- work with others to enable effective patient/client outcomes
- advancement of interdependent working relationships among all participants
- facilitation of effective team processes
- facilitation of effective decision-making
- establishment of a climate for collaborative practice among all participants
- co-creation of a climate for shared leadership and collaborative practice
- application of collaborative decision-making principles
- integration of the principles of continuous quality improvement to work processes and outcomes (p. 15)

Ultimately, every individual develops his or her own style of leadership, which is shaped by influencing factors such as past positive and negative leadership/followership experiences. Just as one's career development requires creation of a deliberate plan based on identified goals, leadership development requires conscious thought and effort. Developing a strategic plan for personal and professional leadership growth based on sound analyses of one's leadership capacity is a good practice. It enables such growth and the likelihood of positive outcomes in practice.

The most effective approaches to leadership development involve the individual, potential informal and formal mentors and guides within the interprofessional team, and the workplace organization. On an ongoing basis, individuals are encouraged to consider their own perspective on leadership, their lifetime experiences with leadership and followership (both within their professional lives and in other less formal roles), and what they perceive as important contributions they can make in this area. Beginning with a focus on self-exploration allows the individual to create a personal action plan that focuses on developing and strengthening necessary competencies.

A number of opportunities emerge routinely from which we can continue to develop our own leadership capacity and leadership skill set. These include, but are not limited to:

- learning about leadership through reading and critical reflection/thinking,
- observing in our workplace or educational environments for demonstrations of effective leadership,

- learning to enact leadership through simulation activities such as practice in a lab setting where coaching and feedback may be provided,
- learning to enact leadership through real-world practicum experiences, including clinical placements and internships,
- reflecting on leadership,
- demonstrating leadership through modelling, and
- nurturing leadership and passing it on by engaging in active teaching (Canadian Nurses Association, 1995; Dickson, 2008; RNAO, 2013a).

Two key resources that health care professionals and teams can use to support leadership development are the RNAO's *Developing and Sustaining Nursing Leadership Best*

Table 7.4 RNAO Framework Recommendations and Example Behaviours

Recommendation	Example Behaviours
Develop personal resources for effective leadership.	■ Exhibit strong professional identity. ■ Reflect upon and take responsibility for growth and development of leadership expertise. ■ Cultivate professional and social supports. ■ Develop leadership skills and build support network.
Build relationships and trust.	■ Reflect on values and goals, sharing them openly. ■ Participate in professional development activities. ■ Communicate with others to determine needs and changes.
Create empowering work environment.	■ Critically reflect on personal use of empowering behaviour. ■ Foster opportunities for individuals to think and learn.
Create a culture that supports knowledge development and integration.	■ Engage with other health care professionals to improve efficiency in existing organizational processes.
Lead and sustain change.	■ Reflect on personal attitudes and skills on change and change management. ■ Critically apply evidence to change initiatives.
Balance competing values and priorities.	■ Separate personal values from professional responsibilities. ■ Be sensitive to multiple pressures including finances, power, and politics. ■ Acknowledge and name conflicting perspectives; understand that cultural diversity influences perspectives.

Source: Registered Nurses' Association of Ontario (RNAO). (2013b). *Developing and sustaining nursing leadership best practice guideline* (2nd ed.). Retrieved from http://www.rnao.org/Storage/16/1067_ BPG_Sustain_Leadership.pdf.

Practice Guideline (BPG) (2013) and the *LEADS in a Caring Environment Capabilities Framework* (Dickson, 2008). Both resources present a research-based model for individuals to use to develop the leadership competencies, attributes, and skills need to address the challenges inherent in providing care as members of IPP teams. The LEADS framework focuses on the capabilities that individuals involved in care at various levels (e.g., health professionals at the point of care) need in order to manage complex issues and situations and to create transformative changes at all levels of the system. Similarly, the RNAO BPG (2013b) focuses on how leadership behaviour can promote healthy work environments and healthy outcomes for the patient/client, the health care provider, the team, the organization, and the system. While the guideline focuses on nursing, analysis of the two models and subsequent further development of the BPG shows that the two models address the same dimensions of leadership and related capabilities.

The RNAO framework (2013b) also outlines a comprehensive approach to leadership development that can be utilized by all health care professionals, not just nurses, to develop their leadership capacity and take action as autonomous practitioners or as part of a team. Table 7.4 lists the personal and leadership recommendations from the RNAO BPG (RNAO, 2013b) and identifies examples of behaviours and attributes of each competency area. Helpful Tools 7.2 lists a number of specific strategies that can help professionals begin to develop and demonstrate the behaviours associated with the evidenced-based leadership practices identified by the RNAO framework. Mentoring and role modelling, two of the most common approaches to leadership development, are worthy of particular note.

Helpful Tools 7.2

Examples of Strategies to Develop Leadership Practice

- Complete formal courses, programs, or workshops focused on leadership development.
- Participate as a member of an action or change project, which integrates leadership and leadership development.
- Attend networking opportunities and conferences (particularly those with a leadership focus) to gain information and referrals and develop contacts to individuals who may be able to provide mentoring and coaching. Networks are often specific to practice or topic areas. Networks may offer support, understanding, and empathy. Conferences, while less intimate, and short-term, offer opportunities to learn, access information, and make new contacts.
- Take the opportunity to observe effective leaders and model your leadership on their evidence-based leadership practice. Review the literature on leadership and reflecting upon leadership experiences.
- Seek feedback from others about your leadership capabilities.
- Identify individuals who demonstrate effective and evidence-based leadership practices and are able to support your own development broadly or within a particular domain. Invite them to be your mentor or coach.

Mentoring and Role Modelling Mentoring and **role modelling** are two of the most common approaches discussed in the literature related to leadership development. Mentors and role models/guides have the potential to provide support as an individual "tries on" leadership opportunities and learns through the process. Role modelling is a form of learning from the experience of others that allows the learner to adopt new behaviours without the trial and error of doing things for him- or herself. Learning in this context occurs by observation and imitation (Murray & Main, 2005).

Role modelling can occur either on its own or as an aspect of **mentoring**, defined as a process involving an experienced individual who provides guidance to a less experienced person. In mentorship, the *mentor* invests considerable time and effort to help the *mentee* advance and grow. This relationship is deliberate and purposeful, and can extend over a number of years. Mentors provide counsel and encouragement, while also challenging mentees toward excellence. They teach by example and modelling, acting as a partner and/or sponsor and providing honest feedback, both positive and constructive.

Interprofessional mentoring is a professional relationship that takes place between various health care providers (or providers and students) who are from different disciplines or health professions. Learning in this context is aimed at helping mentees learn about the roles of other professions and how to work together to provide patient-centred care. Interprofessional mentorship is a relatively new approach to the creation of mentoring relationships. As such, it may at times raise concerns about role conflict and role confusion. It is important to recognize that interprofessional mentoring differs from profession-specific leadership and mentoring, and is not intended to replace these processes and relationships fundamental to professional development. Rather, it is intended to support leadership development for IPP and model the types of collaboration required for team-based practice. Both profession-specific mentorship and mentorship by members of the interprofessional team are critical supports that can make a difference in whether or not someone is willing to accept a leadership role and, just as importantly, in their experience in enacting that role.

Regardless of the approach to leadership in health care practice, the integration and development of leadership competencies as part of the broader process of implementing IPP cannot occur effectively without support at the organizational level and beyond. Ensuring that there are structures and processes within the workplace that allow for leadership opportunities is essential. This type of support and guidance to those seeking to develop leadership skills not only benefits the seekers, but creates a much more cohesive organization overall.

CONCLUSION

The evidence from the vast body of literature related to leadership and human systems leaves very little doubt that leadership is integral to providing quality care and sustaining a health system. The focus on IPP and IPP teams, coupled with the increasing complexity of providing care, has generated cause for consideration of leadership within the health system. Of particular interest is the kind of leadership necessary to drive change and optimize outcomes for patients, practitioners, organizations, and the system. The emerging consensus is that leadership must move beyond traditional perspectives toward theory and practice that is more aligned with the complexities of the concept itself and of the contexts in which it must be enacted.

In the context of IPP and IPP teams, effective leadership must reflect elements such as relationship, partnership, cooperation, and shared decision making. The personal and professional leadership development of IPP team members forms the foundation for interprofessional leadership. This chapter outlines a number of contemporary theories and perspectives about leadership such as the shared leadership framework and the quantum science paradigm. Although they may differ in one respect or another, the complementary nature of these ideas creates an overarching framework and toolkit to support interprofessional leadership practices.

SUMMARY

- Leadership is both important and necessary to interprofessional team functioning. Developing a common conceptualization of leadership in IPP contexts may be challenging given barriers such as professional socialization, professional boundaries, and the division of work among health care professionals.
- Leadership is process-oriented and requires the collective effort of all team members. It involves guiding, organizing, directing, coordinating, supporting, and motivating others. Leadership in health care generally takes the form of either leadership by virtue of being appointed/elected to a specific role (e.g., unit manager) or shared leadership based on an appreciation of the specific leadership needs within the presenting situation and the leadership competencies available within the IPP team.
- Leadership requires vision, strong communication skills, change, stewardship, and developing and renewing others. Both leadership and followership are important in the process of accomplishing something new.
- Traditional leadership perspectives focus on the innate traits of the individual leaders, whereas more contemporary leadership theory shifts attention to the capacity of the entire team, positing that effective leadership requires different strategies at different times.
- More recently the conceptualization of leadership has shifted to focus on the relational aspects, acknowledging that leadership is process-oriented and requires equal engagement by leaders and followers. Relationship-based theories of leadership include transformational leadership theory, relational leadership theory, and authentic leadership theory.
- The quantum science of leadership is emerging as a framework for leadership in IPP. Within a quantum science perspective, there is recognition that while the

individuals are important, the collective relationship to a system (e.g., health care system) is more critical.

- Effective team members lead, follow, and transition between the two states. Individual practitioners must be aware of their own personal traits and professional values as they embark upon leadership activities. They must also be able to assess their personal skill sets and capitalize on opportunities for personal and professional leadership development.

Key Terms

authentic leadership
change
chaos
contemporary leadership
developing and renewing others
followership
functional or style leadership
interprofessional mentoring
leadership
mentoring
quantum science
relational leadership theory
role modelling
shared leadership
situational leadership
stewardship
traditional leadership
vision

Review Questions

1. Define leadership and followership and describe the relationship between these two concepts.
2. Compare and contrast traditional leadership perspectives with the "new science" or quantum leadership paradigm.
3. Describe several strategies for leadership development.

Application Exercises

1. Consider the health care environment with which you are most familiar, perhaps where you have completed a practicum placement or where you are working. What leadership roles are you able to identify? Are these roles reflective of shared leadership practices, or are the leaders appointed/elected? What do you think might result, both in a positive and a negative way, if these roles were filled in ways other than is current practice?
2. The RNAO BPG on developing and sustaining nursing leadership (RNAO, 2013b) offers a systematic approach to plan leadership development. Using the guidelines along with the LEADS framework and suggested strategies in Helpful Tools 7.2, create a personalized leadership development plan for the upcoming year.

Additional Resources

Websites/Electronic Documents

LEADS in a Caring Environment Capabilities Framework
http://chlnet.ca/wp-content/uploads/leads_genesis.pdf

Additional Readings

Books

Hibberd, J. M., & Smith, D. L. (2006). *Nursing leadership and management in Canada* (3rd ed.). Toronto: Mosby Books.

References

Avolio, B. J., & Gardner, W. L. (2005). Authentic leadership development: Getting to the root of positive forms of leadership. *Leadership Quarterly, 16*, 315–338.

Bass, B. M. (1990). *Bass & Stogdill's handbook of leadership*. Basingstoke, UK: The Free Press, Macmillan.

Bennis, W. (2006). The end of leadership: Exemplary leadership is impossible without full inclusion, initiatives, and cooperation of followers. In W. E. Rosenbach & R. L. Taylor (Eds.), *Contemporary leadership issues* (6th ed., pp. 129–142). Boulder, CO: Westview Press.

Bennis, W., & Nanus, B. (1985). *Leaders: The strategies for taking charge*. New York: Harper & Row.

Buck, K., & McPherson, B. (2006). Co-creating the space for change: Through dialogue, ministry leaders will find confidence to move into the future. *Health Progress, 87*(3), 62–65.

Burns, J. S. (2002). Chaos theory and leadership studies: Exploring uncharted seas. *Journal of Leadership & Organizational Studies, 9*, 42–56.

Campbell, J. S., & Kinion, E. S. (1993). Teaching leadership/followership to RN-to-MSN students. *Journal of Nursing Education, 32*(3), 138–140.

Canadian Interprofessional Health Collaborative (CIHC). (2010). *A national interprofessional competency framework*. Vancouver, BC: Author.

Canadian Nurses Association. (1995). *Preceptorship resource guide. Teaching and learning with clinical role models*. Ottawa: Authors.

Clements, D., Dault, M., & Priest, A. (2007). Effective teamwork in healthcare: Research and reality. *Healthcare Papers 7*(Spec. Issue), 26–34.

Collins-Nakai, R. (2006). Leadership in medicine. *McGill Journal of Medicine: MJM, 9*(1), 68–73.

Cummings, G. G., MacGregor, T., Davey, M., Lee, H. P., Wong, C., Lo, E., Muise, M., & Stafford, E. (2010). Leadership styles and outcome patterns for the nursing workforce and work environment: A systematic review. *International Journal of Nursing Studies, 47*, 363–385.

Dickson, G. (2008). *Genesis of the leaders for life framework*. Retrieved from http://chlnet.ca/wp-content/uploads/leads_genesis.pdf

Duffy, D., Gordon, G., Whelan, G., Cole-Kelly, K., & Frankel, R. (2004). Assessing competence in communication and interpersonal skills: The Kalamazoo II report. *Academic Medicine, 79*(6), 495–507.

Edwards, N., Marck, P., Virani, T., Davies, B., & Rowan, M. (2007). *Whole system change in health care: Implications for evidence-informed nursing service delivery models*. Ottawa: University of Ottawa.

Edwards, N., Rowan, M., Marck, P., & Grinspun, D. (2011). Understanding whole systems change in health care: The case of the Nurse Practitioners in Canada. *Policy, Politics, & Nursing, 12*(1), 4–17.

Erçetin, S. S., & Kamaci, M. D. (2008). Quantum leadership paradigm. *World Applied Sciences Journal, 3*(6), 865–868.

Evetts, J. (1999). Professionalisation and professionalism: Issues for interprofessional care. *Journal of Interprofessional Care, 13*, 119–128.

Foels, R., Driskell, J. E., Mullen, B., & Salas, E. (2000). The effects of democratic leadership on group member satisfaction: An integration. *Small Group Research, 31*, 676–701.

Forsyth, D. R. (2006). *Group dynamics* (4th ed.). Belmont, CA: Thomson/Wadsworth.

Galuska, L. (2012). Cultivating nursing leadership for our envisioned future. *Advances in Nursing Science, 35*(4), 333–345.

Goertzen, B. J. (2013). Chapter 6: Contemporary theories of leadership. In D. T. Foster, C. Nollette, C., F. P. Nollete, & B. J. Goertzen (Eds.), *Emergency services leadership: A contemporary approach* (pp. 83–100). Burlington, MA: Jones & Bartlett Learning.

Goffee, R., & Jones, G. (2006). *Why should anyone be led by you? What it takes to be an authentic leader*. Boston, MA: Harvard Business School Publishing.

Grinspun, D. (2007). Healthy workplaces: The case for shared clinical decision making and increased full-time employment. *Healthcare Papers, 7*(Spec. Issue), 69–75.

Grinspun, D. (2010). *The social construction of caring in nursing* [doctoral dissertation]. York University, Toronto.

Grossman, S. C., & Valiga, T. M. (2009). *The new leadership challenge: Creating the future of nursing* (3rd ed.). Philadelphia, PA: F. A. Davis Company.

Gunderson, L. H., & Holling, C. S. (2002). *Panarchy: Understanding transformations in human and natural systems*. Washington, DC: Island Press.

Hall, P., & Weaver, L. (2001). Interdisciplinary education and teamwork: Long and winding road. *Medical Education, 35*(9), 867–875.

Hall, P., Weaver, L., Handfield-Jones, R., & Bouvette, M. (2008). Developing leadership in rural interprofessional palliative care teams. *Journal of Interprofessional Care, 22*(S1), 73–79.

Kouses, J. M., & Posner, D. Z. (1995). *The leadership challenge: How to keep getting extraordinary things done in organizations*. San Francisco: Jossey-Bass.

Laschinger, H. K. S., & Smith, L. M. (2013). The influence of authentic leadership and empowerment on new graduate nurses' perceptions of interprofessional collaboration. *Journal of Nursing Administration, 43*(1), 24–29.

Lewin, K., Lippitt, R., and White, R. K. (1939). Patterns of aggressive behavior in experimentally created social climates. *Journal of Social Psychology,* 10, 271–301.

Luthans, F., & Avolio, B. J. (2003). Authentic leadership: A positive development approach. In K. S. Camerson, J. E. Dutton, & R. E. Quinn (Eds.), *Positive organizational scholarship* (pp. 241–261). San Francisco, CA: Barrett-Koehler.

Malloch, K., & Porter-O'Grady, T. (2009). *The quantum leader: Applications for the new world of work*. Sudbury, MA: Jones and Bartlett.

Manogaran, M., & Gamble, B. (2011 November). *The role of interprofessional collaboration on the discharge planning process in the neonatal intensive care unit*. Collaborating Across Borders III, 3rd Biennial Interprofessional

Educational Conference, Tucson, AR, November 2011.

Marquis, B. L., & Huston, C. J. (2009). *Leadership roles and management functions in nursing* (6th ed.). Philadelphia, PA: Lippincott, Williams & Wilkins.

Martin, V., & Rogers, A. (2004). *Leading interprofessional teams in health and social care*. London: Routledge.

McCallin, A. (2003). Interdisciplinary team leadership: A revisionist approach for an old problem? *Journal of Nursing Management, 11*(6), 364–370

Metcalfe, S. (2009). *Cengage Advantage Books: Building a speech* (7th ed.). Boston, MA: Wadworth Publishing.

Murray, C. J., & Main, A. (2005). Role modeling as a teaching method for student mentors *Nursing Times, 101*(36). Retrieved from http://www.nursingtimes.net

Myers, S. A., & Anderson, C. M. (2008). *The fundamentals of small group communication*. Thousand Oaks, CA: Sage Publications.

Øvretveit, J. (1990). Making the team work! *Professional Nurse, 5*, 284–288.

Pearce, C. L., & Conger, J. A. (2003). All those years ago: The historical underpinnings of shared leadership. In C. L. Pearce & J. A. Conger (Eds.), *Shared leadership: Reframing the hows and whys of leadership* (pp. 1–18). Thousand Oaks, CA: Sage.

Plsek, P. E., & Greenhalgh, T. (2001). The challenge of complexity in health care. *BMJ, 323*(7313), 625–628.

Porter-O'Grady, T. (2003). A different age for leadership part 2: New rules, new roles. *Journal of Nursing Administration, 33*(3), 173–178.

Porter-O'Grady, T., & Malloch, K. (2007). *Quantum leadership: A resource for health care innovation* (2nd ed.). Sudbury, MA: Jones & Bartlett.

Redfern, L. (2008). The challenge of leadership. *Nursing Management, 15*(4), 10–12.

Reeves, S., MacMillan, K., & van Soeren, M. (2010). Leadership of interprofessional health and social care teams: A sociohistorical analysis. *Journal of Nursing Management, 18*, 258–264.

Registered Nurses' Association of Ontario (RNAO). (2013a). *Developing and sustaining interprofessional health care: Optimizing patient, organizational, and systems outcomes*. Retrieved from http://umanitoba.ca/programs/interprofessional/media/IPC_Summary.pdf

Registered Nurses' Association of Ontario (RNAO). (2013b). *Developing and sustaining nursing leadership best practice guideline* (2nd ed.). Retrieved from http://www.rnao.org/Storage/16/1067_BPG_Sustain_Leadership.pdf

Rogers, A., & Reynolds, J. (2003). Leadership and vision. In J. Sedan & R. Reynolds (Eds.), *Managing care in practice* (pp. 57–82). London: Routledge.

Ross, F., O'Tuathail, C., & Stubberfield, D. (2005). Towards multidisciplinary assessment of older people: Exploring the change process. *Journal of Clinical Nursing, 14*, 518–529.

Sampson, E. E., & Marthas, M. (1990). *Group process for the health professions* (3rd ed.). Albany, NY: Delmar Thompson Learning.

Sergiovanni, T. J. (2007). Leadership as stewardship. In *Rethinking leadership: A collection of articles* (2nd ed., pp. 49–60). Thousand Oaks, CA: Corwin Press.

Sharp, L. F., & Priesmeyer, H. R. (1995). Tutorial: Chaos theory: A primer for health care. *Quality Management in Health Care, 3*(4), 71–85.

Shelton, C. K., & Darling, J. R. (2001). The quantum skills model in management: A new paradigm to enhance effective leadership. *Leadership and Organization Development Journal, 22*(6), 264–273.

Shirey, M. R. (2009). Authentic leadership, organizational culture, and healthy work environments. *Critical Care Nursing Quarterly, 32*(3), 189–198.

Sullivan, T. J. (1998). *Collaboration: A health care imperative*. New York, NY: McGraw Hill.

Thornberry, N. (2006). A view about "vision." In W. E. Rosenbach & R. L. Taylor (Eds.), *Contemporary issues in leadership* (6th ed., pp. 31–43). Boulder, CO: Westview Press.

Uhl-Bien, M. (2006). Relational leadership theory: Exploring the social processes of leadership and organizing. *Leadership Quarterly, 17*, 654–676.

Vicenzi, A. E., White, K. R., & Begun, J. W. (1997). Chaos in nursing: Make it work for you. *American Journal of Nursing, 97*(10), 26–31.

Wheatley, M. (2006). *Leadership and the new science: Discovering order in a chaotic world* (3rd ed.). San Francisco: Berrett-Koehler Publishers, Inc.

Willumsen, E. (2006). Leadership in interprofessional collaboration: The case of childcare in Norway. *Journal of Interprofessional Care, 20*(4), 403–413.

Wirrmann, E. J., & Carlson, C. L. (2005). Public health leadership in primary care practice in England: Everybody's business? *Critical Public Health, 15*(3), 205–217.

Wong, C. A., & Cummings, G. G. (2009). Authentic leadership: A new theory for nursing or back to basics? *Journal of Health Organization and Management, 23*(5), 522–38.

Yuki, G. (2002). *Leadership in organizations* (6th ed.). Upper Saddle River, NJ: Prentice Hall, Inc.

Part III
Issues in Interprofessional Care

Part III of this book builds on foundational concepts presented throughout the first seven chapters. Exploring in greater detail the complexities of interprofessional practice (IPP), our focus shifts to the contexts within which it is taught, practised, and evaluated. Concepts central to IPP are applied to a range of practice situations and involving a wide variety of health care providers, increasingly highlighting the unique aspects of IPP and the potential it holds to positively impact health care delivery and health care outcomes in Canada.

Chapter 8 provides the reader with an important examination of interprofessional education (IPE). While continuing to evolve, IPE is one of the most widely cited areas of development relating to IPP. Understanding the roots of the IPE movement and the directions that show the greatest promise is important in setting the stage for future advances. Chapter 9 shifts gears, exploring policy and regulation for IPP. Within the context of health care in Canada, understanding the very significant implications of a change in practice, such as that encapsulated by IPP, including legal and regulatory implications, is critical for all health care providers. Finally, Chapter 10 focuses on evaluation in the context of IPP and emerging evidence related to health care outcomes. The chapter provides an overview of key concepts related to evaluation in general, and more specifically evaluation methods and approaches that have been applied to IPP settings and situations.

Chapter 8

Interprofessional Education for Interprofessional Practice

Interprofessional rounds are a common practice on the Neonatal Intensive Care Unit (NICU) of a large Canadian teaching hospital. During this weekly meeting, health care professionals on the unit come together to discuss the discharge plans of each infant on a case-by-case basis. In this week's meeting, the staff physician identifies Baby Johnson as ready for discharge.

Carlos Williams (staff physician): Baby Johnson has been doing pretty well this week. All his tests have come back negative and his progress has been pretty steady this week. He is ready for discharge. Please make the necessary preparations.

Heather (occupational therapist): Sorry, excuse me, Dr. Williams, but I'm not sure that Baby Johnson is really ready for discharge this week or next week. I've been monitoring his feeds and he hasn't even reached the halfway mark of his feeding target.

Carlos: Well, I don't think that his feeds should be much of a problem. We have to take into consideration his bigger health issues. Considering he's been steady in those domains, we should discharge him and make room for another infant in need.

Celina (discharge coordinator): According to the resources that he'll need, there's only one pediatric unit close to his hometown that can take him in as a patient. However, their requirement is that his feeds are at the appropriate level. So we really should take into consideration his feeding level before discharging him.

Myuri (social worker): I'm also concerned that we haven't brought the Johnson family into this discussion yet. I don't think they're prepared for his transfer out of the unit this quickly.

Carlos: I hear what you are all saying, but I don't think it should take too long to bring his feeding levels up. We should see improvement this week and be able discharge him next week at the latest. That should give everyone plenty of time to get ready.

Heather: Dr. Williams, I haven't had much luck with him lately and it's taking him a really long time to get used to sucking. I think it will take him a couple more weeks to get anywhere near the half mark. I'm also a little concerned that we're making this decision without input from the whole team. Humberto is the charge nurse today but when I passed him on my way in he was busy helping one of the nurses with a sick baby and didn't think he'd be able to make it in to this meeting. Maybe we should wait until everyone can meet to talk about this discharge?

Carlos: Heather, I think if we all work on Baby Johnson more frequently, this week should be possible for discharge. OK, what's next on the agenda?

Rezsponding to Carlos' prompt, the team moves on to discuss other patient issues. Shortly after the meeting, Heather strikes up a conversation with Celina about the interaction during the meeting related to Baby Johnson's feeding level.

Heather: I can't believe what went on in there. I mean, does he [Dr. Williams] really think the baby will learn to suck and bring his feeding to level in a matter of days?

Celina: I agree with your assessment; however, Dr. Williams seems to believe he has a good sense about the timing to get feedings to level.

Heather: I know. But really, I think I'm the expert on feeding. He should take the time to listen to what I have to say and give consideration to the fact that I have more knowledge in this area than he does. They really need to have education for the physicians on the roles of the different health care professions. It's probably the only way we can set things on the right track and work to eliminate this stress.

Celina: I don't disagree with you, but come to think of it, I don't know if it's just a physician issue. Can any of us on the team seriously say we understand what the other person's role is beyond the generic descriptions of our professions? I think we could all benefit from a little education about each other and how to work together.

Heather: (smiling) Celina, you may be onto something there!

Learning Outcomes

After studying this chapter, you should be able to:

1. **Define interprofessional education.**
2. **Identify key elements of interprofessional education.**
3. **Describe examples of interprofessional education projects in Canada.**
4. **Summarize the benefits and challenges associated with interprofessional education.**

INTRODUCTION

Health and human services systems worldwide are searching for solutions to a number of health system challenges, such as family and community health, infectious disease, noncommunicable diseases, mental illness, humanitarian crises, and the shortage of health human services workers. As we have previously discussed in this book, interprofessional practice (IPP) is seen as key to improving health system performance (Ladden, Bednash, Stevents, & Moore, 2006). The patient or the client is at the centre of IPP (Gilbert, 2005b; Health Canada, 2007) with the goal of improving patient satisfaction and improving patient outcomes. The successful implementation of IPP is dependent upon health and human services workers being properly prepared to meet these challenges today and into the future (Greiner & Knebel, 2003). To this end, changing the way health and human services workers are educated and trained is a key strategy. This being so, many observers have advocated for the formal incorporation of educational approaches that will prepare health professionals with the knowledge and skills necessary to engage successfully in IPP.

At the same time, the education and the training of health and human services workers have become increasingly challenging and complex over the past century (Mitka, 2010). The Flexner Report, released over 100 years ago, served as a catalyst to transform the education of medical students from an apprenticeship model of education to one that incorporated scientific knowledge into a formalized education system. Since that time, education and training programs have evolved to meet the health system challenges and the proliferation of new health care professions (Frenk et al., 2010).

Ideally the scenario in the opening vignette would have been different if all health care workers involved in the care of Baby Johnson were working collaboratively. However, as discussion between Heather, the occupational therapist, and Celina, the discharge coordinator, highlights, health care professionals (HCPs) have historically been trained in silo-based educational models that do not incorporate interprofessional learning and the development of related knowledge and skills. Thankfully the educational silos of yesterday are being dismantled as IPP gains greater acceptance as a best-practice approach to providing quality and safe health care.

Interprofessional education (IPE) provides the opportunity and the tools for learners and practitioners to gain the skills necessary to participate in IPP (World Health Organization [WHO], 2010). An important goal of IPE programs is to provide an environment that promotes the respect and recognition of the knowledge and skills of each HCP. Only then will each professional have an equal opportunity to participate in IPP (Barr & Low, 2011).

The World Health Organization (WHO) (2010) has identified the following educational benefits of IPE:

- students have real world experience,
- staff from a range of professions provide input into an educational program development,

- students learn about the work of other health and human services workers,
- IPE fosters respect among the workers, eliminates harmful stereotypes, and
- IPE evokes a patient-centred ethic in practice.

IPE provides learners with the skills, knowledge, and experience they will need to become part of an IPP workforce.

The aim of this chapter is to foster an introductory understanding of IPE and the processes involved, and an appreciation of the importance of IPE to the IPP agenda. The chapter reviews key concepts related to IPE; explores how IPE programs are developed, implemented, and evaluated; and provides an overview of the issues, challenges, and enablers of the IPE process. Within the chapter a number of examples of IPE programs and initiatives within the Canadian context are also highlighted.

DEFINING INTERPROFESSIONAL EDUCATION

Many different definitions of IPE exist. Table 8.1 provides a sample of the those most common within the literature. The Canadian Interprofessional Health Collaborative (CIHC), a Health Canada–funded initiative that works to promote interprofessional education across Canada (CIHC, 2009), conducted an extensive literature review on IPE and concluded that there was a lack of clarity surrounding the concept of IPE (CIHC, 2007). The report found that while many of the IPE definitions share commonalities, the interchangeability of the terms used often results in different interpretations. Needed is a standard definition to allow for clarity within and across health professions and jurisdictions. On the basis of their findings, the CIHC has adopted the definition of IPE used by the Centre for the Advancement of Interprofessional Education (CAIPE). CAIPE is recognized as an organization that supports the development and implementation of IPE worldwide. CAIPE (2011) defines IPE thus: "two or more professions learn with, from and about each other to improve collaboration and the quality of care" (para. 1). The term "professions" here is meant to be inclusive, recognizing that a variety of health and human services workers are involved in the delivery of interprofessional collaborative practice. The CAIPE definition is recognized worldwide and is used as the standard definition in this book.

Defining IPE is a key step in developing an understanding of IPE; however, it is also important and helpful to be clear about what does not represent IPE. The following are examples of situations, activities and/or initiatives that are not considered IPE:

- A classroom made up of learners from different professional streams receiving the same learning experience without reflective interaction (Freeth, Hammick, Reeves, Koppel, & Barr, 2005)
- An educator from a different professional background than learners (e.g., physiotherapist educator speaking to a class of nursing students) leading a learning experience without relating how the professions would collaborate to deliver care (Buring et al., 2009)

Table 8.1 Definitions of Interprofessional Education

Source	Definition
Centre for the Advancement of Interprofessional Education (CAIPE, 2011)	"Two or more professions learn with, from and about each other to improve collaboration and the quality of care" (para. 1).
World Health Organization (1988)	"The process by which a group of students or workers from the health-related occupations with different backgrounds learn together during certain periods of their education, with interaction as the important goal, to collaborate in providing promotive, preventive, curative, rehabilitative, and other health-related services" (p. 769).
American Association of Colleges of Pharmacy (AACP) Interprofessional Education Task Force (2009) [Buring et al.]	"Interprofessional education involves educators and learners from 2 or more health professions and their foundational disciplines who jointly create and foster a collaborative learning environment. The goal of these efforts is to develop knowledge, skills and attitudes that result in interprofessional team behaviors and competence. Ideally, interprofessional education is incorporated throughout the entire curriculum in a vertically and horizontally integrated fashion" (para. 5).
George Brown College (2013)	"Interprofessional Education (IPE) involves learning about, from and with each other, and sharing our different perspectives while learning together in areas of common interest in the practice of health care."

Sources: Definition from "*Interprofessional Education*". Published by Centre For The Advancement Of Interprofessional Education (CAIP), © 2011.

Reproduced with the permission of the publisher, from Report of a *WHO Study Group on Multiprofessional Education of Health Personnel*, World Health Organization Technical Report Series, Geneva, World Health Organization, 1998. (http://whqlibdoc.who.int/trs/WHO_TRS_769.pdf)

Definition from *Interprofessional Education: Definitions, Student Competencies, and Guidelines for Implementation*, American Journal of Pharmaceutical Education Volume 73 Issue 4 Article 59. Copyright © 2009 by American Journal of Pharmaceutical Education. Used by permission of American Journal of Pharmaceutical Education.

- Learners participating in clinical training led by a clinical educator from a profession not representative of those participating in the training without discussing shared decision making or an approach to collaborative practice (Greiner & Knebel, 2003)

It is also important to understand the difference between *interprofessional* and *intraprofessional* practice. A number of profession-specific groups have expanded to include support workers (e.g., Occupational Therapist Assistants), specialty areas of practice (e.g., specialties in medicine: emergency medicine, family medicine, etc.), and changing division of labour within a profession (e.g., Registered Nurses and Registered Practical

Nurses). Intraprofessional collaborative practice occurs when health workers from the same professional group collaborate to provide patient-centred care. For example, Occupational Therapists collaborate with Occupational Therapist Assistants to enhance the quality of occupational therapy services (Dillon, 2002). Similar education and training opportunities are required for both interprofessional and intraprofessional practitioners to enhance the understanding of each other's roles and to describe their own scope of practice to colleagues and the general public (Greiner & Knebel, 2003).

INTEGRATING OF INTERPROFESSIONAL EDUCATION IPE INTO THE LEARNING PROCESS

The CAIPE definition of IPE implies that it is process-driven. Integrating IPE into learning processes in academia and practice environments requires attention to a number of key considerations and the processes of planning, implementing, and evaluating programs and initiatives.

Timing of Interprofessional Education

Debate surrounds when is the best time to introduce IPE into the curriculum and the learning experience (Carlisle, Cooper, & Watkins, 2004; Margalit et al., 2009). Historically, training and educational models for the health professions have been designed to train each profession separately (i.e., **uni-professional education** or *silo education*) (University of British Columbia [UBC], n.d.). Each professional group is socialized into a particular area of expertise and knowledge, and to varying degrees learns to become protective of its role (Downes, 2001; Hall, 2005). Some observers suggest that for IPE to be successful it is important that students first develop a professional identity and role clarity prior to engaging in IPE and, subsequently, IPP. Other scholars and practitioners have argued that IPE should be incorporated into the learning experience at the very beginning of educational and training programs. Proponents of this perspective believe this helps prevent the establishment of negative stereotypes of other health care workers and resistance to IPP (WHO, 2010). The view taken in this text is that IPE is an ongoing process that ideally begins once an individual enters an educational program for training in the chosen discipline and continues throughout his or her entire career. Thus, IPE may be introduced to students newly admitted into a professional program or within practice environments and situations such as the scenario in the opening vignette. Further, regardless of when IPE is introduced, it is important that other factors influencing successful integration, such as support and the use of tools to guide the process, are taken into consideration.

Support for Interprofessional Education

Within the Canadian context there is growing support and commitment for IPE from all levels of government and education and practice sectors. Building on the momentum generated by a number of important works such as Commissioner Roy Romanow's report

Building on Values: The Future of Health Care in Canada, in 2003 the federal government, as part of a broader health human resources strategy, committed funding to an interdisciplinary education for collaborative patient-centred practice (IECPCP) initiative (Herbert, 2005). The IECPCP initiative was "designed to facilitate and support the implementation of an approach to interprofessional education for collaborative patient-centred practice across all health care sectors. The overall goals of the initiative [were] to contribute to improved patient satisfaction, increase patient and provider satisfaction and, ultimately, improved patient outcomes" (Herbert, 2005, p. 2). A total of 20 initiatives were funded across Canada for a period of five years. While these projects varied, the majority focused on integrating IPE into curricula in university and college programs (CIHC, 2009).

Since the closing of the IECPCP initiative, there has been a steady increase in IPE programs, initiatives, and focused activities, some funded, in academia and in practice environments. Across Canada it is now commonplace to find IPE programs and initiatives at varying levels of integration in academic institutions and health care settings of all jurisdictions (see examples within the chapter and in the Additional Resources section at the end of this chapter).

Frameworks for Interprofessional Education

A number of frameworks have been proposed to advance the integration of IPE into curricula and practice environments. D'Amour and Oandasan (2005) have developed a framework for IECPCP that focuses on the interdependent relationship between IPE and IPP. The IECPCP framework describes the main factors, determinants, and elements of IECPCP at three conceptual levels (micro, meso, and macro) and represents interprofessional educational processes and IPP as separate but interconnected components (D'Amour & Oandasan, 2005). The appeal of the IECPCP framework is that it "provides a necessary foundation to consider ... the determinants and processes necessary for moving IECPCP forward across international borders" (Oandasan & Reeves, 2005, p. 45). The IECPCP framework has also been useful as an evaluation tool to map and classify outcome measurement strategies (CIHC, 2007).

With regard to the development of educational programs and initiatives, Oandasan and Reeves (2005) have described a conceptual framework for educators and administrators to use during planning and implementation. The framework is situated within the broader IECPCP framework and focuses on the learner as the centre of the IPE process, with the educator directly influencing the learner. The conceptual framework's inclusion of internal (values and belief) and external (the context) factors emphasizes that IPE initiatives must take these factors into consideration and address them in the planning process of a program or initiative (Oandasan & Reeves, 2005).

Moving beyond the conceptual level, other frameworks have been proposed that provide a blueprint for IPE project and program planning and implementation. For example, Nasmith, Oandasan, and colleagues (as cited by the Centre for Interprofessional

Education, University of Toronto, 2010) developed a series of questions intended to assist developers design their IPE projects (see Additional Resources), and D'Eon (2004) has described several approaches to interprofessional learning.

Development of Interprofessional Education Programs and Initiatives

Several key elements are necessary for the successful development, implementation, delivery, and evaluation of IPE programs: (a) identification of the principles or goals of the IPE program, (b) establishment of the curriculum, (c) identification of effective methods of delivery, (d) definition of the educational needs of the trainers, and (e) evaluation of the IPE programs.

Identification of Principles A first step is to define a set of principles (or goals) that create the foundation for the IPE program. To support academia- and workplace-based initiatives in this critical first step, CAIPE has established IPE principles that draw upon the literature in this area and its members' experiences, and focus on values, process, and outcomes (Barr & Low, 2011).

Establishment of Curricula The curriculum design and assessment of an educational program for health care professionals should be based on competency-based models (Greiner & Knebel, 2003) that "capture the knowledge, the skills, and the attitudes and behaviours" (CIHC, 2010, p. 7) required to become a successful practitioner in the context of IPE. Competencies for uni-professional education are generally well defined, measurable, and incorporated into profession-specific curricula. However, as noted, this type of culture is not well suited to developing the competencies and knowledge necessary to work collaboratively. In fact, silo-based educational models foster attitudes (e.g., professional tribalism) that hinder IPP by establishing unequal power relations and negative stereotypes about collaborative practice with other professionals (Fagin & Garelick, 2004).

As a result, a competency-based model of IPE is needed (Barr, 1998) to inform and build IPE curricula (CIHC, 2010). The identification and the establishment of IPP competencies have proven to be challenging. A number of different institutions and associations have established lists of interprofessional competencies. While similarities do exist, the lack of standardization in how the competencies are presented can lead to different interpretations. These differences can be largely attributed to "discipline-specific goals and variations in terminologies used" (CIHC, 2007, p. 15).

In Canada, the CIHC National Interprofessional Competency Framework is emerging as a useful practical tool for developing interprofessional education programs and activities (e.g., Bainbridge, Nasmith, Orchard, & Wood, 2010). The CIHC competency framework builds on a number of Canadian jurisdictional competency frameworks, integrating the best evidence and practice literature in this area of study (CIHC, 2010). As previously discussed in this book, the CIHC competency framework identifies six interprofessional competency domains: interprofessional communication; patient, client, family, or community-centred care; role clarification; team functioning; collaborative leadership; and interprofessional conflict resolution. Within the framework, the domains of interprofessional communication and patient, client, family, or community-centred care support and influence the other four domains. Unlike other such frameworks, competence in the CIHC framework is determined not by a list of objective and observable behaviours but by the ability to integrate knowledge, skills, attitudes, and values in arriving at judgments (CIHC, 2010). Additionally, the structure of framework makes it adaptable to the context of the learning experience, building on the level of experience and expertise of the learners.

Identification of Effective Delivery Methods The implementation of IPP competencies into curricula can be accomplished through a variety of learning opportunities including but not limited to problem-based learning (PBL), special study modules, self-directed learning, clinical practicums, simulation laboratories, and case studies (HealthForceOntario, 2010). As noted previously, IPE may take place pre- and post-licensure. Accordingly, where and when IPE occurs can also vary (e.g., basic training programs, postgraduate programs, continuing professional development, and learning for quality service improvement). In a growing number of health care settings, particularly those with a teaching focus, IPE departments have been established that coordinate and collaborate with other workplace educational departments (e.g., nursing and medical education) to provide continuing education opportunities. Assuming that the hospital in the opening vignette has established an IPE department, Heather, the occupational therapist, and Celina, the discharge coordinator, with the team's support, might initiate the involvement of this department to help address the IPP challenges highlighted in the scenario.

Definition of Trainers' Educational Needs The education and the training of health care professionals involves both in-classroom instruction and on-the-job training in clinical placements in hospitals, the community, and the home settings. As a result, there is a need for faculty and health care professional staff development initiatives and activities so that these trainers have the information and skills needed to plan IPE programs and facilitate IPE (Steinert, 2005; WHO, 2010). This is especially true for those responsible for clinical training. In a study focusing on the perspectives of physical therapy clinical instructors (CIs) about IPE, Chau, Denomme, Murray, and Cott (2011) found that CIs felt they lacked knowledge about the educational institution's IPE curriculum, support, and direction regarding the expectation for IPE in the clinical environment. One way to address the needs of in-class and clinical faculty is to provide—independently or as part of existing orientation and professional development programs and initiatives—structured and topic-focused continuing education opportunities and sessions (Reeves, Goldman, & Oandasan, 2007). These might be delivered as a joint venture between academic programs and clinical placement environments such as teaching hospitals. Spotlight 8.1 provides an example of an educational opportunity for trainers working within a community context.

Spotlight 8.1

Training the Trainer

Faculty at the University of Ontario Institute of Technology, funded by a HealthForceOntario (2010) grant, developed and delivered a series of workshops for community managers/leaders. The objective was to build capacity and develop strategies needed to optimize IPP for the delivery of senior care in the community. Key to the success of the workshops was the use of simulation-based case studies, open discussion with guiding questions supplemented by presentations, and peer-reviewed articles to help frame the challenges and benefits of IPP at the provider, the organizational, and the policy levels. Participants after completion of the workshops were able to identify potential solutions to inter/intra-professional boundaries and the competencies necessary to implement IPP. These skills were then used by participants to complete projects specific to the implementation of IPP in the community.

Evaluation of Programs A successful IPE program allows learners to recognize, value, and engage with the difference arising from the practice of an array of health professionals (McPherson, Headrick, & Moss, 2001). Ongoing evaluation of educational programs is necessary to ensure the educational methods employed are meeting stated goals and objectives. Program evaluation provides the opportunity to expand knowledge, develop new strategies, and continue to adapt existing programs as the need arises. Evaluation is an important part of the planning process. Freeth, Reeves, and colleagues (2005) stress this point, noting that although there is mounting evidence to support IPE based on evaluation data, a number of studies within the literature miss opportunities to add to this body of knowledge because they use poor evaluation methodologies inappropriate to address the questions being asked. During IPE program planning it should be decided what will be evaluated and how to conduct the evaluation. To support evaluation planning, a number of excellent resources are readily available through the Internet and other sources. Helpful Tools 8.1 provides a list of some of these excellent resources.

Accreditation and Interprofessional Education

Accreditation is described as an educational process that benefits staff, facilitates team building, and provides an organization with access to valuable advice from outside experts. The accreditation of interprofessional education is in its infancy. In Canada, beginning in 2007, Health Canada has funded the Accreditation of Interprofessional Health Education (AIPHE) initiative. The purpose of this initiative is to begin the process of identifying the principles and practices for incorporating IPE into health professional education accreditation processes. Phase one of the initiative was completed in 2009. Eight national organizations (Accreditation Council of Canadian Physiotherapy Academic Programs, Canadian Association of Occupational Therapists, Canadian Council for Accreditation of Pharmacy

Helpful Tools 8.1

Resources for IPE Program/Initiative Evaluation Planning

The following are examples of the various types of resources readily available to support IPE program evaluation planning.

Guides and Tools

Evaluating Interprofessional Education: A Self-Help Guide. This guide, developed by Freeth, Reeves, and colleagues (2005), can be downloaded from the Higher Education Academy's Health Sciences and Practice Subject Centre website (http://www.hsaparchive.org.uk). It is intended to help educators plan and conduct studies, and consists of sections outlining the evaluation process, ideas, and secondary resources for IPE evaluation.

Professional Websites

University of Toronto's Centre for Interprofessional Education (http://ipe.utoronto.ca). Among many resources and helpful tips and information, the Centre for Interprofessional Education's website includes a section on evaluation that discusses key points for consideration and basic steps for evaluation planning.

Systematic Reviews and Reports

Evaluation of Interprofessional Education. Although this report, from the Centre for the Advancement of Interprofessional Education (CAIPE), focuses on evaluation of IPE programs and initiatives in the United Kingdom, it identifies various evaluation methodologies currently in use and provides assistance to those wishing to reproduce and develop these methods (CAIPE, 2000).

Programs, Canadian Association of Schools of Nursing, Canadian Association of Social Work Education, College of Family Physicians of Canada, Committee on Accreditation of Canadian Medical Schools, and Royal College of Physicians and Surgeons of Canada) responsible for the accreditation of pre-licensure education of six Canadian health professions (i.e., physical therapy, occupational therapy, pharmacy, social work, nursing, and medicine) partnered and established standards for interprofessional education. Phase two, started in 2010, includes the same national organizations in consultation with other key stakeholders responsible for the development of an Interprofessional Health Education Accreditation Standards Guide and Knowledge Exchange Workshop with representatives of accrediting organizations of 26 other health professions (Lackie & Banfield, 2009).

Integrating Interprofessional Education: Canadian Examples

A number of educational institutions in Canada are involved in interprofessional initiatives. Spotlights 8.2 and 8.3 highlight two of these highly successful projects. Table 8.2 further summarizes key elements of the Interprofessional Collaborative Learning Series (IP-CLS).

Spotlight 8.2

Michener Institute of Applied Health Sciences' Readiness to Practice Model

The Michener Institute of Applied Health Sciences (The Michener) in Toronto, Ontario, delivers academic programs that train and educate a variety of allied health care professionals (e.g., Respiratory Therapy, Medical Laboratory Science, Nuclear Medicine, Radiation Therapy, Radiological Technology, Chiropody, Diagnostic Cytology, Genetics Technology, Cardiovascular Perfusion, Ultrasound, MRI, and Anesthesia Assistant). One such program The Michener has developed and implemented is the Readiness to Practice Model, which uses simulation models and the principles of IPE to prepare learners for IPP. The foundation of the model is core competencies that mirror IPE principles (e.g., professional behaviour, communication, time management, problem solving, self-evaluation, responsibility, team work, conflict resolution, and patient advocacy).

Medical simulation is "an imitation of some real thing, state of affairs, or process" for the practice of skills, problem solving, and judgment (Rosen, 2008, p. 157). The Michener program incorporates a variety of simulation models (e.g., static manikins, role playing, etc.), including high-fidelity simulation (e.g., high-technology simulation monitors and computers). The model is used as an educational and as an assessment tool.

IPE principles are incorporated into both full-time programs for new learners and continuing education programs for professionals already practising their discipline. The Michener model offers the opportunity for a continuum of learning throughout one's career.

Spotlight 8.3

College of Health Disciplines at the University of British Columbia's Interprofessional Collaborative Learning Series (IP-CLS)

The College of Health Disciplines (CHD) was created in 1997 to work with 15 health and human services programs to incorporate IPE into their existing curriculum and to facilitate and provide opportunities for learning together. Some of the learning opportunities combine theory and clinical, while others do not.

The primary goal of CHD is to "advance interprofessional education, practice and research" (CHD, n.d.). To accomplish these goals, CHD provides interprofessional courses for seven affiliate faculties (Applied Science, Arts, Dentistry, Education, Land and Food Systems, Medicine, and Pharmaceutical Sciences) that either represent a health discipline or support programs for health disciplines. CHD fosters interprofessional activities in the academic setting and in the community with partnerships in urban and rural settings. Partnerships with British Columbia's health authorities have been seen as key to establishing student placements.

CHD also supports an Interprofessional Collaborative Learning Series (IP-CLS) (see Table 8.2) for faculty and practitioners. IP-CLS provides an opportunity for practitioners to obtain the knowledge and skills necessary for interprofessional collaboration and to teach using an interprofessional approach.

Table 8.2 Key Elements of Interprofessional Collaborative Learning Series (IP-CLS)

Element	Description
Context-relevant	The IP-CLS is developed such that it can be adapted to various contexts and types of participants (frontline professionals, teams, managers, etc.). This allows for a number of participant needs, factors, and circumstances to be taken into consideration. Each session is about a half-day to a full day in length. The sessions are designed to be delivered a month apart; however, users can modify these timelines to meet their needs and constraints.
Patient-centred	In each of the sessions of the IP-CLS, participants focus on a patient/family case and follow the patient/family through a number of stages as they learn. Cases, depending on population focus, are often presented in a story format.
Train-the-trainer model	The IP-CLS is designed according to a train-the-trainer model. It is intended to build participant capacity to train others; with each successive session, participants take increased responsibility for their learning.

Source: College of Health Disciplines (CHD). (2011). *Interprofessional collaborative learning series (IP-CLS).* University of British Columbia, Centre for Health Services and Policy Research..

CHALLENGES TO IMPLEMENTING INTERPROFESSIONAL EDUCATION

When developing and delivering interprofessional educational programs, a number of challenges and barriers may be encountered. Parsell and Bligh (1999) classify these barriers as structural (e.g., external professional requirements, time and scheduling); professional/disciplinary (e.g., boundary issues, language and nomenclature, lack of knowledge about other professionals); attitudinal (change aversion, lack of support and commitment); curriculum/pedagogy (curriculum structure, approach to teaching, faculty knowledge and skills). Oandasan and Reeves (2005) outline factors at the micro, meso, and macro levels that can be either barriers or facilitators of IPE.

Micro Level Factors

- Professional socialization processes influence the attitudes, beliefs, and stereotypes that members of a profession hold in relation to their role and how they view their profession, creating a common professional culture. These effects either support interprofessional collaboration or lead to isolation of professional groups from each other. IPE provides an opportunity to influence these processes and possibly minimize the formation of negative stereotypes between the health professions.

Meso Level Factors

- Administrative processes refer to the various responsibilities to be assigned and the numerous tasks that must be accomplished in order to make IPE possible within a given educational setting or program. Pirrie et al. (1998) describe inhibitors to IPE that are both internal (e.g., differences in timetables, numbers of students in classes) and external (e.g., accreditation requirements). Ensuring that all relevant health profession stakeholders are part of the planning process is crucial for IPE success.
- Institutional and political leadership is necessary for IPE success. Leadership within academic institutions often translates into support from administrators to ensure that educational policies and resources are in place to promote IPE.

Macro Level Factors

- Institutional and political support may lead to the creation of "incentives" for IPE to take place (Freeth, 2001). Government funding or policy directions, for example, may influence the development of curriculum at a macro level. Curriculum overview processes, such as accreditation mechanisms, may also influence what is taught and how it is approached, significantly influencing whether IPE takes place.

More recently, the WHO (2010) has identified a number of challenges for IPE programs. Curricular challenges relate to issues around (a) shared objectives, (b) learning principles, (c) program content, (d) logistics and scheduling, (e) assessment, and (f) participation. Challenges specific to educators include (a) commitment from the managerial staff, (b) establishment of learning outcomes for the IPE program, (c) support from the educational institution in terms of resources, (d) providing training for academic staff to develop, deliver, and evaluate IPE programs, and (e) identifying champions for the implementation of IPE who will lead the way.

A major barrier to implementing IPE is convincing faculty, learners, and practitioners of its value. Paramount for implementation is breaking down professional barriers that prevent IPP (Carlisle, Cooper, & Watkins, 2004). IPE requires a cultural shift. Profession-specific educational programs need to change curricular content to reflect IPE and to restructure the delivery of programs to accommodate the incorporation of educational strategies that address the goals of IPE. Only then can health care workers think about and interact with one another (WHO, 2010).

As discussed above, one of the first challenges is to identify an agreed-upon definition of IPE. Agreement must be sought across the professions involved in the IPE program. Only then can IPE programs establish agreed-upon goals that can then be applied to the development of educational strategies.

IPE requires a different approach to learning. The traditional learning model for health professionals can be best characterized as "see one, do one, teach one." This approach has raised concerns regarding not only patient safety within teaching hospitals but also a as model that is not conducive to interprofessional learning. IPE requires a constructivist approach in which learning is based on interaction with other learners across professions, and learners construct and develop meaning for themselves. Shifting from a didactic role to a more interactive facilitating role requires time and the acquisition of new skills.

Gilbert (2005a) notes that the implementation of IPE requires a joint partnership between educational institutions and the health care system across jurisdictions. Gilbert suggests (2005b) that in order for this to happen the following structural changes are necessary in colleges, universities, and the health care system:

- different admission requirements for discipline-specific educational programs,
- variation in the length of educational programs,
- the extent and use of community and hospital resources for clinical placement,
- timetabling conflicts and scheduling across discipline-specific educational programs,
- restriction in the selection of courses for students,
- different administration structures across discipline specific educational programs,
- addressing faculty teaching loads and research interest, and
- investing power in the leadership of faculties to influence change (e.g., appointing faculty to develop curricula).

Lastly, the context in which IPE programs are to be implemented is an important consideration. Educators and health and human services institutions/providers will need to consider what approach best suits and benefits their jurisdiction.

EFFECTIVENESS OF INTERPROFESSIONAL EDUCATION

Although there has been considerable movement toward providing IPE in professional education institutions and within health and social service work environments (Freeth, Reeves et al., 2005), it is too early to draw any definitive and generalizable conclusions IPE's effectiveness. Nevertheless, there is some indication, albeit limited, that IPE has a positive impact on the broader IPP agenda. Table 8.3 outlines a number of systematic reviews of the literature conducted in the past decade on this topic.

These reviews point up the need for more longitudinal and multi-method research studies on the effectiveness of IPE using rigorous data collection methods. Such investigations should also reach beyond learner attitude and knowledge changes to include evaluation of behavioural changes; the impact on IPP teams, organizations, and the community; and the benefits to patients/clients.

Table 8.3 Systematic Reviews of the Effectiveness of Interprofessional Education

Review	Results
Zwarenstein, Reeves, Barr, Hammick, Koppel, & Atkins (2000)	Zwarenstein et al. conducted a Cochrane Library review of effectiveness of IPE in improving IPP among health care professionals and/or patient outcomes. None of the 89 studies identified met the Cochrane review criteria and methodological quality standards. According to these standards (e.g., randomized control trials) and the criteria applied, the studies were not rigorous enough to answer the question of IPE's effectiveness.
Barr, Freeth, Hammick, Koppel, & Reeves (2000)	Barr et al. conducted a review of research about the effectiveness of IPE in health and social care the United Kingdom. The authors identified 19 studies evaluating IPE that met their inclusion criteria. They found that few outcomes beyond knowledge and skill acquisition were evaluated, and recommended improving and extending the methodologies used to evaluate the effectiveness of IPE.
Cooper, Carlisle, Gibbs, & Watkins (2001)	Cooper et al. assessed the evidence of the effectiveness of IPE in undergraduate health professional programs. Their analysis suggested that IPE was more effective in producing attitudinal and knowledge changes and less effective in producing behavioural changes and impacting care outcomes. The authors note that these findings may be the result of the outcome measures evaluated (or not) rather than an indication of a limitation of IPE in undergraduate health professional education.
Zwarenstein, Reeves, & Perrier (2005)	Zwarenstein et al. reviewed four studies and compared effectiveness of IPE pre- and post-professional registration. They found that there was some, although inconsistent, evidence that post-registration IPE had positive effects. The study concluded that the effectiveness of pre-registration IPE was unknown.
Clifton, Dale, & Bradshaw (2006)	Clifton et al. conducted a review of the international literature about the effectiveness or impact of IPE in primary care. They found that methodological rigour of the studies reviewed was poor. These limitations notwithstanding, the results strongly supported the effectiveness of IPE in primary care within educational institutions and workplace environments. The authors add that the measures of effectiveness and impact were simple, such as change in knowledge and behaviour of learners, with a smaller portion of the studies evaluating patient outcomes.

FUTURE DIRECTIONS

IPE in health and human services programs remains at the mercy of fashion and expediency unless a coherent body of knowledge (scholarship) develops on which teaching, learning, and practice can be based, assessed, and evaluated. Convincing both faculty and students of IPE's value is a major barrier to making interprofessional teamwork and collaboration seem like desirable goals. Although significant headway has been made on these two fronts, they remain areas for future innovation, research, and debate.

Simulation is viewed as a possible solution to a number of current health care issues (e.g., reduction of adverse events), a way to better prepare learners for clinical training, and a powerful tool to advance IPE and IPP (Baker, Pulling, McGraw, Dagnone, Hopkins-Rosseel, & Medves, 2008; Willhaus et al., 2012). Simulation has been shown to be an effective tool for the interprofessional education of both students (e.g., Baker et al., 2008; Mikkelsen Kyrkjebø, Brattebø, & Smith-Strøm, 2006) and health care professionals (e.g., Prentice, Taplay, Horsley, Payeur-Grenier, & Belford, 2011). The Michener Institute's model of IPE suggests that simulation can also be used for evaluation of IPE programs. As educational programs and technology become more sophisticated, use of simulation will provide the opportunity for educators and practitioners to create innovative tools to foster IPE.

While the state-of-the-art of simulation for IPE is growing, with promising evidence emerging, work is needed to address the barriers and challenges to using simulation in IPE such as insufficient infrastructure and resources, logistical and planning issues, and lack of robust methods to evaluate effectiveness (Willhaus et al., 2012). There is also much variability in the models and approaches to using simulation to support IPE. Additionally, gaps in knowledge in simulation-enhanced IPE exist including a paucity of outcomes research that is methodologically rigorous and uses validated evaluation strategies (Willhaus et al., 2012; Zhang, Thompson, & Miller, 2011). Notwithstanding the gaps and challenges, ongoing development of and research into health care simulation can only serve to further advance IPE and IPP.

CONCLUSION

One of the most widely accepted definitions of IPE describes conditions under which "two or more professions learn with, from and about each other to improve collaboration and the quality of care" (CAIPE, 2011, para. 1). IPE is a lifelong learning focus for health care professionals. Much work has begun to define and develop IPE, but there are challenges to this approach, including the necessary human and financial resources. However, the emerging data that suggests potential benefits provides a compelling rationale to continue to develop and evaluate this educational focus.

SUMMARY

- Interprofessional education (IPE) provides the opportunity and the tools for learners and practitioners to gain the skills necessary to participate in IPP. Although there are a number of definitions of IPE within the literature, the CAIPE's definition is widely adopted across Canada.

- The CAIPE defines IPE as "two or more professions learn with, from and about each other to improve collaboration and the quality of care" (para. 1). Interprofessional education should be conceptualized as an ongoing process that begins once an individual enters a professional educational program and continues throughout his or her career.
- Integrating IPE into curriculum or health and social care workplace environments requires careful planning and systematic implementation and evaluation.
- Interprofessional education initiatives and programs should incorporate the following key elements/steps: (a) identification of the principles or goals of the IPE program, (b) establishment of the curriculum, (c) identification of effective methods of delivery, (d) definition of the educational needs of the trainers, and (e) evaluation of the IPE programs.
- One of the fundamental challenges for IPE programs will be finding the resources both human and financial to support development, implementation, and evaluation.
- For IPE educational programs to be successful they will need to partner with health and human services institutions/providers to teach using a constructivist approach. This endeavour will require learners, educators, and practitioners to think differently and to incorporate the principles of IPE into educational models both within and across professions.
- IPE is not solely focused on health professionals but includes those workers who contribute to the health and well-being of individuals across the continuum of care.

Key Terms

accreditation

interprofessional education (IPE)

medical simulation

uni-professional education

Review Questions

1. What is the purpose of interprofessional education?
2. Identify learning scenarios that do not represent examples of interprofessional education.
3. When should learners and health and human services workers engage in interprofessional learning?
4. How is interprofessional education different from uni-professional education? What are the pros and cons of each?
5. Describe the challenges of implementing interprofessional education.
6. What changes are needed to ensure the successful implementation of interprofessional education?

Application Exercises

You are a student enrolled in a health educator program, offered collaboratively between a Canadian university and college. Within the two academic settings, other health-related programs include medical laboratory science, nursing, paramedics, social work, personal support worker, dental hygiene, occupational therapy and occupational therapy aid, physiotherapy and physiotherapy aid, and addiction counselling. A town hall meeting is scheduled in the near future to provide an opportunity for student input into the idea of moving interprofessional education opportunities into the curriculum. You have been asked by your student group to provide a summary of what you see as the pros and cons of both (a) increasing IPE opportunities and (b) continuing with the current model of uni-professional education.

On the basis of the information presented in this chapter, how would you respond to this task?

Additional Resources

Articles

Barr, H. (2001). Interprofessional education: Yesterday, today and tomorrow. Learning and Teaching Support Network, Centre for Health Science and Practice. Retrieved from

http://www.hsaparchive.org.uk/rp/publications/occasionalpaper/occp1.pdf

Verma, S., Paterson, M., & Medves, J. (2006). Core competencies for health care professionals: What medicine, nursing, occupational therapy and physiotherapy share. *Journal of Allied Health, 35*, 109–115

Websites

Accreditation of Interprofessional Health Education (AIPHE)

http://www.afmc.ca/projects-aiphe-e.php

Canadian Interprofessional Health Collaborative (CIHC)

http://www.cihc.ca

Centre for the Advancement of Interprofessional Education (CAIPE)

http://www.caipe.org.uk

Health Human Resource Strategy and Internationally Educated Health Professionals Initiative 2008/09 Annual Report

http://www.hc-sc.gc.ca/hcs-sss/pubs/hhrhs/2009-ar-ra/index-eng.php

Northern Alberta Institute of Technology School of Health Sciences Interprofessional Education Program

http://www.nait.ca/66403.htm

The McGill Educational Initiative for Interprofessional Collaboration

http://www.interprofessionalcare.mcgill.ca/projectmembers_workgroup.htm

University of Toronto Centre for Interprofessional Education

http://www.ipe.utoronto.ca

World Health Organization: Framework for Action on Interprofessional Education and Collaborative Practice

http://www.who.int/hrh/resources/framework_action/en

References

Bainbridge, L., Nasmith, L., Orchard, C., & Wood, V. (2010). Competencies for interprofessional collaboration. *Journal of Physical Therapy Education, 24*(1), 6–11.

Baker, C., Pulling, C., McGraw, R., Dagnone, J. D., Hopkins-Rosseel, D., & Medves, J. (2008). Simulation in interprofessional education for patient-centred collaborative care. *Journal of Advanced Nursing, 64*(4), 372–379.

Barr, H. (1998). Competent to collaborate: Towards a competency-based model for interprofessional education. *Journal of Interprofessional Care, 12*(2), 181–187.

Barr, H., Freeth, D., Hammick, M., Koppel, I., & Reeves, S. (2000). *Evaluation of interprofessional education: A UK review of health and social care*. Centre for the Advancement of Interprofessional Education (CAIPE)/The British Educational Research Association (BERA). Retrieved from http://www.caipe.org.uk

Barr, H., & Low, H. (2011). *Principles of interprofessional education*. Centre for the Advancement of Interprofessional Education. Retrieved from http://www.caipe.org.uk

Buring, S. M., Bhushan, A., Broeseker, A., Conway, S., Duncan-Hewitt, W., Hansen, L., & Westberg, S. (2009). Interprofessional education: Definitions, student competencies, and guidelines for implementation. *American Journal of Pharmaceutical Education, 73*(4). Retrieved from http://www.medscape.com

Canadian Interprofessional Health Collaborative (CIHC). (2007). *Interprofessional education & core competencies: Literature review*. Retrieved from http://www.cihc.ca/files/publications/CIHC_IPE-LitReview_May07.pdf

Canadian Interprofessional Health Collaborative (CIHC). (2009). *What is patient-centred care?* Retrieved from http://www.cihc.ca/files/CIHC_Factsheets_PCC_Feb09.pdf

Canadian Interprofessional Health Collaborative (CIHC). (2010). *A national interprofessional competency framework* [PDF document]. Retrieved from http://www.cihc.ca/files/CIHC_IPCompetencies_Feb1210.pdf

Carlisle, C., Cooper, H., & Watkins, C. (2004). "Do none of you talk to each other?": The challenges facing the implementation of interprofessional education. *Medical Teacher, 26*(6), 545–552.

Centre for Interprofessional Education. (2010). *Planning interprofessional education initiatives*. University of Toronto. Retrieved from http://ipe.utoronto.ca/educators/framework.html

Centre for the Advancement of Interprofessional Education (CAIPE). (2000). *Evaluation of interprofessional education*. Retrieved from http://www.caipe.org.uk

Centre for the Advancement of Interprofessional Education (CAIPE). (2011). *Defining IPE*. Retrieved from http://www.caipe.org.uk/about-us/defining-ipe

Chau, J., Denomme, J., Murray, J., & Cott, C. A. (2011). Inter-professional education in the acute-care setting: The clinical instructor's point of view. *Physiotherapy Canada, 61*(3), 65–75.

Clifton, M., Dale, C., & Bradshaw, C. (2006). *The impact and effectiveness of interprofessional education in primary care: An RCN literature review*. London, UK: The Royal College of Nurses. Retrieved from http://www.rcn.org.uk

College of Health Disciplines (CHD). (2011). *Interprofessional collaborative learning series (IP-CLS)*. University of British Columbia, Centre for Health Services and Policy Research.

College of Health Disciplines (CHD). (n.d.). *What we do*. Retrieved from http://www.chd.ubc.ca/about-us/what-we-do

Cooper, H., Carlisle, C., Gibbs, T., & Watkins, C. (2001). Developing an evidence base for interdisciplinary learning: A systematic review. *Journal of Advanced Nursing, 35*(2), 228–237.

D'Amour, D., & Oandasan, I. (2005). Interprofessionality as the field of interprofessional practice and interprofessional education: An emerging concept. *Journal of Interprofessional Care, 19*(S1), 8–20.

D'Eon, M. (2004). A blueprint for interprofessional learning. *Journal of Interprofessional Care, 19*(S1), 49–59.

Dillon, T. H. (2002). Practitioner perspectives: Effective intraprofessional relationships in occupational therapy. *Occupational Therapy in Health Care, 14*(3–4), 1–15.

Downes, M. (2001). *Changing professions: Inter-professional collaboration in health care education: Report of the proceedings of the staff development seminar.* London, UK: Southern England Consortium for Credit Accumulation and Transfer (SEEC).

Fagin, L., & Garelick, A. (2004). The doctor–nurse relationship. *Advances in Psychiatric Treatment, 10*, 277–286.

Freeth, D. (2001). Sustaining interprofessional collaboration. *Journal of Interprofessional Care, 15*, 37–46.

Freeth, D., Hammick, M., Reeves, S., Koppel, I., & Barr, H. (2005). *Effective interprofessional education: Development, delivery and evaluation.* Malden, MA: Wiley-Blackwell.

Freeth, D., Reeves, S., Koppel, I., Hammick, M., Barr, H. (2005). *Evaluating interprofessional education: A self-help guide* [PDF document]. Higher Education Academy. Retrieved from http://www.hsaparchive.org.uk/doc/mp/04-16_hughbarr.pdf

Frenk, J., Chen, L., Bhutta Z. A., Cohen, J., Crisp, N., Evans, T., ... & Zurayk, H. (2010). Health professionals for a new century: Transforming education to strengthen health systems in an interdependent world. *Lancet, 376*(9756), 1923–1958.

George Brown College. (2013). *Interprofessional education (IPE) at George Brown College.* Retrieved from http://www.georgebrown.ca/ipe

Gilbert, J. H. V. (2005a). Interprofessional learning and higher education structural barriers. *Journal of Interprofessional Care, 19*(S1), 87–106.

Gilbert, J. H. V. (2005b). Interprofessional education for collaborative, patient-centred practice. *Nursing Leadership, 18*(2), 32–38.

Greiner, A., & Knebel, E. (Eds.). (2003). *Health professions education: A bridge to quality*. Washington, DC: The National Academies Press.

Hall, P. (2005). Interprofessional teamwork: Professional cultures as barriers. *Journal of Interprofessional Care, 19*(S1), 188–196.

Health Canada. (2007). *Interprofessional education on patient centered collaborative practice (IECPCP).* Retrieved from http://www.hc-sc.gc.ca/hcs-sss/pubs/hhrhs/2006-iecps-fipccp-workatel/index-eng.php

HealthForceOntario. (2010). *Implementing interprofessional care in Ontario: Final report of the Interprofessional Care Strategic Implementation Committee.* Retrieved from http://www.healthforceontario.ca

Herbert, C. (2005). Editorial. Changing the culture: Interprofessional education for collaborative patient-centred care in Canada. *Journal of Interprofessional Care, 19*(S1), 1–4.

Interprofessional Education Consortium. (2002). Volume III. *Creating, implementing, and sustaining interprofessional education* [PDF document]. Retrieved from http://matrixoutcomesmodel.com/MatrixFiles/stuart/Volume3.pdf

Lackie, K., & Banfield, V. (2009). *Action strategy: Leading organizational approaches to sustain IPE in the post-secondary education sector.* Vancouver, BC: Canadian Interprofessional Health Collaborative (CIHC).

Ladden, M. D., Bednash, G., Stevents, D. P., & Moore, G. T. (2006). Educating interprofessional learners for quality, safety and systems improvement. *Journal of Interprofessional Care, 20*(5), 497–505.

Margalit, R., Thompson, S., Visovsky, C., Geske, J., Collier, D., Birk, T., & Paulman, P. (2009). From professional silos to interprofessional education: Campuswide focus on quality of care. *Quality Management in Healthcare, 18*(3), 165–173.

McPherson, K., Headrick, L., & Moss, F. (2001). Working and learning together:

Good quality care depends on it, but how can we achieve it? *Quality Health Care, 10*(S2), 46–53.

Mikkelsen Kyrkjebø, J., Brattebø, G., & Smith-Strøm, H. (2006). Improving patient safety by using interprofessional simulation training in health professional education. *Journal of Interprofessional Care, 20*(5), 507–516.

Mitka, M. (2010). The Flexner report at the century mark: A wake-up call for reforming medical education. *JAMA, 303*, 1465–1466.

Oandasan, I., & Reeves, S. (2005). Key elements of interprofessional education. Part 2: factors, processes and outcomes. *Journal of Interprofessional Care, 19*(S1), 39–48.

Parsell, G., & Bligh, J. (1999). Interprofessional learning. *Postgraduate Medical Journal, 74*, 89–95.

Pirrie, A., Wilson, V., Harden, R. M., & Elsegood, J. (1998). AMEE Guide No. 12: Multiprofessional education. Part 2: Promoting cohesive practice in health care. *Medical Teacher, 20*, 409–416.

Prentice, D., Taplay, K., Horsley, E., Payeur-Grenier, S., & Belford, D. (2011). Interprofessional simulation: An effective training experience for health care professionals working in community hospitals. *Clinical Simulation in Nursing,7*(2), e61–e67.

Reeves, S., Goldman, J., & Oandasan, I. (2007). Key factors in planning and implementing interprofessional education in healthcare settings. *Journal of Allied Health, 36*(4), 231–235.

Rosen, K. R. (2008). The history of medical simulation. *Journal of Critical Care, 23*, 157–166.

Steinert, I. (2005). Learning together to teach together: Interprofessional education and faculty development. *Journal of Interprofessional Care, 19*(S1), 60–75.

University of British Columbia (UBC). (n.d.). *Interprofessional continuing education: Resources.* Retrieved from http://www.interprofessional.ubc.ca/resource_organizations.asp

Willhaus, J., Plagnas, J., Manos, J., Anderson, J., Copper, A., Jeffries, P., ... Mancini, M. E. (2012). *Interprofessional education and healthcare simulation symposium.* Society for Simulation in Healthcare (SSH), National League for Nursing (NLN), & Josiah Macy Jr. Foundation.

World Health Organization (WHO). (1988). Learning together to work together for health. Report of a WHO study group on multiprofessional education of health personnel: The team approach. World Health Organization Technical Report Series. Geneva: World Health Organization, 769, 1–72.

World Health Organization (WHO). (2010). *Framework for action on interprofessional education and collaborative practice* [PDF document]. Retrieved from http://www.who.int/hrh/resources/framework_action/en

Zhang, C., Thompson, S., & Miller, C. (2011). A review of simulation-based interprofessional education. *Clinical Simulation in Nursing, 7*(4), e117–e126.

Zwarenstein, M., Reeves, S., Barr, H., Hammick, M., Koppel, I., & Atkins, J. (2000). Interprofessional education: Effects on professional practice and health care outcomes. *The Cochrane Database of Systemic Reviews, 3*.

Zwarenstein, M., Reeves, S., & Perrier, L. (2005). Effectiveness of pre-licensure interprofessional education and post-licensure collaborative interventions. *Journal of Interprofessional Care, 19*(Suppl 1), 140–165.

Chapter 9

Interprofessional Health Care Policy and Regulation

Mrs. Robinson is 60 years old and has multiple sclerosis (MS). Her husband, Mr. Robinson, is 75 years old. He retired from the Canadian Forces many years ago due to chronic back problems that have become more debilitating with age. The couple live on Mr. Robinson's veteran's pension, in a province in which doctors, nurses, physiotherapists, occupational therapists, and social workers are all members of separate self-regulating professions. They have one daughter, Mary, who lives in another province.

Mrs. Robinson was recently hospitalized for exacerbation of MS symptoms and received care from an interprofessional team that included nursing, physiotherapy, occupational therapy, social work, and an attending physician. She was discharged after the team held a meeting to discuss the arrangements for continuing care following her hospital stay. Mr. and Mrs. Robinson were not asked to participate in the meeting.

During the meeting, several team members reported on their assessment, discharge planning, and patient teaching interventions. Priya, the physiotherapist, reported that she had been working with Mr. Robinson, who would be fulfilling the role of primary caregiver, to teach him transfer techniques. However, she failed to inform the team of Mr. Robinson's chronic back problems, and team members did not ask about Mr. Robinson's health and capacity to care for his wife. Sharon, the occupational therapist, informed the team that she had completed a home assessment for the Robinsons and made recommendations that railings and transfer bars be installed in the bedroom and bathrooms of the Robinsons' home. Sharon had yet to complete the required follow-up to confirm that the installations were completed; however, she did not mention this to the team. For their part, although team members agreed that these modifications were necessary, none made inquiries about their completion. Kwasi, the social worker, advised the team that although the Robinsons were a low-income family, Veterans Affairs would cover the cost of the installations because of Mr. Robinson's former service in the Canadian Forces. In fact, however, this cost was not recoverable from Veterans Affairs because the installations were intended for Mrs. Robinson's use, not Mr. Robinson's. Nobody asked Kwasi if he had confirmed his opinion with Veterans Affairs.

After Priya, Sharon, and Kwasi had spoken, Dr. Moore responded, "Well, looks like you all have everything in order and we are ready to go." As required by hospital policy, Dr. Moore wrote the order discharging Mrs. Robinson.

Two weeks after discharge, Mrs. Robinson was readmitted to the hospital with a broken hip and a head injury sustained when she fell getting out of her unmodified shower. At the same time, Mr. Robinson was admitted to hospital with a back injury sustained during his effort to help his wife. When their daughter, Mary, arrived from her home out-of-province to find out what went wrong, she quickly learned that although the hospital would do a comprehensive review of its systems and processes, there was no provision for a joint investigation that examined the conduct both of team members and of the team as a whole. She could only get the regulatory bodies for nursing, physiotherapy, occupational therapy, social work, and medicine to look into what happened by filing complaints with each of them, which would trigger a distinct investigation by each regulatory body focusing on their respective members. Mr. and Mrs. Robinson, and each of the members of the interprofessional team, would be expected to participate in each of these investigations.

Learning Objectives

AFTER STUDYING THIS CHAPTER, YOU SHOULD BE ABLE TO:

1. **Define the key terms related to regulation.**
2. **Identify the key aspects of regulation in the context of health care in Canada.**
3. **Demonstrate an understanding of the ways tort law and professional regulation can facilitate interprofessional practice.**
4. **Discuss current thinking about the dynamic interaction of interprofessional collaboration with tort law and professional regulation and the related developments occurring at the provincial and the territorial levels.**

INTRODUCTION

FOR AT LEAST 10 YEARS, MAKING HEALTH CARE AVAILABLE THROUGH INTERPROFESSIONAL health care teams has been a stated priority of Canadian health care policy. In 2003, and again in 2004, the federal and provincial governments (along with those of the three territories) struck two health care accords (First Ministers' Meeting, 2003, 2004). Both promised significant increases in federal health care funding to the provinces and territories. In exchange, the provinces and territories promised their citizens a broad program of health reform to deal (among other things) with waiting times, the affordability of drugs, and the accessibility of home care and primary care. One of the commitments in the 2004 accord was to ensure that at least 50% of Canadians had access to primary care through team-based practice. In this way, Canadian governments, pushed largely by citizen dissatisfaction with access to services, made interprofessional collaboration in the delivery of primary health care a government policy priority within a broader health care reform agenda focused on how the delivery of health care was organized and managed.

This chapter is about one aspect of the implementation of this policy: the role regulation of health care providers can play in either obstructing or enabling the formation and functioning of interprofessional teams. More specifically, it is about the role, whether as barrier or enabler, of two branches of regulation. One is professional regulation, carried out in Canada (with limited exceptions) under legislation that gives the privilege of self-regulation to each profession, including doctors, nurses, physiotherapists, chiropractors, dieticians, and optometrists. The other branch of regulation is **tort law**, the body of common law that courts apply to determine when health care providers and health care facilities are required to compensate patients injured in the course of care or treatment.

We begin with an explanation of why health care is heavily regulated. With in that context, we explain why the operation of professional regulation and of tort law raises concerns that they will inhibit the formation and effective functioning of interprofessional teams. This sets the stage for a discussion about how professional regulation and tort law might actually function as enablers of interprofessional collaboration, especially if policy-makers and regulators took steps to harness their enabling potential while preserving their capacity to protect patients. The chapter concludes with a sketch of some of the policies being pursued in the provinces and territories to bring interprofessional care into reality. Using the vignette and real-world examples from Ontario and Nova Scotia, we also illustrate how professional regulation is evolving both to better align it with interprofessional collaboration and to improve it by making such collaboration a defining attribute of how health providers are regulated.

The goal of this chapter is to enable the reader to see professional regulation and tort law function as part of a complex web of regulation directed at ensuring quality of care and safety of patients. The reader will have gained knowledge of key concepts related to professional regulation and tort law and an understanding of the broader policy and political context within which interprofessional team practice occurs.

REGULATION AND HEALTH CARE PROVISION: AN OVERVIEW

What Is Regulation?

"Regulation" is a vague term capable of being used in many different ways. Although naturally associated with law, it can be used to refer to any system of control, associated with legal regulation or not (Black, 2002). For example, economists will sometimes refer to regulation of business by the laws of supply and demand. Similarly, it might be said that health professionals are regulated by their professional knowledge, by the traditions and culture of their profession, and by the distribution of power within and between health professions. But in neither case is the regulation taking place an example of regulation by law.

In law, the word **regulation** is often used to mean that part of legislation enacted not by the legislature but by Cabinet or an administrative agency authorized to adopt regulations by the statute passed by the legislature. In broad terms, **statutes** set out the general principles of the legislative framework and the regulations fill in many of the important details. For example, if the opening vignette occurred in the province of Ontario, the *Physiotherapy Act*, enacted by the Ontario legislature, confers broad authority on the Ontario College of Physiotherapists to regulate registered therapists (PTs) such as Priya. But the rules governing peer and practice assessments of PTs are set out in Ontario Regulation 532/98 made by the Ontario cabinet under authority conferred on it by the *Physiotherapy Act* to make regulations.

The word "regulation" is also generally used to indicate the administrative work carried out by a regulator to implement or enforce legislation, such as the work of the regulatory bodies for doctors, nurses, and occupational therapists that exist in all provinces and territories. This distinguishes regulatory law from the **common law**, which is formulated and applied by the courts as they decide individual cases brought to them for determination through lawsuits. It also broadly distinguishes regulatory law from criminal law. Like regulatory law, criminal law is mostly legislative law. But criminal law is primarily enforced by the police, not by regulators.

In this chapter, we limit ourselves to regulation carried out under and through law. But we define **legal regulation** broadly to include any law that establishes norms of behaviour and provides a mechanism for enforcing them (Black, 2002; Parker, Scott, Lacey, & Braithwaite, 2004). This definition includes explicitly regulatory law that applies to health care providers, such as professional regulation. But it also includes the common law rules that determine the liability of health care providers for malpractice. Even though the latter are not regulatory in how they are applied, they are regulatory in effect. Indeed, doctors in particular are likely to care about regulation through tort law as much as (or more than) they do about regulation through their self-governing college of physicians and surgeons. This is because doctors, including good ones, are more likely than other health care providers to be sued because of the nature of the care they provide, the critical decisions they must make, and the level and scope of responsibility they shoulder for patients' overall well-being. This point is illustrated in the opening vignette. Although it was the team that determined that Mrs. Robinson was ready to be discharged home as per hospital policy, responsibility for the decision was borne by Dr. Moore as the signing authority.

Regulation and the Provision of Health Care

When regulation is defined as we have defined it above, it is obvious that the provision of health care is heavily, even pervasively, regulated. Just a few examples will make this point. The applicable regulations include those administered by Health Canada to decide which drugs and which medical devices can be used in Canada. They include the regulations under which ministries of health in each province and territory regulate the operation of hospitals, continuing care facilities, and (in some provinces) various kinds of private clinics. They include a range of laws that regulate the provider–patient relationship, including those under which health care providers must obtain the informed consent of patients to treatment and those under which patients can give advance directives for how they wish to be treated in the event they become incapacitated. And of course, the regulation that applies to health care also includes the two kinds of regulation that this chapter is concerned with: health professions regulation and tort law.

The layers of regulation applicable to provision of health care reflect the fundamental fact that although the essence of health care is to help people, it can cause harm. This is because of the risk inherent in the services being provided and the vulnerable situation of those receiving them. To address this potential for harm, regulation defines the care that can and cannot be provided by specific categories of providers. It defines the process providers must follow in providing care to particular patients. It defines the nature and scope of accountability required of providers for staying within their legally defined boundaries and for providing care in accordance with the standards defined in law or defined by those with legal authority to determine standards. Regulation also defines the processes through which this accountability for compliance with the law is applied when problems arise in the provision of care. For example, a drug company that breaches the terms and conditions under which a drug is approved for market might be prosecuted and fined. A nurse who provides substandard care may have a complaint brought against her by her patient and have her licence to practise restricted or revoked if her regulatory body determines that patient's complaint is warranted.

All regulation of health care must strike a balance between, on the one hand, protecting patients from harm and providing redress when harm occurs, and on the other, enabling and supporting providers not only in avoiding harm but in providing care that maintains and restores health. For example, in deciding which drugs to approve for use in Canada and under what terms and conditions, Health Canada must clearly protect patients from drugs that can cause serious and unjustified side effects. At the same time, however, it is the responsibility of Health Canada to approve drugs that may be the only hope for dying patients with diseases that cannot otherwise be treated. An example from professional regulation is the delicate balance a regulatory body must strike in handling concerns about the competency of members who have addiction or other health issues (Bailey & Jeffries, 2012). A strict approach of removing all such providers from practice would protect the safety of the patients they might otherwise care for; but it might also reduce the access of patients to the services of the profession—to say nothing of damage to the careers and rights of affected providers.

The balance health care regulation must strike between protecting patients and contributing to access to beneficial care must in large measure be defined and maintained by how regulators deal with specific cases. This is especially true in tort law, since it is largely determined by how courts decide individual cases. But in professional regulation, the balance struck between protecting patients and enabling developments in health care also depends on the broader legislative framework within which regulation operates. This framework will define the mandate of regulators, their powers, and the processes through which they are required to work.

For this reason, consideration of regulation's role as either barrier or enabler to interprofessional care must pay attention not only to the work regulators perform but also to the decisions made at the policy level. Therefore, in the balance of this chapter, we pay considerable attention to the role health care policy does and can play in defining and maintaining the balance that regulation must strike between protecting patients from harm and enabling interprofessional care delivery.

HEALTH PROFESSIONAL REGULATION AND TORT LAW

Before turning to a more detailed consideration of health professional regulation and tort law, it is worth noting that these are not the only kinds of regulation that may be in tension with a health care model based on interprofessional collaboration.

- The regulation that governs the administration of hospitals or continuing care facilities may contain provisions that require certain decisions to be taken or approved by a member of a specified profession despite the competency of others to make those decisions in some circumstances. For example, under the "Hospital Management Regulations" made under Ontario's *Public Hospitals Act*, treatment and diagnostic procedures must be performed under the written order of a doctor, nurse, midwife, or dentist. In addition, workplace rules, like those codified in collective agreements or organizational policies, may have more significance in how work is allocated among employees than do the statutorily defined scopes of practice that apply to the employees as members of regulated professions.
- In primary care, the funding of the system in accordance with the *Canada Health Act* (R.S.C. 1985, c. C-6) under provincial laws and administrative systems that provide for funding for primary care when it is delivered by physicians but not when it is provided by others has been a significant regulatory barrier—many would say the most important regulatory barrier—to collaborative interprofessional teams. It can seriously constrain the role that other kinds of providers, such as nurse practitioners, can play.

Here, however, we focus on professional regulation and tort law, because they have received most if not all the attention in Canada's recent emphasis on interprofessional delivery of health care. In this section, we concentrate on the how these two fields are thought to cause problems for interprofessional collaboration.

Professional Regulation

Provincial Jurisdiction In Canada, **health professions regulation** is a provincial jurisdiction under Canada's federal constitution. This means that every province (and each of the three territories) deals separately with the regulation of their health professions.

Despite this, health professional regulators across Canada administer a consistent process of regulation. In summary, the core elements of this process are as follows:

1. determining educational and other criteria for licensure (or registration or certification);
2. applying these criteria in deciding who is admissible to the profession;
3. establishing the code of ethics and the standards of practice members of the profession must follow;
4. helping members competently and ethically discharge their professional responsibilities through programs of continuing professional learning and development; and
5. dealing with concerns about members, particularly when a patient makes a complaint against (for example) her or his doctor, nurse, therapist, practitioner of traditional Chinese medicine, or (where regulated) paramedic.

The fact that health professional regulation is a provincial (and territorial) responsibility does, however, mean there is considerable variation across provinces and territories in how regulation is legislatively structured. For example, the list of health occupations that are regulated differs from jurisdiction to jurisdiction. So, while doctors, nurses, pharmacists, and dentists are regulated in all provinces and territories, paramedics, audiologists, midwives, and medical radiation technologists (and others) are regulated in some provinces or territories but not in others.

Umbrella Legislative Model The more significant difference is between jurisdictions that have "umbrella legislation" and those that do not. In Quebec, Ontario, Manitoba, Alberta, and British Columbia, all or most regulated health professions are governed by a common statute and by legislation (either a separate statute or regulations made under the common statute) that applies only to them. For example, in Ontario occupational therapists are governed by both the *Regulated Health Professions Act* and the *Occupational Therapy Act*. The idea is to ensure that the regulatory body for each profession is established and operated under a common legislative framework except to the extent that professional differences justify legislative variation.

In most provinces with this legislative model, the umbrella statute establishes an independent advisory body that advises the Minister of Health on policy questions, such as the design and functioning of the legislative framework, and on whether an unregulated occupation should be regulated. For example, in Alberta this body is called the Health Professions Advisory Board (HPAB) and in British Columbia the Health Professions Council.

Another feature of the umbrella legislation model is what is called either the *controlled acts* or the *restricted acts* model of licensing. Under this approach, the **legislated scope of practice** for each profession describes the work that can be performed by members of the profession but it does not limit the work performed by other regulated or unregulated providers. These enabling scopes of practice operate in conjunction with a list of acts (called the *controlled* or *reserved* acts) that everyone is prohibited from performing unless he or she is a member of a regulated profession that has authorization under the umbrella statute to perform the act in question. The idea is to limit the restrictiveness of the regulatory system on the patient's choice of provider to the specific acts truly capable of causing harm if not provided by specific kinds of providers.

Traditional Legislative Model In jurisdictions that do not have umbrella legislation, each regulated profession is exclusively governed by its own statute. There is therefore no overarching legislative framework for the overall system of health professions regulation. There is also no independent body advising the Minister of Health on health professional regulation on an ongoing basis. The controlled-acts or restricted-acts approach is also inapplicable. Instead, the statute for each profession will define its scope of practice and provide for either licensing or certification of members to provide services falling within that scope. Where licensing is applied, only members of the profession can provide those services within the profession's scope of practice. In contrast, certification grants authority to provide services within the scope of practice to those who are certified but it does not preclude provision of the service by others. For example, in Nova Scotia, all regulated professions are licensed. In other provinces, some are licensed and some certified. But licensing is the norm in both Nova Scotia and the provinces that make use of certification for the traditionally self-regulating professions, including medicine, dentistry, pharmacy, and nursing. The result is a regulatory framework that has the potential to be quite restrictive as to which providers can perform many health care services.

Common Elements It is clear that the legislative framework for health professional regulation differs in important ways from one province (or territory) to another, including in ways that seem relevant to the impact it may have on interprofessional collaboration. Despite these differences, we can still speak of a Canadian model of health professional regulation and of the obstacles that this largely common model poses to interprofessional collaboration.

With limited exceptions, there is a distinct regulatory body for each regulated profession in all jurisdictions. The governance of these regulatory bodies is typically assigned to the members of their respective professions, subject to very limited oversight from ministries of health. Although the responsibility of these regulators is to use the privilege of self-regulation to advance the public interest, pressure from members to instead regulate in the self-interest of the profession can be strong, including when occupational turf seems threatened by expansion in the role of other occupations. This pressure can be stronger when the regulator has a dual mandate of both regulating in the public interest and representing the interests of the profession, as some regulators in some provinces do. In addition, until recently at least, applicable legislation neither required nor enabled the regulatory bodies of health professions to work together in carrying out their regulatory functions. As an example, in the opening vignette, this would mean that if Mrs. Robinson's daughter, Mary, were to complain about her treatment involving providers from multiple professions (such as a doctor, a paramedic, and a nurse), the regulator for each profession would have to carry out its own investigation, even though an integrated investigation would be more convenient for the patient (and probably for others) and more likely to arrive at a complete picture of why harm was suffered by the patient.

Umbrella legislation and the controlled- (or restricted-) acts approach to licensing mitigate but do not eliminate the impediments the common Canadian approach to regulation may cause for interprofessional collaboration. For example, Ontario has in recent years made considerable efforts to better align health professional regulation with interprofessional collaboration, even though it has had umbrella legislation since 1991. This is partly due to the fact that under the controlled-acts approach each scope of practice still limits the work that can be performed by the members of the profession to which it applies even if it does not give them exclusive control over that work.

But the tension between interprofessional regulation and a regulatory system that confers the privilege of self-regulation goes deeper than the restrictiveness of scopes of practice. It goes to the very structure of the regulatory system and the reinforcement it gives to the separateness and independence of all health professions. Take continuing professional education as an example. Given the pace of change in health care practice, such education is one of the most important responsibilities of the regulatory bodies for regulated health professions. Under Canada's system of health professional regulation, the tendency has been for each profession to do its own continuing education, even on subject matters of common relevance to multiple professions. This in effect reinforces the professional divisions that have been too characteristic of the education health providers have tended to receive in colleges and universities.

Tort Law

Tort Law as Regulation Courts impose responsibility for wrongful acts that cause harm. In Quebec, this is the law of *delict* and functions under a statute called the Civil Code of Quebec. In the rest of Canada, it is the law of torts, which is part of the common law. This means liability is not based primarily on statute law (written law passed by a legislative body) but instead on law made by the courts as they decide cases by applying to new disputes the principles determined in previous ones. In both systems, however, the law works in essentially the same way. It imposes a duty on health care providers (and institutions) to obtain informed consent from their patients before initiating treatment and a duty to carry out the treatment with the skill expected of a reasonably skilled and prudent practitioner of their profession or specialization within their profession.

To understand the concern that tort law might be a barrier to interprofessional collaboration, it is necessary to understand a little more about how tort law works. Tort law applies where a patient starts a legal action (a lawsuit) against his or her health care provider to recover damages (financial compensation) for injuries sustained in the course of treatment. Overwhelmingly, such proceedings are against doctors, not because doctors are more careless than other providers but because they carry more responsibility for the care provided, including the care that is, by its nature, more likely to go wrong and cause serious harm. Whether the action is against a doctor or another kind of provider, the court will apply principles of tort law, and more specifically of the tort of negligence, to determine whether the provider should be held liable and required to pay damages. The court will order the defendant (the provider) to pay damages to the plaintiff (the patient) for negligence where the plaintiff establishes that his or her injury was caused by lack of appropriate care by the defendant. Damages obviously provide redress to the plaintiff. But they are also expected to deter other providers from failing to provide appropriate care. This is the deterrence function of tort law that is supposed to contribute to the quality and safety of care overall. In other words, it is the regulatory effect of tort law mentioned earlier.

Questions About Tort Law and Interprofessional Teams Tort law aims to place liability for payment of damages on the individual or individuals responsible for causing the injury. Where health care is delivered through collaborative interprofessional teams, questions arise as to which individuals will be held accountable by tort law when things go wrong, as they inevitably will in some cases. For doctors in particular, the question is whether tort law might continue to hold doctors accountable as the ultimately responsible provider, even though overall responsibility for decision making would have shifted, to varying degrees, from the doctor to the team. The distinct but related question raised by doctors is whether they might face lawsuits more frequently if interprofessional collaboration compromised the quality of care precisely because it reduced the control and leadership of physicians. Taken together, the two concerns raise the spectre of an approach to health care delivery that reduces the control of physicians over the management of care while increasing their exposure to liability.

For members of other professions, the concern about tort law is often in the opposite direction: that as they accept responsibility or co-responsibility for functions historically discharged solely by doctors (or by another profession higher in the traditional hierarchy), they would be held accountable by tort law to the standard of conduct the courts would have expected from doctors (or the other profession previously responsible). This would make sense where the standard was necessary for safe and effective care, but not where it was in excess of what was required for safe and effective care.

Joint and Several Liability A third concern for physicians (and some other professions, like nursing) is the reliance of tort law on the doctrine of joint and several liability. This doctrine applies where the proceeding is against multiple defendants, as it often would be when care is delivered by an interprofessional team. It allows successful plaintiffs to recover the full amount of their damages from any one of the defendants found to have contributed to their injury, independently of the court's apportionment of responsibility between defendants. In a team-based care situation such as in the vignette regarding the Robinsons, this would mean that fully insured team members (e.g., Dr. Moore) might be financially responsible for the liability of team members who were not fully insured. This has been a particular concern because some of the professions that would be taking on more responsibility under collaborative interprofessional models have historically been insured either not at all or not to a level commensurate with the elevated responsibility under such models.

Consequences Uncertainty about how tort law would allocate liability in an interprofessional context might lead providers, especially doctors, to resist participation in interprofessional collaboration, except perhaps on teams that might be interprofessional but not truly collaborative. Here, it may be noted that the Canadian Medical Association (CMA), the national advocacy association for physicians, is on record as supporting "collaborative care both in the hospital and in the community, as one of the essential elements of health care delivery in Canada" (CMA, 2008). However, the CMA also states that physicians should assume the role of clinical leader and be ultimately responsible for making definitive clinical decisions within the collaborative care setting.

PROFESSIONAL REGULATION AND TORT LAW IN INTERPROFESSIONAL PRACTICE

Now that we have set the stage in the previous section, the basics of regulation and tort law in relation to health care provision and the nature of health care professional regulation in the context of interprofessional collaboration should now be familiar. In this section we move forward to examine how tort law and professional regulation might function to support interprofessional collaborations in health care practice.

Professional Regulation and Tort Law as Facilitators

The discussion of how professional regulation and tort law function in interprofessional collaborations was brought into focus by Health Canada through an initiative it called Interdisciplinary Education for Collaborative Patient-Centred Practice (IECPCP). This initiative came after the negotiation of health accords in 2003 and 2004 between the Canadian federal government and the provinces and territories that brought interprofessional collaboration into the mainstream discussion of health (see Spotlight 9.1). As the name suggests, the initiative focused largely on the role of education in prompting the changes in attitude and behaviour that Commissioner Roy Romanow and many others said were necessary if collaborative approaches to the delivery of health care were to become widespread. It also asked two of the authors of this chapter (Lahey & Currie, 2005) to write a paper titled "Regulatory and Medico-Legal Barriers to Interdisciplinary Practice," addressing the question of whether professions regulation and tort law might stymie the cultural and behavioural change interprofessional education might otherwise stimulate and drive.

The Lahey and Currie (2005) analysis is outlined in Table 9.1. Their high-level conclusion was that professional regulation and tort law could be, but did not have to be,

Spotlight 9.1

Interprofessional Collaboration and National Health Care Reform

In Canada, the idea that health care could be improved by delivery models based on interprofessional collaboration has been around a very long time. What has been different in the past decade is the extent to which governments have gotten behind the idea, particularly in relation to the reform of primary care.

This was happening before the Prime Minister and the provincial premiers and territorial leaders got together in 2003 and 2004 to negotiate health accords under which the federal government increased its health care funding for the provinces and territories in exchange for commitments the provinces and territories made to health care reform. There is, however, no question that both accords, especially the 2004 Accord, were significant events in bringing interprofessional collaboration into the mainstream of health care reform. In Annex A to the 2003 Accord, governments agreed to develop a performance indicator on the percentage of Canadians "routinely receiving needed care from a multidisciplinary primary health care organization or team" (First Ministers' Meeting, 2003). Then, in the 2004 Accord, governments referred to "significant progress underway in all jurisdictions to meet the objective of 50% of Canadians having 24/7 access to multidisciplinary teams by 2011" (First Ministers' Meeting, 2004). In the aftermath of the Accord, this has been characterized as a commitment to achievement of this objective.

Both accords reflected the longstanding recognition that Canadian health care is relatively weak in primary care, a conclusion validated by benchmarking comparisons of Canada's health care system to those of countries such as the United Kingdom, the Netherlands, Australia, and New Zealand (Commonwealth Fund, 2010). Both accords also reflected the emphasis Commissioner Roy Romanow put, as a one-person Royal Commission on the future of health care in Canada, on primary health care reform and on multidisciplinary collaboration as one of the enablers of that reform (Romanow, 2002).

barriers to interprofessional collaboration. Instead, each could make a contribution to ensuring that it happened and happened effectively. For example, they concluded that the potential obstacle created by a system of professional regulation in which each profession regulates itself might be turned into a source of support for interprofessional collaboration if professional regulators showed leadership by collaborating to ensure alignment between self-regulation and interprofessional collaboration in the delivery of services. Lahey and Currie also suggested that the emphasis tort law puts on clear role definition and clearly documented processes and accountability might help ensure that interprofessional teams were designed, implemented, and operated with the kind of clarity of roles and responsibilities that would be essential to their effectiveness. In other words, continuing compliance with the expectations of tort law would not only minimize the liability that might ensue from circumstances such as that illustrated in this chapter's vignette, but also help ensure that interprofessional teams delivered safe and effective care.

In broad terms, the common denominator for the arguments on professional regulation and tort law was this: that the relationship between both the policy for and the

Table 9.1 Summary of Lahey and Currie's 2005 Paper	
Topic	**Key Points**
Professional regulation	■ There was limited evidence on which to reach precise conclusions about exactly how professional regulation hindered interprofessional collaboration or about the relative seriousness of the barriers caused by professional regulation. There was therefore a need for research to provide the basis for evidence-based reform.
	■ In adjusting professional self-regulation to bring it into better alignment with interprofessional collaboration, it was important to retain three essential strengths of self-regulation: first, the greater knowledge of the regulated activity that a self-regulatory body was likely to have relative to the alternatives of regulation by government or by a regulatory agency mandated to regulate all or most health professions; second, the credibility and therefore the persuasive influence that self-regulators are likely to have with regulated providers precisely because they regulate from within the regulated profession; and third, the role a system based on self-regulation might play in ensuring a level of independence of regulation from government and those who manage health.
	■ The possibility exists that because self-regulators are part of the professions from which collaboration is needed, they have the opportunity to lead by example in their relationships with each other and in the actions they take to enable, facilitate, and encourage collaboration among their members. They might in other words replace the silos of traditional self-regulation with a new model of interprofessional self-regulation by extending the ethos and methods of interprofessional collaboration from health care delivery to the regulation of the delivery of health care.
	■ That policy-makers might encourage or enable the transition to interprofessional self-regulation (or collaborative self-regulation) through a number of measures, including: giving health professions regulators an explicit legislative mandate to facilitate interprofessional practice; creating institutional mechanisms for interprofessional collaboration in regulation; eliminating unnecessary legislative inhibitors to interprofessional collaboration in self-regulation; and considering the wider adoption of more flexible legislative models, such as the controlled acts model of licensure.
Tort law	■ The absence of any indication from case law that the courts would impose liability solely because care was provided through a collaborative interprofessional team or impose a standard of care based on the view of the court as to which provider should have been responsible for a function or service, rather than on the basis of the level of knowledge and skill required for safe discharge of the function or provision of the service.

Table 9.1 Summary of Lahey and Currie's 2005 Paper (*Continued*)

Topic	Key Points
Tort law	■ The likelihood that the issue under tort law would be whether the collaborative approach was properly organized and executed, particularly in the clarity with which roles and responsibilities were defined and communications and decisions documented. This suggested that tort law (like discipline proceedings in professional regulation) might help ensure that interprofessional collaboration was properly implemented. ■ The reliance of courts in malpractice cases on expert evidence presented by the parties through expert witnesses as to what is regarded as standard practice in the defendant's profession meant that the evidence in favour of interprofessional collaboration might be put before courts and help ensure that the expectations of tort law kept pace with the transition of the health care system to interprofessional collaboration. Those who wish to enable this shift might exploit this opportunity by proactively gathering and disseminating the evidence for the efficacy and safety of interprofessional collaboration to maximize the chances of it being presented—and presented effectively—to courts in appropriate cases.

Source: Lahey, W., & Currie, R. (2005). Regulatory and medico-legal barriers to interdisciplinary practice. *Journal of Interprofessional Care 19*(S1), 197–223.

practice of interprofessional collaboration on the one hand and professional regulation and tort law on the other should be understood as dynamic rather than static. Both branches of law could be barriers to implementation of the policy, but sometimes in ways that would be good for the effective development and evolution of the policy and its implementation. Conversely, the evolution of both branches toward alignment with or understanding of interprofessional collaboration could support and reinforce the policy process by helping to validate interprofessional collaboration and to encourage its wider use. In short, the general argument was that interprofessional collaboration needed to engage with law, not ignore it or bemoan its seemingly arbitrary ways.

Collaborative Self-Regulation

Engagement is arguably what Health Canada did when it funded the Conference Board of Canada to write two reports in follow-up to Lahey and Currie's (2005) analysis, one on professional regulation and interprofessional collaboration and the other on tort law and interprofessional collaboration (Conference Board of Canada, 2007a, 2007b). On the basis of a wider reading of relevant literature, such as case law, and engagement with experts, these reports validated and extended upon the conclusions of Lahey and Currie.

Of the two reports, the one on professional regulation did more to outline a plan of action for exploiting the potential of regulation to be an enabler of interprofessional collaboration. At the core of this plan of action was the idea that what was needed was a new paradigm for professional self-regulation (which the authors of the report termed "collaborative self-regulation"). Under this paradigm, the efficacy of professional regulation would come to depend on the extent to which it supported effective interprofessional collaboration among regulated professionals. On this perspective, the goalposts had moved. The objective was not just to make law (or at least professional regulation) amenable to interprofessional collaboration. It was to make interprofessional collaboration one of the core objectives of professional regulation.

This bold vision could not be implemented at the national level. Under Canada's federal constitution, the provinces have jurisdiction over the delivery of health care and, with the exception of federal jurisdiction in relation to health care for Aboriginal Canadians, over the management of the health care system. Their jurisdiction (and that of the three territories under federal legislation) over the regulation of health professions is part of this broader jurisdiction. If professional regulation were to be realigned to be supportive of interprofessional collaboration, it would have to happen at the provincial level.

CONTINUING DEVELOPMENTS

In this section we provide an overview of the emphasis that the provinces have put on interprofessional collaboration in the delivery of health care, especially primary care, since the 2003 and 2004 health accords. We also discuss current thinking about the dynamic interaction of interprofessional collaboration with tort law and professional regulation, and outline the legislative changes being made to better align professional regulation with interprofessional collaboration.

Provincial Health Care Policy and Interprofessional Collaboration

The Uncertain General Picture In 2009, the Health Council of Canada reported that it was unable to determine how many Canadians were receiving team-based care in accordance with the commitments made in the health accords (Health Council of Canada, 2009). More recently, a committee of the Canadian Senate reached the same conclusion as part of a general review of the implementation of the 2004 Accord (Standing Senate Committee on Social Affairs, Science and Technology, 2012). The Committee accepted the evidence of witnesses that "Insufficient progress has been made toward the goal of ensuring that 50 per cent of Canadians have 24/7 access to multidisciplinary teams by 2011." At the same time, both reports documented the range of actions being taken by provinces and territories to expand the role of collaborative interprofessional teams in the delivery of health care, especially primary care.

Interprofessional Teams in Ontario For example, the Health Council of Canada (2009) reported that Ontario had 150 "Family Health Teams"—which Ontario describes as "physicians, nurse practitioners, nurses, social workers and dieticians who work together to provide primary care for a group of patients"—serving 17% of Ontarians, and 54 "Community Health Centres"—which "employ teams of physicians, nurse practitioners, nurses, counselors, community workers and dieticians." There are also "Family Health Networks" in Ontario in which groups of physicians work with an after-hours telephone advisory service staffed by nurses to make 24/7 access to primary care available to their patients. Against considerable physician opposition, Ontario has also created "Nurse Practitioner–Led Clinics" in which Nurse Practitioners are to provide "comprehensive, accessible, and coordinated family health care services to populations who do not have access to a primary care provider (i.e. unattached patients)" through "a collaborative practice approach which includes Registered Nurses, Registered Practical Nurses, collaborating family physicians, and other health care professionals."

At a broader policy level, Ontario has pursued a comprehensive health human resources development process called *HealthForceOntario* that has emphasized interprofessional teams and care. Under this process, the Interprofessional Care Steering Committee issued *Interprofessional Care: A Blueprint for Action in Ontario* in 2007, and the Interprofessional Care Strategic Implementation Committee issued *Implementing Interprofessional Care in Ontario* in 2010. Both reports recognized that wide-scale adoption of interprofessional delivery models depended on active support from many players, including government, regulatory bodies, health care professional organizations, academic institutions, unions, health administrators, insurers, educators, researchers, communities, and patient advocacy groups. Although both reports called for the removal of regulatory barriers, they also, like those produced at the national level, recognized the role that regulation could play in enabling and supporting the effective design and implementation of interprofessional models.

Interprofessional Teams in Nova Scotia Nova Scotia provides another example of provincial approaches to improving health care through interprofessional collaboration. In response to a study of the province's health care system that concluded (among other things) that providers in acute care were spending too much time on duties that did not require their specific qualifications, Nova Scotia launched the Models of Care Initiative to transform the way acute care services were delivered (Province of Nova Scotia, 2008; Tomblin Murphy, Alder, MacKenzie, & Rigby, 2010). A core part of the initiative was the Collaborative Care Model, which was to support providers in working to their optimal scopes of practice through collaboration within interprofessional teams. Subsequently, another study, this one on access to emergency services in small towns and rural communities, concluded that clinics staffed by interprofessional teams were the solution (Ross, 2010). Nova Scotia now has collaborative community emergency centres in various communities, an approach recommended for consideration by other provinces and territories by the Health Care Innovation Working Group of the Council of the Federation, the national organization of premiers and territorial leaders (Health Care Innovation Working Group, 2012).

Policy Influences, Objectives, and Reactions The initiatives launched in Ontario and Nova Scotia—and those being pursued in other jurisdictions—reflect the emphasis put on interprofessional teams by Romanow, the intergovernmental health accords, and the follow-up work done by Health Canada. They also reflect the growing evidence in favour of interprofessional collaboration in the delivery of health care and the continuing pressure on provincial governments to address citizen unhappiness about access to services and continuity of care while finding ways to control growth in health care spending. This combination of policy objectives can lead to suspicion that some applications of the concept of interprofessional collaboration have more to do with the substitution of some professions for others than with true interprofessional collaboration. On these grounds, doctors may resist interprofessional models that put nurse practitioners in the lead, and nurses may resist models that promote a larger role for practical nurses, physician assistants, or paramedics.

Aligning Professional Self-Regulation and Interprofessional Regulation

Ontario's Approach Ontario is one of the provinces to have done the most to better align professional regulation with the policy objective of making care available through interprofessional teams (Lahey, 2012). Much of the work has been done by the Health Professions Regulatory Advisory Council (HPRAC), an advisory body that Ontario's umbrella statute, the *Regulated Health Professions Act*, established to give advice to Ontario's Minister of Health. In 2006, HPRAC concluded that the Act needed to be updated to reflect the new reality of interprofessional collaborative practice (HPRAC, 2006). HPRAC gave two reasons: that fostering interprofessional collaboration among regulated professionals was one of the functions of a high-functioning system of professional regulation, and that professional regulation could not fulfill its mandate of protecting patients unless it responded to interprofessional collaboration as a new and pervasive reality in health care.

This thinking was aligned with the call of the Conference Board of Canada for a new paradigm of self-regulation that emphasized its collaborative dimensions. HPRAC was saying that professional regulation could not effectively ensure the competency of regulated professions if it did not address their readiness to work interprofessionally. Nor could it ensure the accountability of regulated providers if it focused solely on their individualized contributions without regard to their work as members of interprofessional teams. Accordingly, HPRAC believed that professional regulation had to come to terms with the implications of interprofessional care for a wide range of regulatory questions, including "[the rules and procedures for] delegation of controlled acts, overlapping scopes of practice, information sharing, the need for colleges to collaborate on standards of practice for professionals involved in multidisciplinary teams, liability insurance and the handling of patient complaints, investigations and discipline" (HPRAC, 2006).

To respond to these challenges, HPRAC recommended that the statutory objects of Ontario's regulators (called *colleges*) be amended to make them responsible for fostering interprofessional collaboration (HPRAC, 2006). Later, HPRAC recommended expansions in the scopes of practice of nursing in the extended class, pharmacy, midwifery, dietetics, physiotherapy, medical radiation, and laboratory technology, to enable members of these professions to more autonomously work to the full extent of their knowledge and skills (HPRAC, 2008a). Most ambitiously, HPRAC also recommended that it be replaced by a body that would support but also oversee the colleges, to ensure they discharged their responsibilities to collaborate and otherwise achieve regulatory excellence (HPRAC, 2009).

Ontario has followed the advice of HPRAC to make interprofessional collaboration one of the statutory objects of all regulatory bodies (*Health System Improvement Act*, 2007, S.O., c. 10). It has also implemented the scope of practice changes recommended by HPRAC (*Regulated Health Professions Statute Law Amendment Act*, 2009, S.O., c. 26). This presumably has made a regulatory model that was already more enabling of collaboration than other models even more enabling. However, Ontario has not created the oversight body recommended by HPRAC; instead, legislative amendments have given Ontario's Minister of Health and Long-Term Care broad powers to put colleges the Minister determines are not fulfilling their responsibilities under the administration of supervisors appointed by the Minister. Overall, colleges might reasonably conclude that the message is: Collaborate or else! Whether or not that is true, Ontario has clearly ended the neutrality of its health professional legislation on the responsibility of self-regulation to contribute to interprofessional collaboration.

Nova Scotia's Alternative Approach Nova Scotia is an interesting contrasting example to Ontario. Like Ontario, the general question of the changes that may be needed in legislation to align professional regulation with interprofessional collaboration has been directly tackled (Lahey, 2009, 2012). As in the analysis of HPRAC, the rationale for this has been as much what interprofessional collaboration among regulators can do to strengthen regulation as it has been the contribution regulation can make to interprofessional collaboration in the delivery of service. As with the HPRAC analysis, the concern has been the misalignment between regulatory processes limited by professional boundaries and a health care system already increasingly interprofessional. The related and distinctive Nova Scotia rationale for regulatory collaboration has been its potential value in allowing regulators in a small province with 22 regulators to pool resources to deal efficiently and effectively with common priorities (such as training or the development of standards or policies) or with issues that exceed the capacity of a single regulatory body, some of which have only a few employees.

A key difference between Nova Scotia and Ontario is that the Nova Scotia process has been led not by government or a government agency but by the regulatory bodies themselves, acting in collaboration with Nova Scotia's Department of Health and Wellness, through their own network. It is therefore not surprising that the process resulted in a recommendation that Nova Scotia adopt legislation that would give regulatory bodies the option of collaborating when they determine it makes sense and is feasible but that would not impose any obligation to collaborate. This recommendation was acted on in 2012 with the passage of the *Regulated Health Professions Network Act* (S.N.S., 2012, c. 48). It authorizes members of the Regulated Health Professions Network to develop and share regulatory best practices and to collaborate on specific regulatory functions such as investigating patient complaints, conducting appeals from registration decisions, and administering or requesting changes to scopes of practice.

Such an approach may look weaker and more uncertain than the legislated duty to collaborate adopted in Ontario. But the contrary view advocated by the Nova Scotia regulators is that an optional approach is a truly collaborative one that will better foster the collaboration wanted from regulated providers (Nova Scotia Regulated Health Professions Network, 2011). It may also be one that avoids both resistance to collaboration and "collaboration for the sake of collaboration" that might come with a prescriptive approach. Indeed, the approach may yield more collaboration and more quality collaboration precisely because it is voluntary.

It is far too early to tell which approach is better. It may turn out that each is right for the province to which it is being applied. Either way, the difference points up the positive role Canada's federalism can play in advancing health care policy by giving decision makers, scholars, and Canadians the opportunity to compare and evaluate the different approaches provinces take to implementing policy objectives defined as shared national objectives.

Other Provinces Similarly to Ontario, the province of British Columbia now mandates collaboration between regulatory colleges (*Health Professions Act*, 1986, R.S.B.C., c. 183). Meanwhile, other provinces have taken a range of actions that tilt generally in the direction of breaking down or avoiding interprofessional regulatory barriers. For example, Manitoba has implemented umbrella legislation based on the Ontario model (*Health Professions Act*, S.M., 2009, c. 15), while Newfoundland and Labrador has adopted (but not activated) a version that on the one hand is more limited than the Ontario model (it applies only to seven professions) but on the other hand goes further (all seven are brought under the authority of one regulatory body, the Council of Health Professions) (*Health Professions Act*, S.N.L., 2010, c. H-1.02). Prince Edward Island has gone in a similar direction (Prince Edward Island Health and Wellness, 2012). Numerous provinces have adopted or expanded their nurse practitioner legislation. There has also been a general trend toward expanding the scope of practice of pharmacists.

Finally, it is worth noting that the notion of collaborative self-regulation is gaining traction among Canada's health professions self-regulators. For example, the College of Registered Nurses of British Columbia has concluded that it will be vital to the future success of professional self-regulation in health care (College of Registered Nurses of British Columbia, 2012).

Tort Law as a Facilitator of Interprofessional Care

The CMPA Position on Collaborative Care The Canadian Medical Protective Association (CMPA) funds the representation of physicians when civil proceedings are brought against them by injured patients. In 2005, the CMPA affirmed the importance of interprofessional practice to the improvement of Canadian health care. In its policy paper, *Collaborative Care: A Medical Liability Perspective*, the CMPA downplayed fear that interprofessional teams might increase doctor exposure to liability by concluding that negligence law can support collaborative practice without jeopardizing either patient or physician interests (CMPA, 2005). Given the great confidence members of the medical profession across the country have in the CMPA, this ought to have been reassuring to physicians and a significant step forward in removing a barrier to physician participation in interprofessional practice.

It is also noteworthy that the CMPA did not say that doctors managing liability exposure required physician leadership and control of decision making in interprofessional teams. Instead, it said that the choice between interprofessional teams led by physicians who did the decision making and self-managed teams in which such responsibility was shared should be made on the basis of what works best in the circumstances.

The CMPA position was, however, subject to two conditions. The first was that doctors should only participate in interprofessional teams when there is a clear and explicitly documented understanding and agreement among team members regarding the roles and responsibilities of each team member. In other words, the choice between leadership and decision making by the physician or by the team has to be clearly and unequivocally made, with the participation of the patient. This requirement reflects and respects the fact that tort law puts a premium on clarity in roles and responsibilities, not only in health care but in general. Like others, the CMPA was confident that when teams are built on clearly defined roles and strong communication, liability will be minimized and patient care enhanced.

The second CMPA condition to physician participation in interprofessional teams was that all members of the team need to be protected by professional liability insurance or by a mutual protection plan, such as that operated by CMPA, one adequate to pay whatever share of the team's liability might be apportioned to an injured patient. This was to address the concern, described earlier, that a physician (or other adequately insured member of a team) might be held responsible under the doctrine of joint and several liability not only for his or her share of the damages but also for the share of the damages found to be owed to the patient by uninsured or inadequately insured team members. Like the CMPA, the Canadian Nurses Protective Society (CNPS) recommends that nurses only participate in interprofessional teams when all team members are adequately protected against civil liability (CMPA & CNPS, 2005).

Recent Case Law The CMPA position strongly suggests that tort law provides no rationale for physician unwillingness to participate in interprofessional teams provided they are properly constituted. Meanwhile, recent court cases provide reassurance that tort law should also not discourage members of other professions from participating in interprofessional teams. As explained above, the concern for members of these professions has been that as they share in responsibilities that would otherwise belong exclusively to medicine (or to another more qualified profession), they might be held accountable under tort law for meeting the standards of medicine (or of the other more qualified profession) rather than those of their own profession. The 2006 decision of the Alberta Queen's Bench in *Gemoto v. Calgary Regional Health Authority* (see Spotlight 9.2) illustrates why this concern is unfounded. In that case, although the court found that both the doctors and the nurses were negligent relative to the collective failure to chart the child's vital signs for an extended period of time, they were each negligent under the distinct standards of care of their respective professions. This was not altered by the fact that the doctors and nurses were working as part of a team. Indeed, the court recognized that teamwork was essential in health care and that effective teamwork depended on each member of the team fulfilling the standard of care of his or her own profession.

The *Gemoto* case and others strongly suggest that when patients are injured by the care they receive from interprofessional teams, courts will determine the responsibility of

Spotlight 9.2

Gemoto v. Calgary Regional Health Authority (Alberta Children's Hospital), Court of Queen's Bench, Alberta

Chad was seven-and-one-half months old when his parents took him to the hospital's emergency department with fever, vomiting, and diarrhea. He had elevated heart and respiration rates and tests showed he had critically high potassium levels. Six hours after admission he went into cardiac arrest. After another three hours, he died of acute peritonitis secondary to a ruptured appendix. His parents sued the hospital and various physicians and nurses who were part of Chad's health care team. They were successful in proving the team failed to take reasonable care in their son's case.

The hospital records showed that for a considerable period of time prior to Chad's arrest, vital signs were not charted by either the child's attending physician or by nurses. There was also failure to chart a distended abdomen, which was a change in condition. Failure to chart this information was contrary to both hospital policy and good care. Adequate charting, observed the court, is particularly important in a team-based approach to care. Notwithstanding oral testimony from the physician and nurses that vital signs were checked and the distended abdomen was detected, the court found that the pediatric emergency physician failed to monitor and assess Chad properly and emergency nurses failed to bring necessary information to the physician's attention. Because greater care had not been taken, Chad's deteriorating condition was not noticed early enough to institute treatment that would save his life.

The court highlighted in this case the importance of teamwork by referring with approval to the following comments found in a previous case: "The healthcare system in Canada mandates that these professionals work as a team.... Each person must carry out their role within their appropriate standard of care and each of these professionals is entitled to rely upon (and must rely upon) the others to fulfill their respective individual responsibilities" (*Bauer v. Saeger*, 2000).

The court was careful to note in Chad's case that the specific standard of care owed by physicians to a patient is not the same as that owed by nurses to a patient even though similar principles might be shared. The court conducted separate reviews of the duties of the physician and of the nurses in the circumstances. The standard of care applied to the emergency department pediatrician was that of a reasonable emergency department pediatrician. The standard of care applied to the emergency department nurses was that of reasonable emergency department nurses. In Chad's case, both the physician and the nurses were liable for failing to meet the requisite standard of care required of them according to their own professional standards of competence.

each member of the team by asking if individual members met the standard of care expected of them by their own separate profession, including that inherent in their role as members of interprofessional teams. For example, in the vignette of this chapter, if Mary, the daughter of Mr. and Mrs. Robinson, on behalf of her mother sued the hospital and members of the health care team (Dr. Moore, the physician; Priya, the physiotherapist; Sharon, the occupational therapist; and Kwasi, the social worker), the court would expect each team member named in the suit to meet the standard of care of reasonably prudent members of their respective professions.

CONCLUSION

This chapter has shown how health care reform at both the provincial and the national levels has identified interprofessional collaboration as a key policy lever for improving care delivery. It has shown how this focus has concentrated attention on the role health professions regulation and tort law can play as barriers to the successful adoption and implementation of collaborative approaches to care delivery. One result has been analysis that questions the true nature and extent of the barriers and that suggests positive roles professional regulation and tort law might play in enabling interprofessional collaboration.

For health professions regulation, the positive contribution includes the role interprofessional collaboration in regulation might play in enabling parallel collaboration in the delivery of health care while maintaining and improving the effectiveness of professional self-regulation in protecting patients and ensuring they receive quality health care. For tort law, the positive contribution lies in the premium it puts on role definition and clear allocation of responsibilities among collaborative team members and on liability insurance commensurate with the increased responsibilities members of various professions accept under collaborative team-based care.

Currently, there is a convincing argument, supported by court decisions, that tort law is not an impediment to interprofessional care. Meanwhile, a range of approaches are being taken among the provinces to make the legislative framework of health professional regulation less restrictive of collaboration and to either require or enable interprofessional collaboration among professions regulators. If nothing else, this suggests that the focus on interprofessional collaboration within health care reform has increased and broadened the attention given to tort law and to health professional regulation in health care policy-making. It also means that future consideration of interprofessional collaboration in health care reform at both the national level and in particular the level of provinces and territories can be informed by the experience of the provinces in pursuing common and largely shared objectives through a range of different approaches.

SUMMARY

- In Canada, IPP in the delivery of primary health care has been made a government policy priority within a broader health care reform agenda focused on how the delivery of health care is organized and managed. The role played by regulation has been a key aspect of this change in policy direction.
- Regulation, defined broadly, refers to any law that establishes norms of behaviour and provides a mechanism for enforcing those norms when they are breached (Black, 2002; Parker et al., 2004).
- Tort law and health professions regulation are two branches of regulation in health care that have specific implications for IPP and the functioning of IPP teams.

- Professional regulation refers to legislation that gives the privilege of self-regulation to each regulated profession.
- Tort law is the body of common law that courts apply to determine when health care providers, as well as health care facilities, are required to compensate patients injured in the course of care or treatment.
- Although tort law and health professions regulation can be obstructive of interprofessional team formation and functioning, these forms of regulation better function as useful enablers of interprofessional collaboration.
- For example, health professions regulation might be a source of support for IPP if professional regulators collaborated to ensure alignment between self-regulation and IPP. Continued compliance with the expectations of tort law related to role definition and role clarity can help ensure that interprofessional teams are designed, implemented, and operated with the kind of clarity of roles and responsibilities that would be essential to their effectiveness, minimize liability, and ensure that interprofessional teams delivered safe and effective care.
- Since the 2003 and 2004 health accords, provinces and territories have emphasized interprofessional collaboration in the delivery of health care, especially primary care. Ongoing developments at the provincial and territorial levels include legislative changes to better align professional regulation with interprofessional collaboration.

Key Terms

common law
health professions regulation
legal regulation
legislated scope of practice
regulation
statutes
tort law

Review Questions

1. What is the balance that all regulation of health care must strike and maintain? How does the need for this balance at least partly explain the tension between professional self-regulation and tort law and the reform of health care through interprofessional collaboration in the delivery of health care services?
2. What concerns have been raised about the role that professional self-regulation and tort law might each play relative to the wider adoption and beneficial functioning of interprofessional collaboration across the health care system?
3. In what ways might professional self-regulation and tort law be viewed as potential enablers of effective and accountable interprofessional collaboration?
4. What does it mean to say that the relationship between regulation (through tort law and professional self-regulation) and interprofessional collaboration should be viewed as dynamic rather than static? More precisely, to the extent that regulation does present obstacles to

interprofessional collaboration, how might such collaboration be part of the solution for overcoming these obstacles?

5. What are the common objectives of the Ontario and Nova Scotia approaches to improving professional self-regulation through interprofessional collaboration? What are the essential differences in how these objectives are being pursued in the two provinces? How do both processes nevertheless reflect the influence of health policy thinking at the national level?

Application Exercises

1. It's important that all health professionals have an accurate understanding of legal and regulatory issues related to interprofessional practice. In this exercise, you will be asked to debate the following statement:

   > Interprofessional practice will never be fully realized in Canada because of the challenges of regulatory and legal issues faced by health care workers.

   Working in small groups, decide on who will work on creating an argument either (a) in support of this statement or (b) opposing this statement. Once your arguments have been developed, debate the positions, presenting the ideas developed and responding to each other's position.

2. Building on the discussion in this chapter, consider how scope of practice legislation can be changed to facilitate interprofessional practice.

Additional Resources

Websites/Electronic Documents

Canadian Interprofessional Health Collaborative
http://www.cihc.ca

Canada's Health Care System, Health Canada, Government of Canada
http://www.hc-sc.gc.ca/hcs-sss/pubs/system-regime/2011-hcs-sss/index-eng.php#a15

Federation of Health Regulatory Colleges of Ontario
http://www.regulatedhealthprofessions.on.ca/EVENTSRESOURCES/interprofessional.asp

Interdisciplinary Education for Collaborative Patient-Centred Practice: Research and Findings Report, February 20, 2004
http://www.ferasi.umontreal.ca/eng/07_info/IECPCP_Final_Report.pdf

Legislation and Guidelines, Health Canada, Government of Canada
http://www.hc-sc.gc.ca/ahc-asc/legislation/index-eng.php

Additional Readings

Health Professions Regulatory Advisory Council (HPRAC). (2008b). *An interim report to the Minister of Health and Long-Term Care on mechanisms to facilitate and support interprofessional collaboration among health colleges and regulated health professionals: Phase II, Part I.* Toronto: Author.

References

Bailey, T., & Jeffries, C. (2012). *Physicians with health conditions: Law and policy reform to protect the public and physician-patients*. Edmonton, AB: Health Law Institute, Faculty of Law, University of Alberta.

Bauer v. Saeger, 2000 MBQB 113.

Black, J. (2002). Critical reflections on regulation. *Australian Journal of Legal Philosophy, 27*, 1–37.

Canada Health Act (R.S.C. 1985, c. C-6).

Canadian Medical Association (CMA). (2008). *Achieving patient-centered collaborative care*. Ottawa: Author. Retrieved from http://policybase.cma.ca/dbtw-wpd/Policypdf/PD08-02.pdf

Canadian Medical Protective Association (CMPA). (2005). *Collaborative care: A medical liability perspective*. Retrieved from https://oplfrpd5.cmpa-acpm.ca/-/collaborative-ca-1

Canadian Medical Protective Association (CMPA) & Canadian Nurse Protective Society (CNPS). (2005). *CMPA/CNPS joint statement on liability protection for nurse practitioners and physicians in collaborative practice*. Retrieved from http://www.cnps.ca/index.php?page=29

College of Registered Nurses of British Columbia. (2012). *Underlying philosophies and trends affecting professional regulation*. Retrieved from https://www.crnbc.ca/crnbc/Documents/783_framework.pdf

Commonwealth Fund. (2010). *The Commonwealth Fund 2010 international health policy survey in 11 countries*. Retrieved from http://www.commonwealthfund.org/Surveys/2010/Nov/2010-International-Survey.aspx

Conference Board of Canada. (2007a). *Liability risks in interdisciplinary care: Thinking outside the box*. Retrieved from http://www.conferenceboard.ca/e-library/abstract.aspx?did=1979

Conference Board of Canada. (2007b). *Achieving public protection through collaborative self-regulation: Reflections for a new paradigm*. Retrieved from http://www.eicp.ca/en/toolkit/regulation/achieving_public_protection.pdf

First Ministers' Meeting. (2003). *First Ministers' meeting on health care renewal, February 5, 2003, Doc. 800-039*. Retrieved from http://www.hc-sc.gc.ca/hcs-sss/delivery-prestation/fptcollab/2003accord/index-eng.php

First Ministers' Meeting. (2004). *A ten-year plan to strengthen health care, September 16, 2004, Doc. 800-042*. Retrieved from http://www.scics.gc.ca/CMFiles/800042005_e1JXB-342011-6611.pdf

Gemoto v. Calgary Regional Health Authority, 2006 ABQB 740.

Health Care Innovation Working Group. (2012). *From innovation to action: The first report of the Health Care Innovation Working Group*. Retrieved from http://www.councilofthefederation.ca/pdfs/HealthInnovationReport-E-WEB.pdf

Health Council of Canada. (2009). *Teams in action: Primary health care teams for Canadians*. Retrieved from http://www.dsrf.org/media/teamsinaction.pdf

HealthForceOntario. (2007). *Interprofessional care: A blueprint for action in Ontario*. Retrieved from http://www.healthforceontario.ca/UserFiles/file/PolicymakersResearchers/ipc-blueprint-july-2007-en.pdf

HealthForceOntario. (2010). *Implementing interprofessional care in Ontario*. Toronto: Author. Retrieved from: http://www.healthforceontario.ca/UserFiles/file/PolicymakersResearchers/ipc-final-report-may-2010-en.pdf

Health Professions Act, 1986, R.S.B.C., c. 183.

Health Professions Act, S.M., 2009, c. 15.

Health Professions Act, S.N.L. 2010, c. H-1.02.

Health Professions Regulatory Advisory Council (HPRAC). (2006). *Regulation of health professions in Ontario: New directions*. Toronto: Author.

Health Professions Regulatory Advisory Council (HPRAC). (2008a). *An interim report to the Minister of Health and Long-Term Care on mechanisms to facilitate and support interprofessional collaboration among health colleges and regulated health professionals*. Toronto: Author.

Health Professions Regulatory Advisory Council (HPRAC). (2009). *Critical links: Transforming and supporting patient care*. Toronto: Author.

Health System Improvement Act, 2007, S.O., c. 10.

Lahey, W. (2009). *Collaborative self-regulation and professional accountability in Nova Scotia's health care system*. Halifax: Dalhousie Health Law Institute. Retrieved from http://hli.law.dal.ca/Files/WG_Document_Nov_4_2009.pdf

Lahey, W. (2012). Interprofessional and collaborative self-regulation in the health professions: Two variations on an emerging Canadian theme. In S. D. Short & F. McDonald (Eds.), *Health workforce governance: Improved access, good regulatory practice, safer patients* (pp. 113–143). Surrey, UK: Ashgate Publishing.

Lahey, W., & Currie, R. (2005). Regulatory and medico-legal barriers to interdisciplinary practice. *Journal of Interprofessional Care 19*(S1), 197–223.

Nova Scotia Regulated Health Professions Network. (2011). *Toward collaborative self-regulation*. Retrieved from http://hli.law.dal.ca/Files/WG_Document_Dec_2011.pdf

Parker, C., Scott, C., Lacey, N., & Braithwaite, J. (2004). *Regulating law*. Oxford: Oxford University Press.

Prince Edward Island Health and Wellness. (2012). *Proposed umbrella health professions legislation for Prince Edward Island: Consultation paper*. Retrieved from http://www.gov.pe.ca/photos/original/RHPAEnglish.pdf

Province of Nova Scotia. (2008). *Nova Scotia's new collaborative care model: What it means for you*. Retrieved from http://www.gov.ns.ca/health/mocins/MOCINS_What_it_Means_For_You.pdf

Regulated Health Professions Act, 2009, S.M., c. 15.

Regulated Health Professions Network Act, 2012, S.N.S., c. 48.

Regulated Health Professions Statute Law Amendment Act, 2009, S.O., c. 26.

Romanow, R. J. (2002). *Building on values: The future of health care in Canada—Final report*. Ottawa: Commission on the Future of Health Care in Canada.

Ross, J. (2010). *The patient journey through emergency care: A prescription for new medicine*. Retrieved from https://www.gov.ns.ca/dhw/publications/Dr-Ross-The-Patient-Journey-Through-Emergency-Care-in-Nova-Scotia.pdf

Standing Senate Committee on Social Affairs, Science and Technology. (2012). *Time for transformative change: A review of the 2004 health accord*. Retrieved from http://www.parl.gc.ca/Content/SEN/Committee/411/soci/rep/rep07mar12-e.pdf

Tomblin Murphy, G., Alder, R., MacKenzie, A., & Rigby, J. (2010). *Model of care initiative in Nova Scotia (MOCINS): Final evaluation report*. Retrieved from http://novascotia.ca/dhw/mocins/docs/MOCINS-evaluation-report.pdf

Chapter 10

Practice Outcomes and Measuring Success with Interprofessional Practice

Brookhaven Family Practice Team (FPT) is situated within a small community one hour from a major Canadian city. The FPT, a relatively new team of primary care practitioners, has taken advantage of a startup grant initiative that is part of an overall strategy to improve access to primary health care. In addition to funding support, the initiative provides a number of resources to guide potential FPTs through the process of creating their teams within the community.

The main activities currently facing the Brookhaven FPT in its final planning stage are (a) hiring the health care providers they need to deliver the services they will be providing and (b) building and maintaining an interprofessional practice (IPP) team.

Today, the health care providers who have been hired thus far and the administrative staff are meeting to continue their planning. During their discussion, Susan, a nurse practitioner, raises the issue of evaluation.

Susan (nurse practitioner): I'm concerned that in our planning we've left out how we will evaluate our progress and the outcomes we are interested in achieving.

Don (registered nurse): I'm not sure I understand what you are saying. We've already set out objectives that we are aiming for, such as high levels of team member satisfaction and patient satisfaction. We plan to look at measuring these things a little further down the road and make changes as we go along.

Susan: You make my point exactly, Don. We've spent a lot of time carefully planning the implementation of this FPT and determining how we are going to build our team. But from my perspective, we haven't figured out how we will concretely assess both the impact of what we're doing and the effectiveness of how we're going about it. For example, we haven't identified what we think is the best way to measure our satisfaction and our patients' satisfaction. I think we need to develop a detailed and systematic plan for how we will evaluate our team's development and the impact of our practice.

Marta (physician): I think Susan is right. If we want to ensure that the care we provide is based on best available practices, I think we should apply the same level of attention to evaluation as we have been to other aspects of this FPT implementation process.

Kida (manager): I agree. I recently read about a project or maybe it was a program. (Pause) Anyway it was intended to help teams like ours implement collaborative team practice and evaluate their efforts. Oh, I remember ... it was called TIPS. Maybe we can use something like that to get us started in the right direction in terms of developing our evaluation strategy.

Susan: If it's OK with everyone else, I'd like to take the lead on this and do some research about where we should be going in terms of evaluating team practice and outcomes. Kida, maybe we can connect about that TIPS program?

Team Members: Sure!

Kida: That sounds like a plan!

Learning Outcomes

AFTER STUDYING THIS CHAPTER, YOU SHOULD BE ABLE TO:

1. **Describe the significance of evaluating IPP.**
2. **Define key terms related to evaluating IPP, including formative and summative evaluation, reliability and validity, evidence-based practice, and outcomes research.**
3. **Summarize emerging evidence related to outcomes of IPP.**
4. **Apply an evaluation framework to an IPP or IPE situation.**

INTRODUCTION

AS INDICATED IN CHAPTER 1, THE TRANSITION FROM A HEALTH CARE APPROACH IN WHICH professions are operating in silos to one that embraces interprofessional practice (IPP) is challenging and complex. Thus, it is important that initiatives related to both IPP and interprofessional education (IPE) be carefully evaluated to determine the impact of team-oriented approach on quality of care, health outcomes, and patient and provider satisfaction. Specifically, this focus on evaluation is critical in order to determine the potential value to health care recipients and providers of IPP and IPE. Evaluation also enables us to identify the most efficacious and efficient means by which this type of practice and education should happen. Finally, evaluation is critical because it allows us to monitor progress both in the care we provide and in the way we practise interprofessionally.

The opening vignette for this chapter highlights the kind of discussion that would be beneficial to health care teams at all stages of development. The situation involving the Brookhaven FPT is somewhat ideal in that the team is just forming and is simultaneously building in plans for evaluation. While this may not always be possible, it is essential to remember that the approach to evaluation must always be systematically designed no matter what point in a team's development it is considered. The Building Positive

Inter-Professional Relationships in Health Care: A Collaborative Initiative for Patient Safety and Quality Work Environments (TIPS) project referenced in the vignette provides an evaluative approach to IPP and IPE. As we will see later in this chapter, teams can use it as they engage in measuring their team practice and associated outcomes (see the Additional Resources section at the end of the chapter).

Our goal in this chapter is to assist the reader in developing a greater understanding of the importance of evaluating IPP, and knowledge about the processes and methodologies involved. It consists of three main sections. In the first section, a very brief overview of relevant research and evaluation concepts in health care is provided. In the second section, a brief overview of health research basics is addressed in order to more effectively frame the discussion of specific evaluation related to IPP. The third section provides a summary of emerging evidence related to IPP.

RESEARCH AND EVALUATION CONCEPTS

Evaluation may be defined as the systematic acquisition and assessment of information to provide useful feedback about some object (Trochim, 2006). This definition highlights a number of elements of evaluation that are consistent across the literature:

- "*Systematic.*" Evaluation is a systematic, stepwise, and orderly process.
- "*Acquisition and assessment of information to provide useful feedback.*" Evaluation involves collecting information, analyzing data in order to reach an opinion about the quality of that information, and making inferences about the item to which the information is referring.
- "*About some object.*" The "objects" of evaluation can vary. Programs, activities, tools and resources, and needs, to name a few, can all be the object of an evaluation (Creswell, 2012; Trochim, 2006).

While the purposes and types of evaluation may differ, it is widely believed that the use of multiple types of available evaluation tools and methods is generally the most effective (Kahan, 2008). Regardless of the purpose and type of evaluation, the methods by which we conduct our investigation must be rigorous and representative of the most current and relevant data available. They must also hold up to external scrutiny. This chapter includes a review of broad ideas underpinning evaluation in health care. These concepts are important to understanding the specific approaches to and methods of IPP evaluation.

Health Care Research

All sciences, including health care sciences, are based on a foundation of research. While historically focused on controlled studies in laboratory settings, health care research and health care system research, which are of particular interest in this discussion, now commonly take place directly within practice settings. Research essentially involves a series of steps taken to collect and analyze information in order to develop or increase our understanding of something (Creswell, 2012). In its simplest representation, Creswell describes three steps in the basic research process: (a) posing a question, (b) collecting data to find the answer to that question, and (c) presenting the answer.

Creswell's article highlights common approaches to research to illustrate how various phenomena in health care can be examined and better understood. Health research that takes place in a laboratory may focus on how a particular type of cell, for example a cancer cell, responds to a specific drug. Research in a health care setting may involve a randomized control trial to determine how patients respond to this treatment. These studies involve **quantitative research methods** in that the interventions and outcomes are observable and measurable. Additionally, **qualitative research methods**, which focus on understanding human experience and behaviour, may examine the experience of patients living with a disease or undergoing a specific medical treatment. This understanding is accomplished through processes whereby we ask people to share details of their own experiences, such as their story of their health–illness journey. In this case, the results of the research may be the themes researchers identify as common to the experiences described by patients. Both types of research, quantitative and qualitative, are scientific, but each utilizes different methodologies.

Of particular relevance to this chapter, research in health care settings may also be undertaken specifically for the purpose of evaluation. Research of this kind attempts to determine the impact of a program, a technique, an intervention, or a product on patients, providers, and the organization. An example would be the evaluation of how a specific treatment impacts patient outcomes. Such evaluation can also be extended to examining system impacts, such as overall health outcomes, financial outcomes, professional trends, recruitment, and retention across professions. Program evaluation, which includes elements such as learning and orientation opportunities, fall within this focus. Donabedian (1988) classifies the inferences that can be drawn about the quality of care as (1) *structure*—the facilities, equipment, money, human resources, and organizational structure within a given health care facility, (2) the *process* of giving a receiving care, and (3) *outcomes*, which encompass the effects of care of the health status of individuals and populations.

Regardless of methodology, it is essential to ensure validity and reliability of the research process and outcomes. **Validity** refers to the extent to which we are actually measuring what we say we are measuring in a scientific study. For example, if we design a study to look at the effectiveness of team problem-solving processes, we must ensure that what we are measuring actually is the outcomes of the processes. **Reliability**, on the other hand, refers to how consistent a measure is. For example, if we repeat the test multiple times, do we find approximately the same result? Reliability cannot be calculated exactly; rather, it is estimated in a number of ways.

Outcomes

When focusing on health care delivery approaches, it is important to consider the assessment of outcomes, which are integral to the development of best health care practices. **Care delivery outcomes** are defined as "the observable or measureable effects of some intervention or action. They are focused on the recipient of the service, not the provider, and can be measured at the individual, group, organization, or community level" (Ingersoll, 2004, p. 301). Outcomes measurement occurs when we collect specific data about an observable effect that results from some health care delivery process or health promotion strategy. For example, in the opening vignette, patient satisfaction is one of the outcomes the Brookhaven FPT identified. The team believes patient satisfaction will provide information to help improve team functioning and evidence that their approach has a positive impact. To assess this outcome, the team might use a variety of quantitative and qualitative measures. Through data analysis and interpretation of findings, the team will then be able to draw conclusions about their progress and the impact of their efforts to implement IPP.

Outcomes research is a specific type of research with particular significance when considering implementation of health care system and health care delivery changes. The term is used to refer to scientific research that seeks to understand the outcomes of various practices and interventions by measuring effects, such as changes in patients' condition and health status. Outcomes research results in care delivery standards that rely on evidence-based practice (Agency for Health Care Research and Quality, 2000).

In the most traditional sense, outcome indicators in relation to health and health care often focused heavily on morbidity (rate of illness) and mortality (rate of death). However, health and health care are much more complex than these two indicators can reveal. When considering outcomes, it is important to remember that there are many stakeholders in relation to health care and thus, at times, competing priorities in terms of outcomes. There is undoubtedly general agreement that we are seeking to identify the best possible interventions in order to help recipients of care remain healthy, return to health, adapt to altering health conditions, or experience as little discomfort at possible when facing terminal illness. We are also seeking the means to evaluate systems or methods of care delivery that lead to various outcomes and to identify, if possible, exactly what the relationship between the delivery system (e.g., IPP) and the outcome (e.g., decreased patient mortality or increased satisfaction with health care experience) might be. The last part of this chapter provides an overview of emerging evidence related to outcomes associated with IPP.

Evidence-Based Practice

While the roots of evidence-based practice can be traced to Dr. Archie Cochrane's critique of physicians' lack of critical appraisal and research synthesis skills, in the past two decades the movement has truly taken hold. In fact, it has become so widespread that, not uncommonly, patients seeking health care will question the evidence behind proposed treatment plans. **Evidence-based practice** is a "framework for clinical practice that incorporates the best available scientific evidence with the expertise of the clinician and the patient's preferences and values to make decisions about health care" (Levin, 2006, p. 6). Evidence-based-practice core competencies are now considered essential to the educational curriculum of most health disciplines. When considering IPP, it is important to examine the structures in a health care organization, such as policies, expectations, and tools, that enable a strong IPP approach. **Structure evaluation** refers to assessing the attributes of the setting in which care occurs. It is also important to assess the processes that support IPP, such as communication, decision making, and leadership. In addition, it is critical to examine the outcomes of IPP that focus not only on the provider but also on the patient and the organization. **Process evaluation** refers to measuring how care is being delivered and received. Outcome measures can include those related to patient/provider experience and those related to clinical, health, and quality of life outcomes. The Registered Nurses' Association of Ontario (RNAO), the voice of registered nurses in Ontario, widely known for its work in developing evidence based best practice guidelines (see Additional Resources), has recently published an evidence-based best practice guideline related to interprofessional care. The guideline, titled *Developing and Sustaining Interprofessional Health Care: Optimizing Patient, Organizational, and System Outcomes*, provides evidence-based recommendations related to practice, education, organization, and system policies that will enable effective interprofessional practice (RNAO, 2013). It includes an evaluation matrix featuring structure, process, and outcome indicators related to client, provider, and organization impacts.

Thus far, we have briefly discussed key ideas relevant to the types of evaluation that take place in health care. The concepts described also underpin the processes and practices involved in evaluating IPP and IPE. The next section focuses more specifically on the methods and approaches most applicable to IPP evaluation.

EVALUATING INTERPROFESSIONAL PRACTICE AND PRACTICE OUTCOMES

We have argued that evaluation is a necessary, scientific activity that enables insight into the phenomena of interest. Within the contexts of health care delivery, outcomes, and education and patient/provider experience, the objectives of IPP are to impact safe, quality health care and positive health outcomes. Solid evaluative data will inform us about the nature of IPP in health care, and the resulting impacts on client, provider, and organizational outcomes. The challenge is to develop planned evaluation research related to the many emerging models of IPP using valid and reliable measures to capture their outcomes.

Progress has been made toward amassing resources and tools that researchers, teams, and organizations involved in implementing and maintaining IPP may use. What follows is a discussion of results of the work to date in this area.

Types of Evaluation

Evaluation can be either formative or summative. In IPP evaluation, **formative evaluation** occurs at various points throughout program startup and delivery, and focuses on data that provides feedback on the progress and effectiveness of the efforts being made toward implementing this model of practice. It is often carried out at the team level, with the purpose of improving and shaping the team to better meet their IPP goals. It focuses on structures and processes that enable IPP. The team gathers evidence to support changes aimed toward improving team functioning processes and procedures.

Formative evaluation provides early indication if new approaches are promising. It provides teams with the data to alter course if necessary. Key stakeholders should be involved, so that everyone is informed about and on board with process and structure changes that may have to be made.

Summative evaluation takes place at a predetermined end point in the IPP program and is used to assess outcomes and the overall impact of the intervention or action. It may also include assessment of how well processes, such as interprofessional collaboration, were enacted. Kahan (2008) notes that intervention or program-based evaluations tend to readily combine both formative and summative evaluation. Summative evaluation, because it is used to gain an understanding of the overall impact of an intervention, tends to involve others within organizations and collaborative stakeholders. The decision making that may follow is also likely to have high stakes and involve bodies at the organizational level that determine whether a program will continue.

In the two types of evaluation, similar tools may be used; however, summative evaluation requires more focus on outcome indicators at predetermined end points. In both types, there is a need for rigorous procedures and clear program goals, objectives, and expected outcomes that can lead to development of indicators to direct the evaluation process (Wall, 2011).

Approaches to Evaluation

In the opening vignette, Susan volunteers to review the literature and identify resources and approaches to evaluation that the Brookhaven FPT can use to make decisions about how they will evaluate the development and maintenance of their team and the implementation of IPP. In her review of the literature, Susan is likely to encounter a vast body of information about approaches to evaluation, including those that have been specifically applied to IPP evaluation. In a comprehensive review of evaluation approaches and frameworks, Kahan (2008) concludes that the countless approaches to evaluation necessitate the selection of a carefully thought-out methodology using a set of criteria that are discussed here. The questions to be addressed include:

- What is the intent of the evaluation? (What is to be learned?) (Is it formative or summative evaluation?)
- Who is involved? That is, who are the stakeholders?
- What resources are available?

Depending on the answers, it may be necessary and/or advantageous to use different elements of a number of approaches, combining and/or modifying approaches (Kahan, 2008; Rogers & Fraser, 2003).

Within the literature, there are examples of different approaches to evaluating IPP and IPE interventions (e.g., Canadian Interprofessional Health Collaborative (CIHC), 2008; el Ansari, Phillips, & Hammick, 2001). Kahan (2008) summarizes the approaches to

Helpful Tools 10.1

Choosing an Evaluation Approach

Rogers and Fraser (2003) offer a simple yet effective set of criteria that may be applied when choosing an approach to IPP evaluation. The criteria have been framed as questions to further assist in their use.

- **Plausibility.** How likely is the evaluation approach to be helpful and in what way?
- **Practicality.** Is it possible for the evaluation approach to be successfully implemented? Does the evaluation approach offer enough support and direction?
- **Effectiveness.** What is the evidence that demonstrates that the evaluation approach works? Is the evidence sufficient (Kahan, 2008; Rogers & Fraser, 2003, p. 76)?

evaluation according to eight main categories: (a) goal-based, (b) goal-free, (c) theory-based, (d) utilization, (e) collaborative, (f) balanced scorecard, (g) appreciative inquiry, and (h) other. The category "other" is meant to capture the developmental nature of approaches to evaluation, referring to new approaches emerging as a result of innovation and necessity. Although many of the published evaluations may describe their approaches differently, they are best categorized as collaborative because they tend to focus on "a variety of types of evaluation, with varying degrees of participation and different purposes" (Kahan, 2008, p. 26–27). Helpful Tools 10.1 outlines criteria that can be applied when selecting an approach to IPP evaluation.

Evaluation Frameworks

The application of a framework has been identified as an essential aspect of evaluating IPP and IPE (CIHC, 2008; Haire, 2010). An **evaluation framework** is essentially a road map; it guides the user through the process of evaluation by summarizing and organizing key elements of the type of evaluation being undertaken. Kahan (2008) notes that while at the bare minimum an evaluation framework need only describe an approach or model of evaluation and operational steps, a comprehensive framework should consist of the following components:

- guiding principles,
- concepts,
- models/approaches,
- steps for operationalizing the models or approaches, and
- understanding evaluation in practice: positives to encourage and negatives to avoid, challenges and solutions, and prerequisites for success (p. 5–6).

Using a framework that incorporates as many of these elements as possible enhances the rigour of the IPP evaluation process (Kahan, 2008).

Spotlight 10.1

The Modified Kirkpatrick Model

The Kirkpatrick Model of Evaluation (1967) is commonly used for evaluating educational interventions in general. It consists of four levels (reaction, learning, behaviour change, and results). To evaluate IPE interventions, Freeth, Reeves, Koppel, Hammick, and Barr (2005) modified the model by adding one level to the original model. The levels of the modified model are outlined in Table 10.1. The first is the reaction level. Reaction or satisfaction with a program intervention is relatively straightforward to assess. The second level is learning or the acquisition of knowledge and skills. Freeth et al. (2002) have divided this level into two: (a) changes in perception and (b) acquisition of skills. Oandasan and Reeves (2005) have noted that most studies have measured changes in attitude. Several authors (e.g., Barr, Freeth, Hammick, Koppel, & Reeves, 2000) have noticed a dearth of instruments within the literature for measuring the knowledge and skills of collaborative practice, and urged development of methods to assess all competencies of IPE.

The next levels in the model (behavioural change, change in organizational practice, and benefits to patients) are particularly important for assessing IPP interventions. There is limited research examining these levels (as opposed to exploring indicators of the reaction, attitudinal change, and knowledge acquisition levels), which may be explained by the time and considerable resources, including financial, required to obtain evidence at these levels.

The use of frameworks in the evaluation of IPP and IPE is demonstrated by the findings of the CIHC (2008) analysis of the projects developed through the Health Canada Interprofessional Education for Collaborative Patient-Centred Practice Initiative IECPCP (see Chapter 8). The review found that in all the projects, a framework was used to guide the evaluation of the interventions or programs. The frameworks varied depending on the needs of the project. Of the 13 different models/frameworks identified, the Kirkpatrick Model of Evaluation (1967) was most commonly used. This model will be further explored in Spotlight 10.1 and Table 10.1.

As the CIHC (2008) review demonstrates, there are a number of frameworks to choose from when considering how to evaluate IPP-related initiatives and programs. When deciding which may be most suitable, it is important to recognize the differences between IPP, IPE, and interprofessional organizational (IPO) interventions. To this end, Reeves and colleagues (2011) have provided definitions and a framework to clarify the distinctions among IPP, IPE, and IPO. Furthermore, clear understanding of the objectives of the intervention, program, or initiative being implemented is very important. Accordingly, Reeves et al. have derived the following interprofessional intervention categories:

- IPE interventions that occur when two or more professions learn interactively to improve collaboration and the quality of care,
- IPP interventions that are activities or procedures incorporated into regular practice to improve collaboration and the quality of care, and

Table 10.1 Modified Kirkpatrick Model of Interprofessional Education Outcomes

Evaluation Level	Description
1. Reaction	Learners' views on the learning experience and its interprofessional nature.
2a. Modification of attitudes/perceptions	Changes in reciprocal attitudes or perceptions between participant groups. Changes in perception or attitude toward the value and/or use of team approaches to caring for a specific client group.
2b. Acquisition of knowledge/skills	Including knowledge and skills linked to interprofessional collaboration.
3. Behavioural change	Identifies individuals' transfer of interprofessional learning to their practice setting and changed professional practice.
4. Change in organizational practice	Wider changes in the organization and delivery of care.
5. Benefits to patients/ clients	Improvements in health or well-being of patients/clients.

Source: Excerpt from "Our Model of Outcomes of Interprofessional Education" by Della Freeth, Marilyn Hammick, Ivan Koppel, Scott Reeves and Hugh Barr from *A Critical Review of Evaluations of Interprofessional Education*, Occasional Paper 2. Published by Higher Education Academy, © 2002.

- IPO interventions that are changes at the organizational level (e.g. space, staffing, policy) to enhance collaboration and the quality of care (p. 169).

Although some early frameworks have been described in the literature (e.g., Haire, 2010, p. 10), a clearly articulated and validated one specifically intended for evaluating IPP has yet to emerge. In contrast, a number of frameworks for IPE evaluation have been developed: (a) the IECPCP framework (D'Amour & Oandasan, 2005), (b) the modified Kirkpatrick Model for Interprofessional Education (Freeth, Hammick, Koppel, Reeves, & Barr, 2002) (see Spotlight 10.1), and (c) the W(e)Learn Model (MacDonald, Stodel, Thompson, & Casimiro, 2009; Casimiro, MacDonald, Thompson, & Stodel, 2009) (see Spotlight 10.2). While these and other, similar frameworks are being widely adopted (e.g., CIHC, 2008), they have limitations in that they often only examine knowledge acquisition and changes in values and attitudes (CIHC, 2008; Barr et al., 2000). With this limited focus, they fail to provide for examination of causal relationships between an intervention and patient outcomes (CIHC, 2008).

The development of a comprehensive framework that can be applied to the many IPE and IPP interventions and programs that currently exist and/or are in development across a variety of practice settings and geographic locations is challenging for a number of reasons. As illustrated by D'Amour and Oandasan's (2005) IECPCP framework, IPE and IPP are

Spotlight 10.2

W(e)Learn Model

Originally designed for evaluating online learning (MacDonald, Breithaupt, Stodel, Farres, & Gabriel, 2002), the W(e)Learn Model was specifically modified to incorporate IPE and IPP (MacDonald et al., 2009; Casimiro et al., 2009).

The W(e)Learn framework is unique in its focus on guiding the design, delivery, and evaluation of health care interprofessional education. In addition, it has validated companion evaluation tools to assess programs using the W(e)Learn framework (MacDonald, Archibald, Trumpower, Cragg, Casimiro, & Jelley, 2010). W(e)Learn outlines four critical dimensions of online IPE—structure, content, media, and service—and is grounded in socioconstructivist theories and interprofessionalism.

W(e)Learn is intended to elicit four levels of outcomes, the pinnacle of which is organizational change toward IPE or IPP and the resulting improvement in care delivery that promotes patient well-being. W(e)Learn offers an emergent design process; throughout the design, development, and delivery of IPE or IPP there is ongoing evaluation that enables program adaptation and improvement as necessary.

interdependent and their relationship is complicated by the broad and multifaceted context within which they are situated. Additionally, the CIHC (2008) notes that "linking educational interventions to such health care quality measures is not linear, straightforward or immediate as the interventions often require changes in structures and processes to achieve the desired outcomes" (Future Development, para. 1).

Evaluation Instruments

Evaluation instruments are helpful resources when engaging in any evaluative process. They provide the means to collect the data needed to determine if outcomes have been attained. There are many types of evaluation instruments, which differ in terms of the kinds of information collected and the means by which data is collected. Commonly known examples are surveys and sets of questions to obtain qualitative information using a focus group format.

When choosing an evaluation instrument, its validity (how well it measures what it is intended to measure) and reliability (the degree to which it produces stable and consistent measurements) must be considered. Other possible considerations are the purpose of the evaluation, the type and approach of the evaluation, the framework being used, and resources available.

More and more evaluation instruments are being designed expressly for IPP and IPE evaluation—see, for example, the Interprofessional Collaborative Competencies Attainment Survey (MacDonald et al., 2010). However, many are specific to the projects for which they were designed, and have not been tested for validity and reliability (Freeth, Reeves, Koppel, Hammick, & Barr, 2005). Additionally, the majority of published evaluation instruments are limited to evaluating IPE interventions at the level of learner perceptions (Gillan, Lovrics, Halpern, Wiljer, Harnett, 2011).

In an analysis of evaluation plans used in the Health Canada–funded IECPCP projects, the CIHC (2008) highlights a number of important needs related to evaluation instruments:

- the need for a variety of evaluation instruments and outcome measures to capture the range of experiences, contexts, and audiences, with sensitivity to cultural and local situations,
- the need for validated evaluation instruments that allow comparisons across projects, and
- the need to create support for evaluating IPE in order to continue to improve interprofessional education.

The call for more validated instruments to evaluate IPP is identified in the literature (Gillan et al., 2011; Thannhauser, Russell-Mayhew, & Scott, 2010). To assist evaluators to identify valid and reliable tools, Thannhauser, Russell-Mayhew, and Scott provide a detailed list of 23 validated measures that have been used to evaluate IPP and IPE. For each tool, the authors identify the instrument's validity and reliability (if available) and the sample size used.

Evaluating the Process

In addition to evaluating the outcomes of IPP implementation (summative evaluation) and collecting information along the way in order to make decisions to refine and improve IPP initiatives and programs, it is important to evaluate the process of IPP implementation. Process evaluation is undertaken to determine what influences both how an initiative or program is operating and how it is able to achieve desired goals (Dehar, Casswell, & Duignan, 1993). Dehar, Casswell, and Duignan stress the importance of process evaluation, noting that it provides (a) indication of the progress being made in reaching the intended ends of a program or intervention and (b) information and insights that can inform how outcome evaluation is carried out, the interpretations of outcomes, and the development of similar endeavours in the future. For example, evaluating the process of implementation can help evaluators judge and contextualize positive and negative outcomes.

Teams and teamwork are integral to IPP implementation. Therefore, process evaluation must include examination of team building and maintenance, in terms of both team functioning and whether a team is meeting its professional mandate. Prior to this evaluation, IPP teams must ensure they have laid the groundwork to potentiate success in the evaluation process. Figure 10.1 depicts a simple but effective framework to support teams in building and maintaining themselves, while establishing the foundation for evaluating their processes. This framework is a component of the Building Positive Inter-Professional Relationships in Health Care: A Collaborative Initiative for Patient Safety and Quality Work Environments (TIPS) program touched upon in the opening vignette of the chapter (see Spotlight 10.3). The components are detailed in Helpful Tools 10.2.

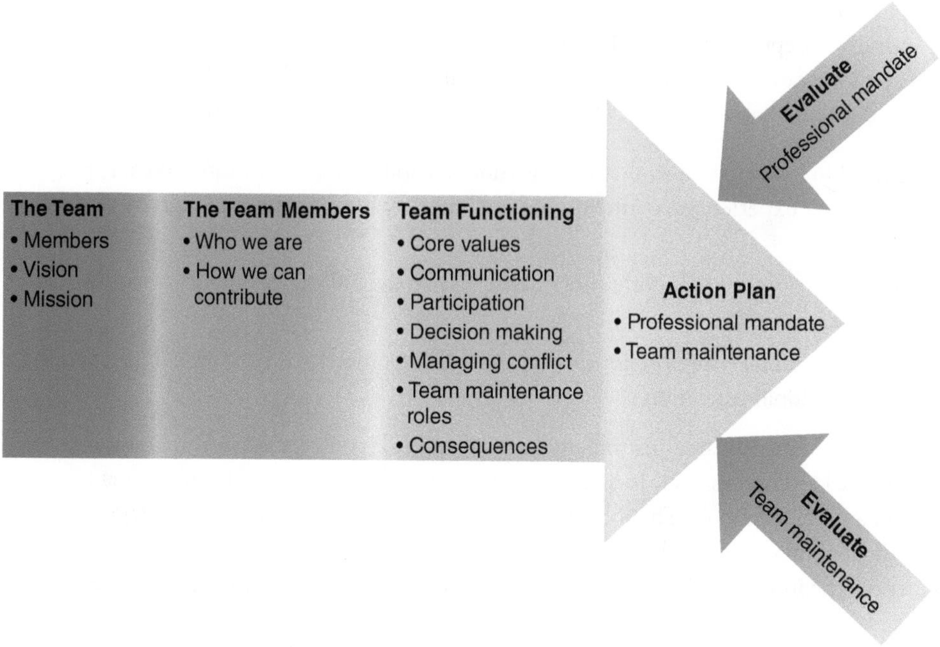

The Team
- Members
- Vision
- Mission

The Team Members
- Who we are
- How we can contribute

Team Functioning
- Core values
- Communication
- Participation
- Decision making
- Managing conflict
- Team maintenance roles
- Consequences

Action Plan
- Professional mandate
- Team maintenance

Evaluate Professional mandate

Evaluate Team maintenance

Figure 10.1 Evaluating Team Progress

Source: "eTIPS: Enhancing teams of interprofessional staff," retrieved from http://www.eworkplacehealth.com/?etips.

Spotlight 10.3

Building Positive Inter-Professional Relationships in Health Care: A Collaborative Initiative for Patient Safety and Quality Work Environments (TIPS)

Building Positive Inter-Professional Relationships in Health Care: A Collaborative Initiative for Patient Safety and Quality Work Environments (TIPS) was a HealthForceOntario-funded project that provided interprofessional education for practising clinical professionals to facilitate the adoption and implementation of interprofessional practice (IPP). The objectives of TIPS were to

- increase clinical professionals' knowledge and skills related to IPP—their ability to work together effectively in health care teams (i.e., understand the roles of others; demonstrate trust in the others' decision making ability; communicate openly; and implement conflict resolution strategies)
- ensure individual attitudes are such that they enhance team effectiveness applying new knowledge and skills, so that incremental performance improvements are realized for common problems in clinical practice

Spotlight 10.3 *(Continued)*

- improve interprofessional communication skills and practice among health care teams
- develop functioning health care teams to improve clinical practice, job satisfaction, patient care and safety, and quality of life

Over the eight months of the project, all teams progressed in relation to their team development, their attitude about the value of effective teams, and their feelings of confidence in promoting and supporting team development within the project team and others to which they belonged. On the basis of the team's current stage of functioning, team development necessarily reflected different needs for each team. Participation in TIPS involved attendance at three two-day training sessions, during which participants, grouped in their interprofessional health care teams, participated as teams in activities to explore practical applications of team development strategies. Specific content areas explored through presentations by experts and opportunities for application included critical conversation methodology, appreciative inquiry, cultivating a teamwork culture, developing a team plan, engaging in difficult conversations, and conflict resolution. Each team had the assistance of an advisor/mentor to guide the process of developing a team action plan. Participants received a workbook that consisted of the objectives of the entire project, each two-day session, and each content area. In addition, reference material, application exercises, and critical resources were included. Two RNAO Healthy Work Environment Best Practice Guidelines related to leadership and collaborative practice were included (RNAO, 2005, 2006). Throughout the program, teams presented updates on their plan development, outcomes related to team building milestones, team outcomes, and even perceived client outcomes. The sessions culminated with teams presenting their plans, accomplishments, and impacts at a final summit. During this summit, each team had an opportunity to document and discuss their journey to creating an effective interprofessional team. Both during the two-day sessions and the final summit, teams had time to engage in formal and informal team building and networking activities to bond with each other and build relationships.

One of the reasons for the success of the TIPS program was the effective use of formative evaluation during the eight-month program. A comprehensive evaluation was conducted during each of the three TIPS two-day sessions. The data were analyzed and results shared both formally and informally with the program facilitators. The teams appreciated the opportunity to share their views through focus groups and completing survey questionnaires during the evaluation process. Moreover, learners seemed to enjoy the style used during the evaluation and felt they were respected and that the researchers made them feel like they were the experts on what would work best in learning how to create and work within an effective team. Making evaluation part of the learning process appeared to motivate teams and validate their accomplishments.

Findings from the evaluation of the TIPS IPP program (Bajnok, Puddester, MacDonald, Archibald, & Kuhl, 2012; MacDonald, Archibald, Puddester, & Bajnok, 2011) further support recent literature that indicates effective teamwork has positive outcomes for patients, health care professionals, and health care organizations.

Key outcomes of the TIPS IPP teams were:

- pride in their teamwork,
- understanding the importance and value of taking time to develop the team,
- recognizing that teamwork enhances clinical outcomes and job satisfaction,
- an understanding of others' roles and responsibilities,
- valuing colleagues from other professionals,
- improving communication procedures, and
- new strategies and mechanisms to improve the workplace environment and patient care.

Helpful Tools 10.2

Creating a Team Agreement

Before evaluating IPP team progress, it is important to develop a team agreement, which helps ensure that all members are clear about the team's expectations. Team agreements should set the ground rules for how members will communicate and work together to fill their mandate. They also establish consequences for members who do not follow these mutually-agreed-upon rules. Such an agreement increases the likelihood that IPP will be successful. It should define elements such as the team, team members, and team functioning (www.eworkplacehealth.com).

Developing an Action Plan

Bajnok and colleagues (2012) underscore the importance of creating clear goals—in other words, of expressing outcomes in terms of specific results. These authors advocate action plans that incorporate goals connected to the interprofessional competencies (which will address team maintenance and functioning) as well as goals required to meet the team's professional mandate.

MacDonald and colleagues (2010) have devised a team contract and an accompanying exemplar that serve as a template for teams to identify goals, strategies, and outcomes under the six competencies of interprofessional practice identified by the National Interprofessional Competency Framework (CIHC, 2010). The six competencies, discussed at length in other chapters of this text, are communication, collaboration, roles and responsibilities, collaborative patient-family centred approach, conflict management/resolution, and team functioning. In addition to creating an action plan for interprofessional competencies, it is suggested that teams also create an action plan for the team's professional mandate that will help teams work effectively and efficiently toward meeting the team's objectives. Teams can use a template similar to the team contract. Finally, there should be ongoing review of action plans by the team to assess what goals have been met and which need to be addressed.

To evaluate team members' development of interprofessional competencies, there are validated survey tools, such as the Interprofessional Collaborative Competencies Attainment Survey (MacDonald et al., 2010), that may be used.

The review of approaches, methods, and issues related to evaluating IPP presented in this section is by no means intended to be exhaustive. As IPP uptake expands and receives greater acceptance, new knowledge and innovation related to its evaluation is developing. In this context, the content presented should be thought of as foundational knowledge to be built upon, and as a lens through which the current available evidence, discussed in the next section, may be considered.

OUTCOMES OF INTERPROFESSIONAL PRACTICE

As the movement toward IPP continues to build momentum, our understanding of the outcomes of collaborative practice is also growing. Having reviewed the importance of evaluation and some methods that may be applied, the final section of this chapter provides a more in-depth description of the emerging consensus around IPP outcomes. While IPP, and hence IPP evaluation, is relatively new, a decade of research evaluating the outcomes of collaborative practice among health care professionals has identified positive outcomes classified at the (a) patient/family/client level, (b) health care provider level, and (c) systems/organizational level.

Enhanced teamwork through IPP has been shown to benefit virtually all stakeholder groups (see Spotlight 10.4). Evidence points to shorter wait times for care, increased satisfaction with care provided, greater access to a broader range of services, and better health outcomes for patients. Providers report increased job satisfaction, decreased stress and burnout, increased staff retention, improved working environments, improved efficiency, and the opportunity to work within their full scope of practice. Health care organizations describe increased efficiency and greater capacity to provide quality care for more patients, improved staff recruitment and retention with decreased turnover, and better patient safety. Within the health care system as a whole, evidence reveals increased access to the system, better ability to develop quality improvement and accountability measures, and increased potential to coordinate all aspects of health care.

Spotlight 10.4

Positive Outcomes with Interprofessional Practice

Positive patient outcomes include:

- increased patient satisfaction with care and a more positive experience with care received,
- increased access to service across Canadian jurisdictions and shorter wait times for patients,
- better coordination of patient care and more comprehensive care,
- enhanced self-care and health condition knowledge and skills,
- better health outcomes (e.g., blood pressure control, diabetes control, health status, quality of life) and improved client self-management of care, and
- decreased emergency room and hospital visits.

Positive provider outcomes include:

- improved provider attitudes toward interprofessional collaboration and more positive perceptions and attitudes toward the value of teams,
- increased provider satisfaction, and expression of a more positive work experience than those working in uni-professional models,
- enhanced provider knowledge and skills, and
- significant improvement in providers' awareness and understanding of roles and scopes of practice.

Positive system outcomes include:

- increased health care system efficiency and
- improved access to and coordination of health care services.

Source: Barrett, Curran, Glynn, & Godwin, 2007; Oandasan, Ross Baker, Barker, Bosco, D'Amour, Jones, ... & Way, 2006.

Table 10.2 Evidence of Outcomes of Interprofessional Practice from Systematic Reviews

Study	Objectives	Authors' Conclusion
Malone, D., Newton-Howes, G., Simmonds, S., Marriott, S., & Tyrer, P. (2007). Community mental health teams (CMHTs) for people with severe mental illnesses and disordered personality. *Cochrane Database of Systematic Reviews, 2,* CD000270.	To evaluate the effects of community mental health team (CMHT) treatment for anyone with serious mental illness compared with standard non-team management.	Community mental health team management is not inferior to non-team standard care in any important respects and is superior in promoting greater acceptance of treatment. It may also be superior in reducing hospital admission and death by suicide. The evidence for CMHT-based care is insubstantial considering the massive impact the drive toward community care has on patients, careers, clinicians, and the community at large.
Mitchell, G. K., Tieman, J. J., & Shelby-James, T. M. (2008). Multidisciplinary care planning and teamwork in primary care. *Medical Journal of Australia, 188*(8), S61.	To examine policy and implementation issues around multidisciplinary care planning (MDP) as a means of improving outcomes for patients with chronic disease and/or complex care needs.	While MDP improves many functional outcomes, widespread implementation of MDP in standard practice will require complex and targeted strategies. Devising and testing such strategies is a prerequisite for widespread, routine use of MPD in chronic disease management.
McAlister, F. A., Stewart, S., Ferrua, S., & McMurray J. J. (2004). Multidisciplinary strategies for the management of heart failure patients at high risk for admission. *Journal of the American College of Cardiology, 2004, 44*(4), 810–819.	To determine whether multidisciplinary strategies improve outcomes for heart failure patients.	Multidisciplinary strategies for the management of patients with heart failure reduce heart failure hospitalizations. Those programmes that involve specialized follow-up by a multidisciplinary team also reduce mortality and all-cause hospitalizations.
Joshi, C., Russell, G., Cheng, I. H., Kay, M, Pottie, K., Alston, M., ... Harris, M.F. (2013). A narrative synthesis of the impact of primary health care delivery models for refugees in resettlement countries on access, quality and coordination. International *Journal of Equity Health, 12*(1): 88.	To identify the components of primary health care service delivery models for refugees that are effective at improving access, quality, and coordination of care.	Access to care is improved by multidisciplinary staff and use of interpreters and bilingual staff, and other factors.

Table 10.2 *(Continued)*

Study	Objectives	Authors' Conclusion
Simmonds, S., Coid, J., Joseph, P., Marriott, S., & Tyrer, P. (2001). Community mental health team management in severe mental illness: A systematic review. *The British Journal of Psychiatry, 178*, 497–502.	To assess the benefits of community mental health team management in severe mental illness.	Community mental health team management is superior to standard care in promoting greater acceptance of treatment, and may also reduce hospital admission and avoid deaths by suicide. This model of care is effective and deserves encouragement.
Zwarenstein, M., & Bryant, W. (2000). Interventions to promote collaboration between nurses and doctors. *Cochrane Database of Systematic Reviews*, (1), CD000072.	To assess the effects of interventions designed to improve nurse–doctor collaboration.	Increasing collaboration improved outcomes of importance to patients and to health care managers. These gains were moderate and affected health care processes rather than outcomes. Further research is needed to confirm these findings. Interventions other than nurse–doctor ward rounds and team meetings should also be tested.

Evidence Supporting Interprofessional Practice

According to the Canadian Health Services Research Foundation policy synthesis (Oandasan, Ross Baker, Barker, Bosco, D'Amour, Jones, ... & Way, 2006, p. i), "a health care system that supports effective teamwork can improve the quality of patient care, enhance patient safety, and reduce workload issues that cause burnout among health care professionals." While there is widespread consensus that the future of Canadian health care design and delivery must reflect IPP approaches, it is essential that we systematically evaluate the potential benefits of this type of care.

High-quality evidence is available that reveals positive outcomes for patients, providers, and the system in general when IPP is applied to care of patients in specialized areas such as mental health and chronic disease prevention and management. To date, IPP approaches in chronic disease management have been most commonly targeted to management of diabetes, coronary artery disease, and depression. The World Health Organization's *Framework for Action on Interprofessional Education and Collaborative Practice* (2010) highlights six systematic reviews examining the outcomes of IPP that provide high-quality evidence in relation to the introduction or utilization of IPP. Table 10.2 summarizes these findings.

The body of evidence related to IPP is growing and beginning to influence models of collaborative practice in Canada. However, more knowledge and systematic research, including evaluative research, is needed to fully understand the value of IPP within Canada's changing health care context, which reflects a greater focus on primary care, health promotion, and a health-outcomes orientation (RNAO, 2012). In all the initiatives described in this chapter, one theme emerges: the need for clarity around IPP and specific direction in terms of not only how to implement it, but critically, how to evaluate it. As we embark on this period of change, in which health care professionals move away from traditional individualistic, uni-professional approaches toward an era of greater collaboration, creating/identifying models and methods for evaluating IPP will be essential to future success.

CONCLUSION

As methods and approaches to IPP continue to expand, so too must our repertoire of evaluation tools. Understanding the importance of evaluation approaches and processes will help practitioners, organizations, and the system effectively engage in IPP and monitor the results in order to ensure IPP is having the desired effects on our health system goals. This chapter provided an overview of general research and evaluation concepts that are particularly relevant to health care settings and situations. Additionally, specific evaluation approaches that may be applied to IPP were reviewed. Finally, a summary of emerging evidence related to the implementation of IPP approaches was presented.

SUMMARY

- Evaluation of IPP is important to ensuring the successful transition to a collaborative model of practice in health care and to the overall outcome of quality health care. Measuring IPP outcomes serves a number of purposes, including determining the most effective and efficient ways to engage in IPE and IPP. Evaluation also enables us to identify what ongoing changes need to be made as we strive for excellence in client-centred care.

- Evaluation in IPP is situated within the broader evidenced-based health care practice context and is focused on developing best practices related to supporting IPP and patient, provider, and health care outcomes. Thus, the evaluation of IPP programs and initiatives must be rigorous and based on sound research methodologies, so that findings are valid and reliable.
- IPP may be evaluated at the level of the patient/client/family, the health care provider, and the organization/system. Several frameworks have been developed to support and add rigour to the IPP evaluation process.
- The evaluation of IPP may be formative or summative, focusing on structures, processes, and outcomes. All evaluation is directed by a set of goals, objectives, expected outcomes, and indicators of success that will aid in determining what to measure, and how to measure it. Formative evaluation of IPP requires that IPP teams invest in team building and maintenance that involves developing action plans and goals/objectives translatable into measurable outcomes for use during the evaluation phase.
- The emerging consensus about IPP based on the evaluations that have been completed and the systematic reviews of these evaluations is that IPP results in positive patient, provider, and health care system outcomes. These are most evident in specialized care areas such as mental health and chronic disease management.
- The reported positive outcomes of IPP notwithstanding, there is a continued need for high-quality longitudinal evaluative investigations using systematic and rigorous research methods, as IPP programs and initiatives continue to grow.

Key Terms

care delivery outcomes
evaluation
evaluation framework
evidence-based practice
formative evaluation
outcomes research
process evaluation
qualitative research methods
quantitative research methods
reliability
structure evaluation
summative evaluation
validity

Review Questions

1. Describe the key differences between IPE, IPP, and IPO.
2. Define formative and summative evaluation and describe how each is integral to evaluating IPP and IPE. Include in your definitions the terms *structure*, *process*, and *outcome evaluation*.
3. Summarize the evidence describing how IPP improves health care outcomes.

Application Exercises

eTIPS is an offshoot of the Building Positive Inter-Professional Relationships in Health Care: A Collaborative Initiative for Patient Safety and Quality Work Environments (TIPS) project that provides interprofessional education and includes a host of helpful tools to support team development and teamwork.

1. Visit the eTIPS website at http://eworkplacehealth.com and review the content and resources.
2. Identify a team that you are currently involved in (e.g., study group, IPP team) and analyze how the team developed on the basis of the three phases of building and maintaining an interprofessional team.

   Has your team progressed through the three phases?
3. Use the resources provided to create a team agreement, develop an action plan, and consider how you will evaluate team progress and functioning.

Additional Resources

Websites and Electronic Documents

Canadian Interprofessional Health Collaborative
http://www.cihc.ca

eTIPS: Enhancing Teams of Interprofessional Staff
http://eworkplacehealth.com/?etips

Registered Nurses' Association of Ontario (RNAO) Best Practice Guidelines
http://www.rnao.org

Team contract templates and exemplars that can be used in the process of developing an action plan, available in French and English
http://www.ennovativesolution.com/WeLearn/IPE-Instruments.html

W(e)Learn
http://www.ennovativesolution.com/WeLearn

References

Agency for Health Care Research and Quality (AHRQ). (2000). *Outcome research: Fact sheet*. Retrieved from http://www.ahrq.gov/clinic/outfact.htm

Bajnok, I., Puddester, D., MacDonald, C.J. Archibald, D., & Kuhl, D. (August 2012). Building positive relationships in health care: Evaluation of the TIPS interprofessional education program. *Contemporary Nurse, 43*(2).

Barrett, J. (2007). *Analysis and synthesis report PHC: Interprofessional collaboration, chronic disease management, and health promotion and disease prevention, activities, processes and tools*. Toronto, ON: Ontario Ministry of Health and Long-Term Care.

Barr, H., Freeth, D., Hammick, M., Koppel, I. & Reeves, S. (2000). *Evaluations of interprofessional education: A United Kingdom review for health and social care*. London, UK: Centre for the Advancement of Interprofessional Education (CAIPE) & the British Educational Research Association. Retrieved from https://caipe.org.uk/silo/files/evaluations-of-interprofessional-education.pdf

Barrett, J., Curran, V., Glynn, L., & Godwin, M. (2007). *CHSRF synthesis: Interprofessional collaboration and quality primary healthcare*. Ottawa, ON: Canadian Health Services Research Foundation.

Canadian Interprofessional Health Collaborative (CIHC). (2008). *Program evaluation of interprofessional education: A mapping of evaluation strategies of the 20 IECPCP projects*. Retrieved from http://www.cihc.ca/files/publications/CIHC_EvalMappingStrategiesReport_Sept08_Final.pdf

Canadian Interprofessional Health Collaborative (CIHC). (2010). *A national interprofessional competency framework*. Vancouver, BC: Author.

Casimiro, L., MacDonald, C. J., Thompson, T. L., & Stodel, E. J. (2009). Grounding theories of W(e)Learn : A framework for online interprofessional education. *Journal of Interprofessional Care, 23*(4), 390–400.

Creswell, J. W. (2012). *Educational research: Planning, conducting, and evaluating quantitative and qualitative research* (4th ed.). Upper Saddle River, NJ: Pearson.

D'Amour, D., & Oandasan, I. (2005). Interprofessionality as the field of interprofessional practice and interprofessional education: An emerging concept. *Journal of Interprofessional Care, 19*(S1), 8–10.

Dehar, M., Casswell, S., & Duignan, P. (1993). Formative and process evaluation of health promotion and disease prevention programs. *Evaluation Review, 17*(2), 204–220.

Donabedian, A. (1988). The quality of care. How can it be assessed? *JAMA, 260*(12), 1743–8.

el Ansari, W., Phillips, C. J., & Hammick, M. (2001). Collaboration and partnerships: Developing the evidence base. *Health & Social Care in the Community, 9*: 215–227.

Freeth, D., Hammick, M., Koppel, I., Reeves, S., & Barr, H. (2002). *A critical review of evaluations of interprofessional education*. London, UK: Interprofessional Education Joint Evaluation Team (JET).

Freeth, D., Reeves, S., Koppel, I., Hammick, M., & Barr, H. (2005). *Evaluating interprofessional education: A self-help guide*. Working paper. London, UK: Higher Education Academy Learning and Teaching Support Network for Health Sciences and Practice. Retrieved from http://www.health.heacademy.ac.uk/doc/mp/04-16_hughbarr.pdf/at_download/file.pdf

Gillan, C., Lovrics, E., Halpern, E., Wiljer, D., & Harnett, N. (2011). The evaluation of learner outcomes in interprofessional continuing education: A literature review and an analysis of survey instruments. *Medical Teacher*, 33(9), e461–470.

Haire, B. (2010). *Interprofessional care: A model of collaborative practice*. Retrieved from http://peihsc.ca/wp-content/uploads/IP_care.pdf

Ingersoll, G. I. (2004). Generating evidence through outcomes management. In B. M. Melnyk & E. Fineout-Overholt (Eds.), *Evidence-based practice in nursing and health care: A guide to best practice* (pp. 299–332). Philadelphia, PA: Lippincott, Williams, & Wilkins.

Kahan, B. (2008). *Excerpts from review of evaluation frameworks*. Saskatchewan Ministry of Education.

Kirkpatrick, D. L. (1967). Evaluation of training. In R. L. Craig & L. R. Bittel (Eds.), *Training and development handbook* (pp. 87–112). New York, NY: McGraw-Hill.

Levin, R. (2006). Evidence-based practice in nursing: What is it? In R. F. Levin & H. R. Feldman (Eds.), *Teaching evidence–based practice in nursing* (pp. 5-13). New York, NY: Springer Publishing.

MacDonald, C. J., Archibald, D., Puddester, D., & Bajnok, I. (2011). Renewal through team development: Experiencing an emerging program design in interprofessional education for health care practitioners. *Journal of Health Administration Education,* Spring, 1–18.

MacDonald, C. J., Archibald, D., Trumpower, D., Cragg, E., Casimiro, L., & Jelley, W. (2010). Quality standards for interprofessional health care education: Designing a toolkit of bilingual assessment instruments. *Journal of Research in Interprofessional Practice and Education, 1*(3), 1–13.

MacDonald, C. J., Breithaupt, K., Stodel, E. J., Farres, L. G., & Gabriel, M. A. (2002). Evaluation of web-based educational programs: A pilot study of the demand-driven learning model. *International Journal of Testing, 2(*1), 35–61.

MacDonald, C. J., Stodel, E. J., Thompson, T.-L., & Casimiro, L. (2009). W(e)Learn: A framework for interprofessional education. *International Journal of Electronic Healthcare, 5*(1), 33–47.

Malone, D., Newton-Howes, G., Simmonds, S., Marriott, S., & Tyrer, P. (2007). Community mental health teams (CMHTs) for people with severe mental illnesses and disordered personality. *Cochrane Database of Systematic Reviews, 2,* CD000270.

McAlister, F. A., Stewart, S., Ferrua, S., & McMurray, J. J. (2004). Multidisciplinary strategies for the management of heart failure patients at high risk for admission. *Journal of the American College of Cardiology, 44*(4), 810–819.

Oandasan, I., & Reeves, S. (2005). Key elements of interprofessional education. Part 2: Factors, processes and outcomes. *Journal of Interprofessional Care, 19*(S1), 39–48.

Oandasan, I., Ross Baker, G., Barker, K., Bosco, C., D'Amour, D., Jones, L., ... & Way, D. (2006). *Teamwork in healthcare: Promoting effective teamwork in healthcare in Canada. Policy synthesis and recommendations.* Ottawa, ON: Canadian Health Services Research Foundation.

Reeves, S., Goldman, J., Gilbert, J., Tepper, J., Silver, I., Suter, E., & Zwarenstein, M. (2011). A scoping review to improve conceptual clarity of interprofessional interventions. *Journal of Interprofessional Care, 25*, 167–174.

Registered Nurses' Association of Ontario (RNAO). (2005). *Developing and sustaining nursing leadership.* Toronto, ON: Author.

Registered Nurses' Association of Ontario (RNAO). (2006). *Collaborative practice among nursing teams*. Toronto, ON: Author.

Registered Nurses' Association of Ontario (RNAO). (2012). *Primary solutions for primary care.* Toronto, ON: Author.

Registered Nurses' Association of Ontario (RNAO). (2013). *Developing and sustaining interprofessional health care: Optimizing patient, organizational, and system outcomes.* Toronto, ON: Author.

Rogers, P. J., & Fraser, D. (2003). Appreciating appreciative inquiry. *New Directions for Evaluation, 100*, 75–83.

Simmonds, S., Coid, J., Joseph, P., Marriott, S., & Tyrer, P. (2001). Community mental health team management in severe mental illness: A systematic review. *The British Journal of Psychiatry, 178,* 497–502.

Thannhauser, J., Russell-Mayhew, S., & Scott, C. (2010). Measures of interprofessional education and collaboration. *Journal of Interprofessional Care, 24*(4), 336–349.

Trochim, W. M. K. (2006). Evaluation research: Introduction to evaluation. In *Research methods knowledge base*. Retrieved from http://www.socialresearchmethods.net/kb/intreval.php

Wall, D. (2011). Evaluation: Improving practice, influencing policy. In T. Swanwick (Ed.), *Understanding medical education: Evidence, theory and practice* (pp. 336–351). Oxford, UK: Wiley-Blackwell.

World Health Organization (WHO). (2010). *Framework for action on interprofessional education and collaborative practice.* Geneva, Switzerland: Authors.

Zwarenstein, M., & Bryant, W. (2000). Interventions to promote collaboration between nurses and doctors. *Cochrane Database of Systematic Reviews, 1,* CD000072.

Part IV
Future Directions

Throughout the first 10 chapters of this text, readers have been exposed to key concepts related to interprofessional practice (IPP). In Part I, the focus was on setting the stage for IPP through a description of the evolution of the Canadian health care system and the challenges currently faced in providing health care to Canadians. We also described a framework by which the reader could deconstruct health care situations, exploring process, relationship, and task dimensions, along with contextual factors. In Part II of this book, we further explored central concepts essential for an understanding of IPP. These included teams and teamwork; professional roles and relationships; collaboration; conflict, problem-solving, and negotiation; and leadership. In Part III, we turned our focus to the contexts within which IPP is taught, practised, and evaluated. In Part IV of this text, we expand the conception of IPP even further, arguing that the next logical step in the evolution of IPP is intersectoral collaboration. Through a review of past and present practices, an analysis of health care gains and challenges over the last number of years, and a review of key policy and regulatory documents, the case is made for collaboration that moves beyond individual health care practitioners—and even beyond the collaboration of health care teams. Rather, we argue for collaboration between all of the players involved in the wide range of sectors that are part of health as it is viewed within the Canada context, as a fundamental resource for living and a right of all Canadians. To this end, Chapter 11 provides the reader with an opportunity to consider future directions that expand the notion of IPP, while also increasing its impact on individual lives.

Chapter 11

Moving Beyond Interprofessional Practice to Intersectoral Collaboration

Hong is a respiratory therapist (RT) making a home visit to a new client. Brian, his client, is a 23-year-old Aboriginal man who suffered a C4 spinal cord injury in a motorcycle accident two years ago. Hong, in reviewing his client's record prior to this meeting, becomes aware of gaps in information. Most importantly, he realizes that he knows little of Brian's story—who he is and what has led him to this point in his life. However, from medical records and the referral provided to him, he is able to piece together a timeline. After Brian's accident, he underwent multiple surgeries and an extended stay in an acute care facility, followed by a lengthy period of rehabilitation in an agency providing specialized neurological care. Recently, Brian moved from living with his family to a government-run supportive housing residence with assisted living services.

Prior to visiting Brian, Hong decides to call Brian's community case worker.

Hong: Hi Cleo, it's Hong Lee calling. I'm the RT who'll be working with Brian K. I'm heading over to see him today for the first time, and was hoping you could give me some information to fill in the gaps. Why this change in residence, for example?

Cleo (community case worker): Hi Hong, I'm glad you've called. I spoke with Brian yesterday about your visit and he gave me permission to share with you what I know. I'm assuming that you have the medical records. In terms of his family and sociocultural context, Brian is Aboriginal. After discharge from the rehabilitation facility, he initially moved back to the First Nations reserve outside of the city to live with his family for about six months. During that time, he worked hard to increase his independence in whatever way he could. His hope was to be able to once again live independently. While he's nervous about the challenges ahead, he's also very excited about this move to assisted-living housing.

Hong: OK, that's good to know. Can you tell me anything more about the kind of care Brian requires and how that's being accomplished?

Cleo: It's a pretty complicated situation. Brian's spinal cord injury resulted in complete paralysis of his body and legs. He still has fairly good head and neck movement as well as some very limited shoulder movement too. That's important for many of the devices he uses. For example, he uses an electric wheelchair, which he manoeuvres with a chin controller.

Hong: Who else is involved in providing his care?

Cleo: Brian requires complete assistance with transferring in and out of his wheelchair and during mealtimes. There are several personal support workers (PSWs) who assist with these and other activities of daily living, such as washing and dressing, and they've just ordered a new lift device to make the process easier.

Hong: I gather I'm going in to assess his breathing and see where things are at with that?

Cleo: Yes. So far Brian has made good progress in breathing on his own but sometimes he needs help in clearing his secretions. His greatest fear is becoming dependent on a ventilator. One of the PSWs was worried about choking risk yesterday. We were wondering about a swallowing assessment. Let us know if you can do that or if we should make a referral to an occupational therapist.

Hong: OK, thanks, Cleo. This is a good start. I'm on my way over and expect I'll be in touch again soon with more questions. I'd better call the housing administrative personnel so that I can coordinate access before I head over.

Shortly thereafter, Hong arrives at Brian's assisted-living residence. He knocks on the door and is greeted by a gentleman who introduces himself as Percy, one of Brian's PSWs. As Hong enters the apartment, he hears a voice and follows Percy to the living room.

Hilde (technologist): OK, Brian, give me a second here ... The mouth-stick setup you've been working with to enable you to communicate with this computer, move your wheelchair, and do other things seems to be working well. But I think we can adjust it to make it a little more sensitive so you don't have to use as much energy to communicate and operate things.

Percy (PSW): That will be great, won't it, Brian? Even though this device is amazing, I know how tiring it can be for you at times.

Hong: (Waving) Hi Brian, I'm Hong. I'm the RT who'll be working with you starting today.

Brian motions with his head toward the technologist who is still working with his mouth-stick.

Hong (smiling): Got it, I'll wait until you're set up to talk with me.

As Hong waits for the next few minutes, he takes in the surroundings. Amid the family photos, he sees numerous Aboriginal art pieces. In addition to Brian's wheelchair, Hong notices a portable lift device and additional medical equipment. Hong realizes there is so much more he doesn't yet know about Brian's care needs and Brian as a person. Family and cultural contexts will be important to understand. Hong realizes that beyond the immediate health sector, he knows very little about the various sectors, including the broader public sector and housing, that are involved with Brian's health. If he is to provide the best care to Brian, he will need to broaden his understanding of collaboration at the intersectoral level.

Learning Outcomes

AFTER STUDYING THIS CHAPTER, YOU SHOULD BE ABLE TO:

1. **Summarize current trends in the health of Canadians and the Canadian health care system.**
2. **Define intersectoral collaborative practice and intersectoral action for health.**
3. **Discuss intersectoral collaboration in the context of IPP and patient care outcomes.**
4. **Describe social determinants of health and relevant sectors that may impact the health of Canadians.**

INTRODUCTION

AS HAS BEEN DEMONSTRATED THROUGHOUT THIS TEXT, INTERPROFESSIONAL PRACTICE (IPP) is an important part of an overall strategy to reform Canada's health care system so that Canadians get better health care and better value for their investments as taxpayers. In the past decade, IPP and other strategic approaches have helped make inroads in addressing the health needs of Canadians. The various topics addressed in this text highlight the integral nature of IPP in realizing superordinate health sector goals, such as increased access to services and better patient outcomes. Notwithstanding the advancements achieved, recent reports suggest that much more change is needed if greater health impacts (resulting from health reform policies, plans, and projects) are to be felt across the country (Health Council of Canada [HCC], 2013a). The way forward is likely to require a multifaceted approach. Undoubtedly, it must involve broader collaborative efforts spanning all **sectors**—that is, parts of the economy—with a role to play in the health of Canadians (including the health sector).

The opening vignette of this chapter demonstrates that a strong relationship exists between the various parts of the health sector and other sectors. In order to meet the health needs of clients, particularly in the community setting, health care providers and IPP teams must extend their collaborative efforts to include all sectors with which clients interact in order to attain their health goals. For example, in the opening vignette, Hong must interact with professionals from multiple sectors, such as housing. When we think of traditional approaches to health care, only a few members of an IPP team (e.g., a social worker) may focus on this type of collaboration. More germane is Hong's realization that, while he needs to expand his conception of IPP to include professionals outside of the health sector, he has limited knowledge about many of the sectors affecting the health outcomes of his client.

This chapter is meant to encourage and help the reader develop knowledge about the sectors outside of the traditional health care focus that influence health outcomes. It also directs him or her in approaches to engaging collaboratively across sectors and at various levels. The chapter begins with a discussion of Canada's position on the health of Canadians and the health care system. This context is important for expanding our view of IPP beyond the borders of the health sector to include other sectors involved in health outcomes. There follows a review of proposed ways forward that support better health care results for Canadians. Finally, we examine the role intersectoral collaborative action can play in optimizing health care delivery and health outcomes.

HEALTH CARE DIRECTIONS IN CANADA

Canada has pursued the ideal of "health for all" for many decades. To understand what actions and conditions are necessary to achieve this goal, we must first be clear on what is meant by *health*. Early definitions focused on absence of disease. However, from the mid-1900s onward, a broader conceptualization that included a state of physical, mental, and social well-being was adopted. Two important policy documents in the 1970s entrenched this perspective. In 1974, the federal government published a report highlighting the construction of health as including human biology, lifestyle, the social and physical environments in which people live, and the organization of health care (Lalonde, 1974). Additionally, in 1978, an international conference was held in Alma-Ata, Russia, that focused on principles of primary health care. Out of this conference emerged the Alma-Ata Declaration, ratified by Canada, which profoundly changed the focus of health from one of acute-illness intervention to one of health promotion. In the Declaration, health was once again defined as physical, mental, and social well-being, rather than the absence of disease. Additionally, it was identified as a fundamental human right, the attainment of which is a critical global goal requiring the action of many social and economic sectors in addition to the health care sector (Pan American Health Organization, 2003, Clause I). Thirty-five years later, we typically view health in Canada in the context of quality of life and respect for individual choice. It is also seen as a resource individually defined and influenced by life circumstances, our culture, and our social, economic, and physical environments. Over these past 35 years, this emerging definition has developed in parallel with an ever-increasing focus on health promotion as a central pillar of health policy in Canada.

Now, more than ever, efforts to ensure that Canadians are experiencing quality of life and access to health-related resources are challenged by the pace at which the needs of Canadians are evolving. Recent health care reform initiatives, including the move to IPP, have been helpful and will continue to be a major part of the overall health strategy. However, as highlighted in Canada's focus on primary health care and included in the

Alma-Ata Declaration, a broader commitment inclusive of all sectors invested in attaining better health for Canadians must be at the forefront of future efforts. This section provides an overview of current and emerging health care trends reflective of the changing needs of Canadians and driving the impetus for broader intersectoral collaboration.

Checking In on Health and Health Care Trends in Canada

Chapter 1 of this text provided an overview of the health care reform agenda in Canada, which was significantly influenced by the 2003 *First Ministers' Accord on Health Care Renewal* and the 2004 *10-Year Plan to Strengthen Health Care*. One of the noteworthy outcomes was the establishment of the Health Council of Canada to "monitor progress and outcomes against the commitments made in the health accords and to track the impact on health care reform across the country" (Health Council of Canada, 2013a, p. 3). A decade later, as the mandate for the health accords is ending and funding to the Health Council ceases, it falls to us to sum up the progress made to date in terms of the health of Canadians as a relevant exercise.

Despite the promises of health care reform inherent in these national policy directions, recent data reveals that to a large extent, the health needs of Canadians have outpaced system resources. Modest progress has been made in reducing wait times, implementing electronic health records, increasing drug coverage, and forming primary health care reform initiatives. However, in many key areas, Canada lags behind other countries. Additionally, while more than three-quarters of Canadians indicate that the medical care received from their primary care physician is excellent or very good, less than half of those with multiple chronic conditions described their care at this same level (HCC, 2011). Add to this figure the context of our expanding number of Canadians diagnosed with chronic health conditions, which climbed to 31% in 2010, putting Canada in seventh place out of 11 comparators (Commonwealth Fund, 2010).

At the same time, the movement to IPP has led to the creation of more interprofessional teams and new approaches to chronic disease management in particular. However, fewer than half of those Canadians who have primary care providers are likely to be able to get a same-day or next-day appointment if needed. This puts Canada last in a comparison of 10 high-income countries (HCC, 2013b). Early gains in decreasing wait time for high-demand procedures, such as hip and knee replacement surgery, have stalled (HCC, 2013a). Escalating prescription drug costs result in 10% of Canadians either skipping doses or failing to secure their required medication at all (HCC, 2013a). Of special concern is that there are not enough home care services to meet the needs of seniors. At the same time, our population is aging, with a median age of close to 40 years. Compare this figure to statistics from just 40 years ago, showing a median age of 26 years. Factors such as the aging baby boomer generation, decreasing family size, and increased life expectancy have resulted in seniors being the fastest-growing age group in the country, estimates suggesting that by 2050 one in four Canadians will be over age 65. Concurrently, while Canadians are living longer, they are experiencing more chronic illness and disability. In 2009, nine out of ten seniors reported living with at least one chronic condition, while 25% of seniors aged 65 to 79 years and 37% of those over 80 years of age indicated having at least four chronic conditions (Public Health Agency of Canada [PHAC], 2010). There can be no doubt that the aging of our population, concurrent with the increased prevalence of chronic illness being identified, will inevitably increase demand for medical services and procedures, home care services, and chronic-disease-management approaches. The system is under unprecedented strain, and novel approaches to care delivery have become essential.

Future Directions for Better Health Outcomes

Health care expenditures in Canada in 2012 were estimated at $207 billion. This represents a two-thirds increase in funding over the previous decade, with only modest success in stimulating the promised health reform upon which they were predicated (HCC, 2013a). One of the most significant findings out of this experience highlights the futility of attempting to address system-wide health care issues by focusing on individual components separately (HCC, 2013a). This idea is not new. For example, the Ottawa Charter for Health Promotion, one of Canada's central health policy documents, "puts health on the agenda of policy makers in all sectors and at all levels, directing them to be aware of the health consequences of their decisions and to accept their responsibilities for health" (World Health Organization [WHO], 1986).

One newly suggested approach to addressing health system challenges at this broader, health system and/or sector level is the Triple Aim Framework (Institute for Healthcare Improvement, 2013). This framework, which focuses on better health, better care, and better value, has already been applied within a number of Canadian jurisdictions, including Alberta, Saskatchewan, and Ontario. Additionally, both the Canadian Medical Association (CMA) and the Canadian Nurses Association (CNA) have used this framework to identify principles for system transformation (CMA & CNA, 2011). The three central components of the Triple Aim Framework describe:

- better health (focusing on the overall health of Canadians, longevity, lifestyle, and chronic disease prevalence),
- better care (focusing on both the indicators of the quality of care and patient and provider satisfaction), and
- better value (focusing on the value attained within the health care system for the resources required, including looking at efficiency and appropriateness as important indicators) (HCC, 2013a).

Considering the Chapter 1 discussion of the values that underpin the Canadian health care system, the suggestion of a complementary approach that includes a strong focus on equity be applied alongside this framework should not be surprising. **Equity** as it relates to health is defined by Braveman and Gruskin (2003, p. 254) as "the absence of systemic disparities in health (or in the major social determinants of health) between social groups who have different levels of underlying social advantage/disadvantage." Placing this notion of health equity squarely within the agenda for health system reform ensures that Canadian values remain central to changes required to make the system sustainable.

Thus far in this text, the discussion of collaboration has typically focused on individuals, or even teams, working together for a common goal. Often this goal is the best possible health outcome for a particular individual, family, group, or community. But consider now broadening that idea to include collaboration across all of the various players with a stake in the health of Canadians, with the goal of the best possible health outcomes for all. This necessary expansion of interprofessional collaboration, which is at the heart of IPP, to intersectoral collaboration is simultaneously visionary and daunting. It requires that we once again move beyond local perspectives and priorities to create a common vision.

INTERSECTORAL ACTION FOR HEALTH

The emphasis upon structural and policy changes, **determinants of health** (the multifaceted factors that influence health), and intersectional collaboration, along with the health promotion movement, have been slow to translate into significant changes (HCC, 2013a; Smith, Van Herk, & Rahaman, 2012). This finding suggests that addressing the health disparities and inequalities experienced by Canadians may yet prove to be a challenge. The good news is that the health care renewal efforts of the past 10 years, with IPP a central focus, have built momentum. They have also brought once again an acute awareness of the transformation needed to make Canada's health system high-performing and capable of significantly improving national health. At the centre of this transformation is the need for greater attention to intersectoral collaboration at all relevant levels (e.g., legislation and policy, local/community, organizational, programs and projects, teams, and individual professionals).

At the level of the IPP team and individual health professionals, this mandate translates into participation in the kinds of collaborative efforts and interdependent actions to meet health care consumer needs that have been the focus of this text. However, as the opening vignette suggests, many professionals in the health sector require knowledge of how social, economic, or physical environment factors influence health. Also, understanding the role of **social determinants of health** (social, economic, or physical environmental factors that influence the health of individuals and communities) is critical. Realizing the degree to which non-health-sector factors impact the health of individuals, families, and communities is becoming increasingly important. Additionally, IPP teams and their members must expand their conception of collaboration beyond their silos, in order to apply their collaborative skills in working with individual professionals and teams in other sectors.

This section provides an introduction to the concepts of intersectoral collaboration and intersectoral action for health. Additionally, it discusses how IPP teams can collaborate with professionals in other sectors to potentiate positive health outcomes.

Defining Intersectoral Collaboration and Action

Intersectoral collaboration (ISC) is defined as follows:

> A recognized relationship between part or parts of the health sector with part or parts of another sector which has been formed to take action on an issue to achieve health outcomes ... in a way that is more effective, efficient or sustainable than could be achieved by the health sector acting alone. (Danaher, 2011, p. 5)

Intersectoral collaboration can be seen as both a process and a tool, reflecting the underlying realization that health problems are linked to many determinants and are too complex for the health sector alone to address (Danaher, 2011; Public Health Agency of Canada [PHAC], 2007). When action is taken to affect health outcomes as a result of ISC, it is referred to as **intersectoral action (ISA)** (WHO, n.d.).

The concept of intersectoral collaboration originated by way of the primary health care principles introduced in the Declaration of Alma-Ata. In the 1980s and 1990s, subsequent international health promotion conferences elevated the profile of ISC. During this period, efforts to work across sectors for better health outcomes increased, as did knowledge development related to social determinants of health (PHAC, 2007). Today, while the importance of ISC is widely acknowledged and well supported, it has not been broadly adopted in Canada, the vast majority of ISC initiatives being limited to specific populations or settings only (PHAC, 2007). However, the successes of these initiatives are a strong indication of the tremendous untapped potential of ISC to help address health disparities and make the kinds of changes necessary.

From the perspective of the health care consumer, ISC makes sense. Research evidence is increasingly demonstrating that the conditions impacting health are often beyond the provision of health care (WHO Commission on Social Determinants of Health [CSDH], 2008; Reading, 2009). Literature is also emerging that indicates health care consumers are progressively concerned about social determinants of health, such as income, social status, and the physical and social environment, identifying these factors as impacting their health and sense of well-being (e.g., Davidson, Kitzinger, & Hunt, 2006; Davidson, Mitchel & Hunt, 2008; Macintyre, McKay, & Ellaway, 2006; Robert & Booske, 2011). In the opening vignette, it is possible to imagine that, when asked, Brian would include among the determinants of his health the assisted living services he receives, housing, a disability income benefits program, and access to technologies and resources that help him communicate and remain socially connected. All these resources and services are outside the purview of the health sector. Yet, in order to meet Brian's health needs, all of them, including the health sector, must come together in a concerted fashion.

Intersectoral collaboration not only refers to collaborating horizontally across sectors at the point of care or other levels, but also vertically between levels (Danaher, 2011; PHAC, 2007). **Horizontal intersectoral collaboration (horizontal ISC)** is effective in circumstances in which there is a need to bring "together diverse resources, expertise and experiences to solve complex issues whose solutions lay outside the capacity of any one sector" (Danaher, 2011, p. 6). **Vertical intersectoral collaboration (vertical ISC)** occurs between different levels, often involving partnering between the governmental and non-governmental sectors to address broad policy and resources issues (PHAC, 2007; MacLean et al., 2010). The opening vignette involving Brian demonstrates a horizontal ISC effort in which the health sector, represented by Hong, collaborates with non-health sectors such as social services, business, and housing to provide care. In the vignette, Hong recognizes the intersectoral nature of the support Brian requires to meet his health needs.

Impact of Intersectoral Collaboration

Evidence emerging from ISC and ISA initiatives and projects both nationally and internationally, and at different levels, support analysis of the impact of these efforts. This literature also describes the lessons learned, including what conditions act as facilitators and barriers to successful collaboration between subsectors in health and across sectors impacting health (Chomik, 2007; Danaher, 2011; PHAC, 2007). Internationally, ISC and ISA efforts have been shown to have "strengthened economic growth and development, health protection and promotion, public security ... and positively impact crime prevention, education, employment, community development, disease prevention, primary care, public health and social cohesion" (Chomik, 2007, p. 5). Within a Canadian context, Chomik (2007) identified several broad health care and health-specific achievements based on an analysis of ICA and ISA case studies. Systems and process related achievements included (a) mobilization of the community at large, (b) improvements in how information is obtained and shared, (c) development of new and more robust collaborations with partners across sectors, and (d) establishment of new mechanisms and structures to support cooperation across agencies. Among the health-related achievements were "an increased capacity to manage and administer health care services, improved health outcomes and quality of life, and a greater understanding among government departments that health is influenced by a complex set of inter-related factors and conditions" (Chomik, 2007, p. ii).

Facilitators and barriers to ISC and ISA may be grouped into several key categories: relationships among partners, shared vision, leadership, resources, structure, and process (Danaher, 2011). Table 11.1 lists some of the more common facilitators and barriers of ISC and ISA identified within these categories.

Intersectoral Collaboration and Interprofessional Practice

Recall that throughout this text we have described IPP as more than just multiple professionals working on the same issue autonomously and then sharing their results. Similarly, ISC involves more than multiple sectors in the same geographical area providing services to individuals such that specific, individual health needs are met. In this sense, we see a parallel between the conceptualizations of ISC and IPP in that both require, among other things, collaboration, communication, planning, shared accountability, and evaluation. It is also important to note the differences between ISC and IPP. For example, IPP typically occurs at the level of service, whereas ISC can occur at many different levels. Intersectoral

Table 11.1 Facilitators and Barriers of Intersectoral Collaboration and Intersectoral Action

Factor	Description
Facilitators	Clearly delineated and agreed-upon framework/model defining health and how health issues are to be approached.
	Clear rationale for the purpose of working together and engaging key partners at the beginning.
	Clearly defined roles and expectation of each partner (individuals and teams).
	Clear individual and joint goals for all partners involved in the collaboration. Goals and related objectives should be concrete with measurable outcomes.
	Stable teams that are well supported. Emphasis put on shared values, common goals, and interest to build trust and respect among partners.
	Establishment of and support for aspects of collaboration and related skills (e.g., open and clear communication, adequate consultation, shared leadership, accountability, clarity of tasks, and a clearly defined plan of action).
Barriers	Amount of effort, time, and negotiation required to establish both vertical and horizontal ISC where there is agreement and shared understanding of common goals and approaches, roles and responsibilities, and accountabilities.
	Lack of or limited resources; lack of or limited access to resources.
	Lack of interest or support: (a) internally within a team, organization, or community or (b) from prospective subsector or other sector partners.
	Lack of accountability and measures to ensure accountability.

Source: Public Health Agency of Canada (PHAC), 2007; Chomik, 2007.

collaboration is also broader. While ISC can involve collaboration between several IPP teams from different sub-sectors within health, it may also involve collaboration between teams in both health and non-health sectors. Additionally, remember that collaboration can occur outside the context of teams and teamwork. Therefore ISC can occur not only between IPP teams in the health sector but also between individual professionals in non-health sectors or through individual-to-individual collaboration.

To illustrate this last point, let's return to the opening vignette. During Brian's immediate recovery period, there was ISC between his IPP team within the acute care hospital and the IPP team in the rehabilitation centre where he later received care. Now living in the community, Brian is having his health needs met through ISCs between health sector professionals and teams and individuals working in other sectors (e.g., Hilde, the communication technology technician assisting Brian with his devices).

Interprofessional practice teams and their members are most likely to be involved in horizontal ISCs, where they collaborate and function interdependently with professionals or teams from other sectors toward commonly agreed-upon goals. For example, the collaboration between the various players within the sectors involved in Brian's care is demonstrative of horizontal ISC. However, IPP teams should be aware of vertical ISC and ISA, particularly when they might influence their practice and collaborative efforts with other sectors. Additionally, when possible, individuals and teams engaged in IPP should aim to participate in vertical ISC if there is an alignment between goals and approaches that will result in positive outcomes for patient care.

The nature and extent of ISC between IPP teams in the health sectors and other teams or individuals in other sectors is dependent primarily on the needs of the health care service user. Other determining factors relate to the facilitators and barriers discussed in the previous section and include contextual aspects such as the setting, the capacity and skill set of the IPP team to reach across sectors to form relationships, and the interest and resources to do so. In this respect, ISC and ISA are similar to IPP. In both types of endeavours, the elements of collaboration discussed in Chapter 5 of this text, along with skills such as problem solving and negotiation (see Chapter 6), must be well honed if the collaboration and the resulting actions are to be successful.

Spotlight 11.1 provides an example of a successful ISC experience. It should be noted that whether the outcomes of an ISC are successful or fall short of the goals, there is always the opportunity to identify the lessons learned that could support stronger partnerships in the future. Table 11.2 summarizes considerations when engaging in ISC and ISA.

Spotlight 11.1

Successful Intersectoral Collaboration: London InterCommunity Health Centre

Located in Ontario, the London InterCommunity Health Centre (LIHC) provides health and social services to individuals and families, including newcomers experiencing barriers to care. These barriers include poverty, homelessness, language or culture, and complex and/or chronic health conditions such as mental health and addictions. The centre offers a range of programs including diabetes care and self-management groups for those with chronic diseases.

LIHC has developed several ISCs involving local community agencies and organizations (e.g., local churches, community centres, other health sector organizations) aimed at meeting their broad goals and targeting social determinants of health influencing the health of the community. A key ISA strategy used by the centre is to hold within community gathering spaces monthly meetings that provide supportive environments and the opportunity to identify and discuss issues and to obtain specific health information (e.g., chronic disease self-management assistance) and other information and resources.

For more about the centre, visit http://lihc.on.ca.

Table 11.2 Considerations for Intersectoral Collaboration and Intersectoral Action

In designing and implementing ISA and ISC initiatives, consideration should be given to:
■ Contextual factors and conditions that may impact ISC work.
■ The selection of issues to be addressed, particularly when policy and program changes are involved. Decisions should be strategic and based on best practices.
■ The complexity of the issue. Complex issues should be purposefully aligned with an intersectoral approach.
■ Whether there is sound rationale for the intersectoral collaboration and initiative.
■ Which committee structure would best support the goals of the initiative and the conditions under which the project is being undertaken.
■ The accountability mechanisms that will be employed during the initiative. Accountability mechanisms should articulate the goals of the initiative, the outcomes, and how they will be measured.
■ Financial mechanisms to facilitate ISC, particularly resource funding needs.
■ How broad-level (e.g., central agency) guidelines, protocols, and resources can guide and support the ISC initiative.
■ How IPP team mandates, processes, activities and expertise fit into the ISC and how they can be harnessed to support the initiative. Teams and individuals involved should be able to see their place within the initiative and how best they can contribute.

Source: Chomik, 2007.

CONCLUSION

This chapter revisited a key message highlighted in Chapter 1 of this text and reinforced in subsequent chapters focusing on IPP and related developments in health care in Canada. If real and sustained change is to occur that will positively transform the experience of health for Canadians, action is required beyond individual or even team-specific silos of practice. As Canada moves forward with its commitments to improve the health of all citizens, the consensus is clear that efforts must be directed to engage individuals and teams across sectors, at different levels, and certainly beyond the traditional borders of the health sector. Attention must be paid, not only to the biomedical aspects of health and related advancements, but also to the conditions and circumstances broadly identified as social determinants of health.

As discussed in this chapter, IPP and IPP teams are integral to such an approach. However, they are not the sole means to this end. Transformative change for health must involve horizontal and vertical ISC and ISA. Actions taken must include the point-of-care collaborative approaches that IPP teams are currently developing and applying successfully. And they must include other actions and initiatives across sectors, involving policy development, program and service coordination, capacity building, mobilization, and advocacy. These efforts should also take into consideration the participation of health care consumers, families, and communities at the centre of care.

SUMMARY

- Efforts to ensure that Canadians are experiencing better health and access to health-related resources are challenged by the pace at which the needs of Canadians are evolving. In response to these challenges, a health care reform agenda significantly influenced by the 2003 *First Ministers' Accord on Health Care Renewal* and the 2004 *10-Year Plan to Strengthen Health Care* was set.
- Health care reform initiatives implemented over the last decade, including the move to IPP, have been helpful and will continue to be a central component of the overall strategy for moving forward. However, a broader commitment, inclusive of all sectors invested in attaining better health for Canadians, must be at the forefront of future efforts.
- *Intersectoral collaboration (ISC)* refers to the interdependent relationships between the parts of all sectors influencing health that form to take action on an issue affecting health outcomes. The action taken is termed *intersectoral action (ISA)*.
- ISC may occur either horizontally (across sectors at any given level) or vertically (between different levels, often involving government and non-governmental organizations).
- The facilitators and barriers to ISC and ISA are related to relationships among partners, shared vision, leadership, resources, structure, and process.
- The impact of ISCs and ISAs at the international level includes strengthened economic growth and development and positive improvements in public health and disease prevention. Nationally, the outcomes of both large- and small-scale ISCs include increased mobilization of the broader community and improved health outcomes and quality of life.
- Although there may be overlaps, IPP and ISC are not the same. While IPP typically occurs at the level of service, ISC can occur at many different levels. ISC is also broader, extending beyond the health sector and involving collaboration between health and non-health sectors.
- To optimize the care clients receive and enable positive health-related outcomes, IPP teams and their members need to develop an understanding of ISC and related concepts. IPP teams and individual professionals must also extend their collaborative skills beyond the borders of the health sector.
- As part of their mandates to improve health outcomes and meet the goals of their clients, IPP teams may include ISC with other teams or individuals in health or non-health sectors.
- An awareness of the facilitators, barriers, and areas for consideration when engaging in ISC will support IPP teams to successfully plan and implement ISC initiatives.

Key Terms

determinants of health

equity

horizontal intersectoral collaboration (horizontal ISC)

intersectoral action (ISA)

intersectoral collaboration (ISC)

sectors

social determinants of health

vertical intersectoral collaboration (vertical ISC)

Review Questions

1. Define intersectoral collaboration and intersectoral action for health.
2. Identify the various sectors in Canada that are relevant to health care and improving health outcomes. List two or three examples for each of these sectors.
3. Describe what is meant by *determinants of health* and *social determinants of health*.
4. Summarize trends in the health of Canadians within the context of the current Canadian health care system.

Application Exercises

1. Returning to the opening vignette with Hong, Brian, Cleo, Hilde, and Percy, consider all of the relevant personnel, representing the various sectors, that could positively impact Brian's health.
   a. Make a list of the contextual data that you are able to glean from the vignette that reveals information about Brian's life and his health from the broadest perspective.
   b. Create categories for this data (e.g., housing, health, finance, etc.).
   c. Create a list with two columns. In the column on the left, include all relevant personnel involved in Brian's care in the scenario. In the column on the right, include all relevant personnel (and perhaps local/provincial/federal departments and agencies) that may have the potential to contribute to Brian's health.
   d. Create a diagram showing how all of these resources (personnel, departments, and agencies) connect to Brian and to each other using lines with arrows to indicate the direction of the relationship. Along the lines, indicate the focus of the connection (e.g., between a local community housing agency and Brian, you might write "Community-assisted living to promote Brian's goal of independent living").

Additional Resources

Websites & Electronic Documents

Lessons Learned from Canadian Experiences with Intersectoral Action to Address the Social Determinants of Health
www.who.int/social_determinants/resources/isa_lessons_from_experience_can.pdf

Better Health, Better Care, Better Value for All: Refocusing Health Care Reform in Canada
www.healthcouncilcanada.ca

A Cornerstone for Health-for-All in the Twenty-First Century (Report of a Conference on Intersectoral Action for Health)
www.cpha.ca/uploads/progs/infra/intersectoral.pdf

References

Braveman, P., & Gruskin, S. (2003). Defining equity in health. *Journal of Epidemiology & Community Health*, *57*(1), 254–258.

Canadian Medical Association (CMA) & Canadian Nurses Association (CNA). (2011). *Principles to guide health care transformation in Canada*. Ottawa, ON: Canadian Medical Association, Canadian Nurses Association.

Chomik, T. A. (2007). *Lessons learned from Canadian experiences with intersectoral action to address the social determinants of health*. Public Health Agency of Canada (PHAC). Retrieved from http://www.who.int/social_determinants/resources/isa_lessons_from_experience_can.pdf

Commonwealth Fund. (2010). *The Commonwealth Fund 2010 international health policy survey in 11 countries*. Retrieved from http://www.commonwealthfund.org/Surveys/2010/Nov/2010-International-Survey.aspx

Danaher, A. (2011). *Reducing health inequities: Enablers and barriers of intersectoral collaboration*. Toronto, ON: Wellesley Institute. Retrieved from http://www.wellesleyinstitute.com/wp-content/uploads/2011/10/Reducing-Disparities-and-Improving-Population-Health.pdf

Davidson, R., Kitzinger, J., & Hunt, K. (2006). The wealthy get healthy, the poor get poorly? Lay perceptions of health inequalities. *Social Science & Medicine*, *62*(9), 2171–2182.

Davidson, R., Mitchell, R., & Hunt, K. (2008). Location, location, location: The role of experience of disadvantage in lay perceptions of area inequalities in health. *Health & Place*, *14*(2), 167–181.

Health Council of Canada (HCC). (2011). *How do sicker Canadians with chronic disease rate the health care system? Results from the 2011 Commonwealth Fund International Health Policy Survey of Sicker Adults*. Canadian Health Care Matters, Bulletin 6. Toronto, ON: Health Council of Canada.

Health Council of Canada (HCC). (2013a). *Better health, better care, better value for all: Refocusing health care reform in Canada*. Toronto, ON: Health Council of Canada.

Health Council of Canada (HCC). (2013b). *How do Canadian primary care physicians rate the health system? Results from the 2012 Commonwealth Fund International Health Policy Survey of Primary Care Physicians*. Canadian Health Care Matters, Bulletin 7. Toronto, ON: Health Council of Canada.

Institute for Healthcare Improvement (IHI). (2013). *IHI triple aim initiative*. Retrieved from http://www.ihi.org/offerings/Initiatives/TripleAIM/Pages/default.aspx

Lalonde, M. (1974). *A new perspective on the health of Canadians*. Ottawa: Government of Canada. Retrieved from http://www.phac-aspc.gc.ca/ph-sp/pdf/perspect-eng.pdf

Macintyre, S., McKay, L., & Ellaway, A. (2006). Lay concepts of the relative importance of different influences on health; Are there major socio-demographic variations? *Health Education Research, 21*(5), 731–739.

MacLean, L., Clinton, K., Edwards, N., Garrard, N., Ashley, L., Hansen-Ketchum, P., and Walsh, A. (2010). Unpacking vertical and horizontal integration: childhood overweight/obesity program and planning, a Canadian perspective. *Implementation Science, 5*(36), 1–11.

Pan American Health Organization. (2003). *Primary health care: 25 years of the Alma-Ata Declaration*. Washington, DC: Author. Retrieved from http://www.paho.org/English/dd/pin/alma-ata_declaration.htm

Public Health Agency of Canada (PHAC). (2007). Crossing sectors: Experiences in intersectoral action, public policy and health. Retrieved from http://www.phac-aspc.gc.ca/publicat/2007/cro-sec

Public Health Agency of Canada (PHAC). (2010). *The Chief Public Health Officer's Report on the State of Public Health in Canada 2010*. Retrieved from http://www.phac-aspc.gc.ca/cphorsphc-respcacsp/2010/fr-rc/cphorsphc-respcacsp-06-eng.php

Reading, J. (2009). *A life course approach to the social determinants of health for aboriginal peoples for the Senate Subcommittee on Population Health*. Retrieved from http://www.parl.gc.ca/40/2/parlbus/commbus/senate/com-e/popu-e/rep-e/appendixAjun09-e.pdf

Robert, S. A., & Booske, B. C. (2011). US opinions on health determinants and social policy as health policy. *American Journal of Public Health, 101*(9), 1655–1663.

Smith, D., Van Herk, K., & Rahaman, Z. (2012). Primary health care. In L. L. Stamler & L. Yiu (Eds.), *Community health nursing: A Canadian perspective* (3rd. ed., pp. 109–123). Toronto: Pearson Education Canada.

World Health Organization (WHO). (n.d.). *Social determinants of health. Intersectoral action*. Retrieved from http://www.who.int/social_determinants/thecommission/countrywork/within/isa/en

World Health Organization (WHO). (1986). *Ottawa charter for health promotion*. Retrieved from http://www.who.int/healthpromotion/conferences/previous/ottawa/en/index.html

World Health Organization (WHO) Commission on Social Determinants of Health. (2008). *Closing the gap in a generation: health equity through action on the social determinants of health. Final report of the Commission on Social Determinants of Health*. Geneva: World Health Organization.

Glossary

Accreditation: An educational process that benefits staff, facilitates team building, and provides an organization with access to valuable advice from outside experts.

Authentic leadership: "[A] process that draws from both positive psychological capacities and a highly developed organizational context, which results in both greater self-awareness and self-regulated positive behaviour on the part of leaders and associates, fostering positive self-development" (Luthans & Avolio, 2003, p. 243).

Care delivery outcomes: The measureable effects of an intervention that focus on the recipient of the service (Ingersoll, 2004).

Change: The process of making or becoming different.

Chaos: Behaviours so unpredictable that they appear to be random and disorganized (Vicenzi et al., 1997).

Collaboration: A process that requires relationships and interactions between health professionals regardless if they perceive themselves as part of a team.

Common law: Law that is formulated and applied by the courts as they decide individual cases brought to them for determination through lawsuits.

Communication: The transmission of and response to information, including many forms such as verbal, nonverbal, and written communication.

Communication structure: The pattern of communication that exists within a team.

Communication styles: How individuals use both verbal and nonverbal communication to signal to others how they should interpret messages.

Conflict: In the content of IPP, conflict refers to the process that occurs when team members, because of the complex and interdependent nature of teams, engage in a struggle that is rooted in a difference of beliefs, thoughts, attitudes, feelings, and/or behaviours.

Conflict resolution: A range of methods that may be used to address conflict, whether at the interpersonal level, between different groups or teams, or even between countries, in such a way that an acceptable solution may be found.

Contemporary leadership perspective: Describes the notion of leadership as social processes of influence involving relational interactions between leaders and followers.

Contextual factors: Contextual factors may be categorized as practice environment factors, organizational factors, individual factors, sociopolitical factors, and unknown factors. The three core dimensions of the organizing framework for IPP (process, relationship, and task) share a reciprocal relationship with these contextual factors.

Cooperation: The action or process of professionals from various disciplines coming together to work jointly to achieve a common goal or produce an outcome.

Decision making: The selection of an alternative from an existing set of options when no externally correct alternatives exist (Myers & Anderson, 2008); a mechanism that individuals and teams use to make choices and judgments. Involves the process of selecting an alternative from an existing set of options when no externally correct choice exists.

Determinants of health: Factors that combine together to influence the health of individuals and communities. These include genetic endowment; individual behaviour; and social, economic, or physical environment factors.

Developing and renewing others: Involves conscious efforts, such as mentoring, or behaviours that indirectly influence others, such as role modelling (Grossman & Valiga, 2009).

Diversity: Individual and collective differences based on culture, demographics (including gender and age), and cognitive factors (e.g., education preparation and learning styles).

Equity: The "absence of systemic disparities in health (or in the major social determinants of health) between social groups who have different levels of underlying social advantage/disadvantage" (Braveman & Gruskin, 2003, p. 254).

Evaluation: Systemic collection and analysis of information in order to make a determination about the quality of the information being explored.

Evaluation framework: A plan that guides the user through the process of evaluation by summarizing and organizing key elements of the type of evaluation being undertaken.

Evidence-based practice: A "framework for clinical practice that incorporates the best available scientific evidence with the expertise of the clinician and the patient's preferences and values to make decisions about health care" (Levin, 2006, p. 6).

Followership: The act of following a leader; involves many of same attributes that are associated with leadership.

Formative evaluation: An evaluation that focuses on data that provides feedback on the progress and effectiveness of the efforts being made toward implementing this model of practice.

Functional or style leadership perspective: Concerned with the functional capacity level of the individual occupying the role of leader and the style of leadership he or she uses.

Goal: Statement of intention that indicates where the client/team wants to be at the end of the problem-solving process; the intended or desired outcome.

Health care team: An organized system consisting of interdependent health care professionals that, in consideration of the expectations of both the patient(s) being cared for and the organization or system in which care is being provided, engage in processes and develop structures to guide actions and encourage collaborative problem solving and decision making.

Health professions regulation: A process of regulation of health care professions consisting of several core elements that is administered by respective governing bodies. Health professions regulation in Canada is jurisdictional in that every province (and each of the three territories) deals separately with the regulation of their health professions.

Horizontal intersectoral collaboration (horizontal ISC): Intersectoral collaboration that occurs at the same level between subsectors or across sectors. Occurs most often where there is a need to bring "together diverse resources, expertise and experiences to solve complex issues whose solutions lay outside the capacity of any one sector" (Danaher, 2011, p. 6).

Interdependence: The occurrence of and reliance on interactions among professionals whereby each is dependent on the other to accomplish his or her goals.

Intergroup conflict: Disagreement or difference between members of two or more groups or their representatives over authority, territory, or resources.

Interpersonal conflict: Conflict that arises between two or more individuals.

Interprofessional communication: Communication styles, approaches, and techniques between and among various members of the interprofessional team.

Interprofessional education (IPE): "[T]wo or more professions learn[ing] with, from and about each other to improve collaboration and the quality of care" (CAIPE, 2011, para. 1); a process in which two or more professions learn with, from, and about each other to improve collaboration and the quality of care.

Interprofessional mentoring: A professional relationship that takes place between various health care providers (or health care providers and students) who are from different disciplines or health professions. Learning in this context is aimed at helping mentees learn about the roles of other professions and how to work together to provide patient-centred care.

Interprofessional practice (IPP): An approach to practice "designed to promote the active participation of each health care discipline in patient care. It enhances patient and family-centred goals and values, provides mechanisms for continuous communication among caregivers, optimizes staff participation in clinical decision-making within and across health care disciplines, and fosters respect for disciplinary contributions of all professionals."

Intersectoral action (ISA): "[A]ctions affecting health outcomes undertaken by sectors outside the health sector, possibly, but not necessarily, in collaboration with the health sector" (WHO, n.d.).

Intersectoral collaboration (ISC): "A recognized relationship between part or parts of the health sector with part or parts of another sector which has been formed to take action on an issue to achieve health outcomes ... in a way that is more effective, efficient or sustainable than could be achieved by the health sector acting alone" (World Health Organization Conference on Inter-sectoral Action for Health, 1997, p. 3).

IPE: See *interprofessional education.*

IPP: See *interprofessional practice.*

ISA: See *intersectoral action (ISA).*

ISC: See *intersectoral collaboration (ISC).*

Leadership: "[T]he process of influencing others to understand and agree about what needs to be done and how it can be done effectively, and the process of facilitating individual and collective efforts to accomplish the shared objectives" (Yuki, 2002, p. 7).

Legal regulation: Any law that establishes norms of behaviour and provides a mechanism for enforcing those norms when they are breached. Includes professional regulation and common law rules.

Legislated scope of practice: The work according to legislation that can be performed by members of a particular profession. The scope of practice for one profession does not limit the work that can be performed by other regulated or unregulated providers.

Listening: A dynamic process involving receiving, perceiving, and making sense of a message with the aim being to respond.

Medical simulation: "[A]n imitation of some real thing, state of affairs, or process" for the practice of skills, problem solving, and judgment (Rosen, 2008, p. 157).

Mentoring: A process involving an experienced individual who provides guidance to a less experienced person.

Negotiation: "[A] reciprocal communication process whereby two or more parties to a dispute examine specific issues, explain their positions, and exchange offers and counteroffers to reach agreement or achieve mutually beneficial outcomes" (Forsyth, 2006, p. 435).

Non-hierarchical relationships: Relationships within a team that are based upon each member having an equal say or equivalent level of power.

Nonverbal communication: Also sometimes called metacommunication; all other communication than verbal used to create meaning.

Normative pressures: The methods utilized by a team to enforce the norms it has established. Normative pressures encourage compliance, while discouraging deviation from the norms of a team.

Norms: Standards or expectations of behaviour, attitudes, and even perceptions.

Outcomes research: A specific type of research that seeks to understand the outcomes of various practices and interventions by measuring effects, such as changes in patient condition and health status.

Personality traits: An individual's psychological makeup; the culmination of an individual's attitudes, values, beliefs, experiences, and behaviour (Myers & Anderson, 2008).

Person-centred care: The notion that the person or patient is at the centre of health care and is fully involved in the care process to the extent they choose. Key constituents of this concept include respecting clients'/patients' autonomy, listening to the needs of clients/patients and their families, and engaging with clients/patient and families as members of the health care team.

Power distance: The degree to which those who are less powerful accept and expect that power will be unequally distributed. Measures how individuals perceive power differences.

Problem: A situation in which an individual or team has a goal or is required to take action but does not know how to achieve the goal or act.

Problem-focused processes: Processes involving the members of a team coming together to solve a problem or overcome an issue. Problem-focused processes are a core element of the concept of collaboration.

Problem solving: The invention of an alternative solution to a problem that is different from any previously existing option (Frey, 1997; Maier, 1958; Adams & Galanes, 2006).

Process dimension: Describes the "how" of engaging in IPP, encompassing four essential elements in a process: (a) actions, (b) progression of time, (c) change that occurs over time, and (d) outcomes or results.

Process evaluation: Measuring how care is being delivered and received.

Processes: Involve actions that occur in the progression toward some goal and within a given period of time.

Professional identity: Defined by three key elements: (a) a set of beliefs and attitudes an individual holds about his or her profession, (b) an understanding of one's role and the boundaries between professions, and (c) a conception of the ways one should engage with others as members of an interprofessional team.

Professionalization: The process of assuming an occupational identity.

Qualitative research methods: Methods of inquiry that focus on understanding human experience and behaviour and often may examine the experience of patients living with a disease or undergoing a specific medical treatment.

Quantitative research methods: Methods of inquiry that focus on collecting observable, quantifiable data that may be analyzed mathematically.

Quantum science: Concerned with understanding complex and intersecting relationships; "looks at change; how it works, what it means . . . [and is] actively interested in adaptation, integration, interaction . . . and the continuous dynamics of movement" (Malloch and Porter-O'Grady, 2009, p. 2).

Regulation: The part of law enacted by cabinet or an administrative agency authorized to adopt regulations by the statute passed by a legislature.

Relational leadership theory: A social influence process through which emergent conditions (i.e., evolving social order) and change (i.e., new values, attitudes, approaches, behaviours, ideologies, etc.) are constructed and produced (Uhl-Bien, 2006, p. 668).

Relationship dimension: Encompasses variables related to the interpersonal realm of health care practice; the "who" of IPP. Consists of elements such as people, roles, perceptions, emotions, values and beliefs, communication styles, leadership and membership approaches, group dynamics, and group climate.

Reliability: How consistent a measure is.

Role: A set of expected behaviours and responsibilities enacted through both what we say and what we do.

Role clarification: Requires that members of the interprofessional team understand their roles and the roles of other professions, and utilize this knowledge to set and achieve appropriate goals.

Role conflict: Occurs when an individual experiences tension and has negative emotions as a result of competing or conflicting sets of expectations and demands associated with their roles.

Role confusion: Occurs among health care providers or in the relationship between health care providers and patients, and involves a lack of understanding of roles or a failure to recognize the boundaries of roles or relationships.

Role distance: The separation or detachment that exists between individuals and the role they expect to occupy.

Role modelling: A form of learning from the experience of others that allows the learner to adopt new behaviours without the trial and error of doing things for himself or herself. Learning in this context occurs by observation and imitation (Murray & Main, 2005).

Sectors: Parts of the economy.

Self-identity: How an individual perceives, describes, and identifies himself or herself.

Shared leadership: A leadership model where multiple team members formally or informally rotate through leadership activities.

Shared ownership of goals: Mutual responsibility in all aspects of working to reach a goal.

Situational leadership: Focuses on the concept that the situation in which a team is operating influences, if not determines, leadership behaviour.

Social determinants of health: Social, economic, or physical environment factors that influence the health of individuals and communities.

Statutes: Written law passed by a legislative body.

Stewardship: "[I]nvolves placing oneself in service of ideas and ideals and to others who are committed to their fulfillment" (Sergiovanni, 2007, p. 59).

Structure evaluation: Assessing the attributes of the setting in which care occurs.

Summative evaluation: An evaluation that takes place at an end point, such the end of an IPP program, and is used to assess outcomes and the overall impact of the intervention or action. May also include assessment of how well processes, such as interprofessional collaboration, were enacted.

Task dimension: Consists of variables representing the work that needs to be undertaken in order to provide patient care in IPP situations; the "what" of IPP. Variables found within this dimension include actions, behaviours, and desired outcomes.

Team effectiveness: The outcome(s) or product(s) of teamwork in relation to a team's success in meeting the goals it has identified; the components, attributes, and processes we would expect to observe in an effective team.

Team processes: The sets of steps or actions enacted by individuals (e.g., health care professionals) working in teams and engaged in teamwork, resulting in desired outcomes.

Teamwork: A goal-oriented and relationally based process that relies heavily on cooperation and collaboration to promote success in achieving a common goal.

Tort law: The body of common law that courts apply to determine when health care providers and facilities are required to compensate patients injured in the course of care or treatment.

Traditional leadership: Focuses on the notion the leadership is innate and inherent to an individual.

Uni-professional education: An educational model designed to train each profession separately.

Validity: The extent to which we are actually measuring what we say we are measuring in a scientific study.

Verbal communication: The words and phrases we use to create meaning.

Vertical intersectoral collaboration (vertical ISC): Intersectoral collaboration that occurs between different levels. Often involves partnering between the governmental and non-governmental sectors to address issues requiring broad, sustainable, and consistent policy and resources.

Vision: "[A] picture of the results you want to create, an ideal sense of what is possible, a statement of destination" (Rogers & Reynolds, 2003, p. 71).

Index

J

K

L

M

N

O

P